ARTERIAL LESIONS AND ARTERIOSCLEROSIS

Edited

by

H. JELLINEK

Professor of Pathology
Director of the 2nd Department of Pathology
Semmelweis University Medical School, Budapest

PLENUM PRESS · LONDON AND NEW YORK

LQM J

Translated
by
Ilona Koch

Translation edited
by
Andreas A. Ábrahám
The Lankenau Hospital
Division of Research and Pathology
Philadelphia, U.S.A.

ISBN 306-30792-8

Library of Congress Catalog Card Number 74-4249

Printed in Hungary

Contributors

A. BÁLINT
I. HÜTTNER
H. JELLINEK
ANNA KÁDÁR
T. KERÉNYI
ÉVA KONYÁR
Z. NAGY
KLÁRA SZEMENYEI
B. VERESS

All the contributors are members of the staff of the
2nd Department of Pathology
Semmelweis University Medical School, Budapest, Hungary

CONTENTS

7

Chapter 6

EXPERIMENTAL OBSERVATIONS

Chapter 7

CHRONIC LESIONS OF SMALL VESSELS (VASCULAR WALL TRANSFORMATION FOLLOWING ACUTE LESIONS OF SMALL VESSELS)

Chapter 8

INFLUENCE OF DRUG THERAPY ON SMALL VESSEL CHANGES IN EXPERIMENTAL HYPERTENSION. PROBLEMS OF HEALING AND REVERSIBILITY

Appendix

11

PREFACE

This monograph summarizes the results of a fifteen-year vascular pathology research project sponsored by the Hungarian Academy of Sciences. The workers who have participated in this project are indebted to the Academy for financing extensive investigations and visits to institutes abroad, the aims of which were to solve certain problems by international cooperation. The results presented here have been achieved by the collective effort of research teams, each studying a particular problem, but working together to the same end. Mutual discussion of findings and a regular exchange of information between the research groups have contributed to the progress of the investigations. Regular publication of details and mutual criticism ensured that the findings were uniformly interpreted. It is hoped that the fundamental aim of our long-term project, i.e. the selection of the right approach to the complex problem of vascular pathology, has been achieved.

The new approach results from the recognition that since arteriosclerosis finally leads to various kinds of vascular injury, attention should be focussed on the events preceding the development of the lesions rather than on the lesions themselves. This claim has been confirmed by various model experiments in which vascular injury inflicted under different conditions uniformly led to morphologically verified arteriosclerotic change. The recent increase in the incidence of civilization diseases of the vascular system has resulted in a world-wide expansion of arteriosclerosis research. Any contribution elucidating one or another aspect of the condition(s) will promote both the clarification of pathogenesis and the development of preventive measures. We believe that the concept proposed here might change the course of traditional arteriosclerosis research. There are already indications that we have been on the right track, judging from literary reports based on this new experimental approach.

Considerable assistance was given by the contributors to this monograph, A. Bálint, I. Hüttner, Anna Kádár, T. Kerényi, Éva Konyár, Z. Nagy, Klára Szemenyei, B. Veress by their having compiled a number of chapters each embodying their original work. The editor wishes to express his sincere appreciation for their contribution. Since the topics covered are closely interrelated, each chapter includes ample reference to the results of those who have dealt with a certain aspect of the problem and have thus indirectly contributed to one or another part of the monograph.

Elaboration of minor problems in the field of related sciences is indispensable in making the work complete. For their contribution in this respect the authors are indebted to present or former co-workers of the institute, Gy. Gorácz, J. Hintalan, A. Kóczé, F. Lajosi, A. Tóth and Klára Szentágothai.

13

The affiliation of this institute to research groups or centres engaged in similar or related fields has made possible the extension of research activities on a collaborative basis, thus permitting a deeper insight into various possible experimental approaches. Thanks are due for valuable advice and fruitful cooperation to G. Bartos, I. Csillag, I. Földes, M. Földi, Gy. Gábor, R. Gergely, Anna Hartai, M. Iskum, I. Krasznai, R. H. More, Julia Nagy, M. Papp, G. Pogátsa, G. Rona, F. Solti, P. Sótonyi and Ilona Venesz.

The editor is indebted to his very first tutor in science, Professor Ö. Zalka, for his having stimulated an interest in vascular pathology by assigning to him a task of uterine vessel investigation in collaboration with Gy. Szinai. Vascular diseases have been the editor's main concern since that time. Dr. I. Csillag, of the First Department of Surgery, Semmelweis University Medical School Budapest, has been an invaluable collaborator for many years in studies of vascular graft organization and direct vascular wall injury by painting with acid. Dr. L. Haranghy, professor emeritus and former director of this institute was instrumental in helping to provide an Academy of Sciences research grant to support our investigations over many years.

Technical work of a high calibre is an essential prerequisite not only of fruitful research, but also in the preparation of the book. In this sense, every co-worker of this institute has had a share in the compilation of this monograph. The authors are indebted to Mrs. R. Nagyiván for typing the manuscript, to Mrs. Emőke Kádár and the late Mrs. S. Kiss for preparing the colour photographs and to Miss Kinga Gyökössy for taking the electron micrographs; all the preparations used were made by Mrs. Judit Szilas and Miss Gizella Penninger. The high-quality electron microscopic preparations were the work of Mrs. Mária Kerényi and Mrs. Katalin Kottász.

The electron micrographs illustrating this volume were prepared in the First and Second Central Electron Miscroscopy Laboratories, Semmelweis University Medical School, Budapest (JEM 6C and HITACHI HU-10 apparatuses, respectively); the Instrument Service of the Hungarian Academy of Sciences, Budapest; the Department of Pathology, McGill University, Montreal, Canada (Philips EM-300); and the Experimental Pathology Division of the Kennedy Institute of Rheumatology, London. Most ultra-thin sections were counterstained with uranyl acetate and lead hydroxide; if otherwise, it is specified in the legend to the illustration. Sections were cut with LKB II and III ultratomes. Fixation techniques for electron-microscopic investigation and staining methods commonly used for light micrographs are described in the Appendix.

The micrographs are presented as Plates at the end of the volume and reference is made to Plate numbers. Each Plate contains several figures which are numbered consecutively. Plates LXI to LXVIII comprise colour micrographs.

INTRODUCTION

The title of this monograph indicates the range of investigations reported therein. Information emerging from fifteen-year morphological studies of vascular lesions associated with various diseases has led to the conclusion that vascular response to different kinds of injury is essentially uniform and that the morphology of the advanced lesions always resembles that of arteriosclerotic change. Various vascular diseases were analysed morphologically one by one, using experimental models which reproduced the conditions of the human disease, and conclusions were drawn from comparison of the models with one another and with human arteriosclerotic or other vascular lesions. Comparative evaluation of the findings favours that arteriosclerosis as such does not represent an independent morphological entity. The morphological characteristics of human and experimental vascular lesions resulting from different kinds of injury are usually so similar that the tissue changes in themselves are as a rule not conclusive as to the nature of the causative factor. The phenomena of vascular injury are essentially uniform, but they may be modified by the duration of the damage, the structure of the vessel wall and —least of all—by the nature of the injury.

It appears, therefore, that arteriosclerosis represents the final stage of various kinds of vascular change and, accordingly, various factors may play a role in its aetiology. All constituents of the process leading to the characteristic arteriosclerotic lesion can be clearly defined and differentiated from one another in the various stages of the change.

The first chapter of this monograph summarizes present knowledge of the ultrastructure of the mammalian arterial wall.

Description of the normal vascular structure is followed by description and evaluation of model experiments on large elastic-type vessels and small muscular arteries. The model experiments have permitted the follow-up of the acute and chronic stages of vascular change, the latter being understood as a process of regeneration.

Analysis of the various experimental models, some of which have been developed in this institute, has unequivocally affirmed that the mechanism of vascular response to various kinds of injury is essentially the same, and factors such as vascular structure, degree and duration of damage, and duration of the lesion only modify, but do not fundamentally alter the morphological events. Additional proof for this implication has emerged from analysis of the role of elastic vascular wall elements and nutritional and permeability conditions of the vessel wall under normal and pathologically altered circumstances. The following chapters deal with the analysis of human acute or chronic lesions as compared with experimental models, with special regard to arteriosclerotic changes.

Model experiments with high lipid (high cholesterol) diets, discussed in connection with large vessel lesions, have shown that permeability change is the decisive factor in the evolution of the atheromatous plaque, both in human and experimental hypertension.

Now that vascular diseases occupy first place in the mortality statistics of so many countries and still more persevering work than hitherto is urgently required to find at least a partial resolution of the problem, we feel that this little monograph may contribute to the elucidation of the pathogenesis of vascular disease by offering some new information on its pathomorphology. An understanding of morphological changes helps to identify the factors involved in the pathomechanism and aetiology, and no effective prevention and control measures can be established until causation and progression become known in full detail.

On the basis of our experience, we think that in future fundamental preventive measures should be directed toward preservation of the functional stability of the vessel wall. This means the protection of the wall against abrupt changes of nutritional and innervation conditions, i.e. against the microtraumata which bring about seemingly slight changes of severe consequence (e.g. single cell necrosis); vessel wall regeneration always means deformation. Our experiments with chemotherapeutics suggest that drug prevention is possible, although the available preparations could not fully prevent, only ameliorate, the hypertensive vascular changes and the associated symptoms. Drugs suitable for arteriosclerosis prevention are expected to ensure stability of transmural flow and nutritional conditions more adequately than a symptomatic therapy, but such preparations remain to be developed by persevering research work.

The editor and co-authors hope that this monograph will contribute some important data to the elucidation of the morphology, morphogenesis and pathomechanism of vascular lesions, facilitating the clarification of further details, and thereby promoting the preventive approach.

H. Jellinek

CHAPTER 1

THE FINE STRUCTURE OF THE MAMMALIAN ARTERIAL WALL

The normal structure of mammalian arteries has been extensively studied by light- and electron microscopy (Jores, 1924; Benninghoff, 1930; Maximov and Bloom, 1957; Fawcett, 1959; Abramson, 1962; Bader, 1963; Buck, 1963; Hess and Stäubli, 1963a, b; Lang, 1965; French, 1966). The following chapters deal only with those details which are essential to the understanding of the subject of this monograph.

THE STRUCTURAL EFFECT OF VASCULAR PRESERVATION

There is a considerable morphological difference between vessels fixed in a collapsed or physiologically distended state (Meyer, 1958; Pease and Paule, 1960; Wolinsky and Glagov, 1964; Bunce, 1965; Fischer, 1965; Wolinsky, 1967; Gardner and Matthews, 1969). In collapsed vessels, the endothelium is thick, the subendothelial gap appears distended near the nuclei, the internal elastic membrane (IEM) and—in elastic vessels—the elastic fibres are undulating and loosely arranged, and the gaps between them vary in width. The thick, rounded smooth muscle cells lie obliquely between the elastic fibres.

The fibres of the distended elastic-type vessels are straight and the gaps between them are uniformly wide. The oblong muscle cells are circumferential. The distension of muscular-type vessels results in a regular arrangement of the originally irregularly ordered groups of elastic fibres and muscle cells; the latter lie along the vessel's circumference and are accompanied by parallelly-ordered, elastic fibrils. The morphology of the junctions between the endothelial cells depends greatly on changes in the physical and chemical properties of the fixing solution, although the endothelial cells themselves are markedly resistant to such effects (Constantinides et al., 1969).

COMPONENTS OF THE NORMAL ARTERIAL WALL

GENERAL STRUCTURE

TUNICA INTIMA

This is composed of the mammalian artery of endothelium, subendothelial gap and internal elastic membrane. The latter is discontinuous in arteries less than 100 μ in diameter and is entirely absent from the capillaries (Rhodin, 1967).

The basic structure of the intima is found in its simplest form in small mammals, mice and rats (Plate I/1). Large mammals including man possess this form only in foetal and neonatal age, and in small vessels. In the thoracic aorta of young mouse the subendothelial gap is narrow and the internal elastic lamina (IEL) appears as a homogeneous bundle, in places fenestrated. The subendothelial gap becomes distended with age and collagenous fibres or elastic fragments appear in it here and there (Karrer, 1961). Newborn rats have a wider subendothelial gap than mice, containing floccular and fibrillar material (Paule, 1963). The gap is distended further with age, although in places the endothelium lies directly on the fenestrated IEM; at this stage collagenous, elastic fragments are seen in the gap (Keech, 1960; Pease and Paule, 1960; Ham, 1962; Still and O'Neal, 1962).

The aortic intima of rabbits is thickest at the arch and becomes gradually thinner toward the abdominal portion. Microscopically, loose connective tissue is seen to fill the promixal part of the subendothelial gap; its cells resemble fibrocytes, histiocytes, monocytes or lymphocytes. An intimal thickening is present at the origin of the aortic branches (Lautsch and McMillan, 1953; Duff et al., 1957). Electron microscopy has shown that collagenous and elastic fibres embedded in the homogeneous basal structure of the subendothelial gap extend into the media through the fenestrae of the IEL. The elastic fibres form in places a more or less continuous, fenestrated membrane, which passes parallel to the endothelium, dividing the intima into two parts. The superficial layer contains only delicate elastic fibres, some of which are in direct contact with the cytoplasmic membranes of endothelial cells. Cells localizing in the deeper layer resemble partly medial smooth muscle cells, partly fibrocytes (Bierring and Kabayashi, 1963; Still, 1964). The intima of the abdominal aorta is thin and the narrow subendothelial layer contains a small amount of fibrillar substance (Buck, 1958).

The structure of the avian thoracic aorta corresponds to that of elastic vessels. Delicate longitudinal elastic fibres lie in the relatively wide subendothelial gap. The latter is more narrow in the abdominal aorta, and three to four elastic lamellae separate it from the predominantly muscular-type media (Grollmann et al., 1963). Electron micrographs have shown that, in addition to collagenous and elastic fibrils, fibroblast-like cells are present in the subendothelial gap (Prior and Jones, 1952; Karrer, 1960b, Hess and Stäubli, 1963a, b; Laitinen, 1963; Simpson et al., 1967).

In large mammals, the basic structure of the intima can be distinguished only during foetal or early postnatal life. During growth, intimal thickenings appear, initially only at the origin of the aortic branches, later also elsewhere, until it is hard to define what should be regarded as a normal structure. Among domestic animals, the aortic structure of the pig is known in greatest detail (French et al., 1965). The thoracic aorta of this animal is of the elastic type. In the young pig, the subendothelial gap is broad and its transition to the media is indistinct for lack of a definitive IEL; it contains collagenous and elastic fibres in diffuse order. Between these fibres lie either round cells reminiscent of mesenchymal stem cells, or fibrocyte-like cells. The abdominal aorta of the pig possesses a muscular-type media, which is separated from the intima by a distinct, although not continuous, IEL.

The aorta of old swine exhibits intimal thickenings; these appear in the thoracic segment chiefly at the orifices of vessels, while in the abdominal segment they are confluent. The main components of the thickenings are fibrocytes and round cells in the thoracic aorta and smooth muscle cells in the abdominal aorta.

Electron micrographs have shown that in man, a fenestration of the IEL begins already in foetal life; it becomes distinct at birth and develops further in the course of growth. During the first year of life, smooth muscle cells pass from the media into the subendothelial gap to form a longitudinally oriented musculo-elastic layer. Initially, this structure is seen only at the orifices of the aortic branches, later it appears along the entire circumference of the vessels, above all in the abdominal segment. Splitting of the IEL on the one hand, and aggregation of newly formed elastic fibres on the other, gives rise to more or less distinct inner-limiting membrane or hyperplastic elastic layer, which divides the intima into two parts. Later the elastic and cellular elements decrease and the collagenous elements become predominant (Prior and Jones, 1952; Movat et al., 1958; Ahmed, 1967). According to recent polarizing and fluorescent microscopic examinations, the hyperplastic elastic membrane may already correspond to an immature, or incompletely cross-linked collagen (Jackson et al., 1968; Joiner et al., 1968). Electron microscopically, a narrow subendothelial gap is seen to separate the endothelium and IEL of the foetal aorta. Initially this gap contains only a delicate filamentous substance and a few collagenous fibres, later smooth muscle cells appear, forming one or two layers in places. Gaps interrupting the IEL contain collagenous fibres (Laitinen, 1963; Haust et al., 1965a). Examinations of apparently sound parts of adult aorta have shown the presence of smooth muscle cells, collagenous and elastic fibres and round cells in the intima (Laitinen, 1963).

CORONARY ARTERIES

The coronary intima of small mammals shows the characteristic basic structure (Plate II/2). The subendothelial gap is narrow and contains as a rule no connective tissue elements. In rabbits, the endothelium extends filiform cytoplasmic processes into the media, through the fenestrae of the IEL (Parker, 1958).

In large mammals, the intima of the coronary arteries resembles that of man both structurally and in the changes which occur. For example, in the newborn pig it is thin and the narrow subendothelial gap contains a few collagenous fibres and delicate fibrils; the IEL is as a rule intact. Focal thickenings of the intima develop already in the early phase of growth. The IEL becomes fragmented, smooth muscle cells migrate from the media into the subendothelial gap and the metachromatic basal structure increases. Elastin formation by the smooth muscle cells has been observed electron microscopically. During aging, the IEL falls apart and the musculo-elastic or hyperplastic-elastic layer described above develops first only at the vascular orifices, later independently along the entire vascular circumference. Electron micrographs show that in the intimal thickenings the IEL becomes fragmented, smooth muscle cells resembling those of the media aggregate, and collagen and elastin are newly formed (French et al., 1965).

In humans and large mammals as well, the basic structure of the intima of the coronary arteries can be observed only during prenatal life. During growth intimal changes of the above type become established (Prior and Jones, 1952; Moon, 1957; Neufeld et al., 1962).

LARGE AND MEDIUM SIZE ARTERIES

In various small and large mammals, the intima maintains its basic structure during postnatal life (Pease and Paule, 1960; Geer et al., 1961; Stehbens, 1963). In man, intimal thickenings are focal, less distinct than in the aorta and coronary arteries, and also take a longer time to develop (Geer et al., 1961; Hogan and Feeney, 1963a; Stallbrass, 1963; Westman and Nylander, 1965).

SMALL ARTERIES

The identification and determination of small arteries by diameter has presented certain difficulties, because the technique of fixation may considerably alter the structure and size of the vessel. A more reliable differentiation has been offered on the basis of the presence or absence of IEL and by the number of smooth muscle fibres present in the media (Benninghoff, 1930; Movat and Fernando, 1963b; Matthews and Gardner, 1966; Gardner and Matthews, 1969).

Small Arteries with Several Layers of Smooth Muscle Cells and IEL. Endothelial cells, basement membrane and IEL are present in the intima. Delicate collagenous and elastic fibres pass between the basement membrane and the fenestrated IEM. With decrease of the number of smooth muscle cell layers, elastic filaments and fragments become predominant over collagenous ones (Maynard et al., 1957; Rhodin, 1962a; Zelander et al., 1962; Hogan and Feeney, 1963a, b; Movat and Fernando, 1963b; Jacobsen et al., 1966; Matthews and Gardner, 1966; Jorgensen and Thorsen, 1969; Vegge, 1969). Arterioles 100 μ in diameter have still a distinct IEL and two to three layers of smooth muscle cells (Rhodin, 1967).

Small Arteries with One Layer of Smooth Muscle Cells. The smooth muscle cell layers decrease in number in arterioles less than 100 μ in diameter, and only a single layer remains at a diameter of 50 μ. At this stage the IEL has become fragmented and its residues as a rule vanish during the preparation of the material (Movat and Fernando, 1964a; Rhodin, 1967). Two basement membranes, 0.05–0.3 μ distant from one another, separate the endothelium from the medial smooth muscle cells (Rhodin, 1967). With the decrease in calibre of the arteriole—approximately at a diameter of 30 μ—the smooth muscle cells often break through the basement membrane and a membrane-to-membrane contact—myoendothelial junction—occurs at a distance of 45 Å (Rhodin, 1967).

CAPILLARIES

The intima of the capillaries is composed of endothelium, basement membrane and pericapillary layer; the structural variation of capillaries in different species, or in different organs of mammals, arises from the dissimilar properties of endothelium and basement membrane and the presence or absence of a pericapillary layer (Moore and Ruska, 1957; Bennett et al., 1959; Movat and Fernando, 1964b, c).

TUNICA MEDIA

ELASTIC ARTERIES

The main elastic-type vessels are the thoracic aorta, the abdominal aorta, and the innominate, subclavial and pulmonary arteries (Alexander and Jensen, 1963; Seifert, 1963a). The media of these vessels is composed of elastic-collagenous elements and cells. The latter are exclusively smooth muscle cells in most species; the occurrence of fibroblast-like cells as well has been observed in the elastic vessels of birds (Hess and Stäubli, 1963a, b; Takagi and Kawase, 1967; Simpson and Harms, 1968; Takagi, 1969b). Takagi et al. (1967b) and Takagi (1969a) believe that the fibroblast-like cells are the first to appear in the aorta of the developing embryonic chick and some differentiate to smooth muscle cells but only later.

The above elements arrange to form concentric lamellae, so-called lamellar units, in vessels fixed under physiological pressure. The number of these lamellae is directly related to the diameter of the vessel, which again depends on the body weight of the animal. The distance between the fibres is constant within the same species (Wolinsky, 1967). As noted in the foregoing, both the light- and electron-microscopic images of elastic fibres and smooth muscle cells are greatly influenced by the collapsed or distended state of the vessel at fixation. The elastic fibres are in places interrupted by gaps and delicate elastic bundles connect the individual fibres with one another. A direct connection between smooth muscle cell and elastic fibre is often seen; they are separated from one another by a gap only 150–200 Å wide. The collagenous fibres are distributed around the smooth muscle cells and elastic fibres.

MUSCULAR-TYPE VESSELS

Most arteries belong to this category. The muscular layer is composed of circularly arranged smooth muscle cell fibres, around which the elastic fibrils form irregular aggregates if the vessel is collapsed, but assume a regular parallel order if the vessel is distended. An IEL separates this layer from the intima, and an IEL from the adventitia.

HYBRID VESSELS

The external part of the media has an elastic structure and its internal part has a muscular structure in the large branches of the aorta (Mayersbach, 1956; Maximov and Bloom, 1957).

TUNICA ADVENTITIA

The tunica intima is composed of loosely arranged fibroblasts and collagenous fibres, as well as elastin fragments, which are particularly numerous near the media; between the elastin fragments pass nerve fibres and in some cases, also capillaries and lymph vessels. The collagenous fibres are less numerous and the

21

adventitia is richer in cells in young animals than in older ones (Paule, 1963). The nerve fibres are chiefly connected with the adrenergic innervation; they usually do not enter into the media, but form a plexus as the borderline between adventitia and media (Ehinger et al., 1966; Bolme and Fuxe, 1967; Mellander and Indransson, 1968; Gardner and Matthews, 1969). They consist of an unmyelinated axon surrounded by Schwann cells and this complex is enveloped by collagenous fibres. The neuro-effector junctions are those areas from which the Schwann cells are missing and that part of the axon rich in mitochondria, as well as in granulated and non-granulated microvesicles, lies close to one or more smooth muscle cells (Zelander et al., 1962; Ehinger et al., 1966; Gardner and Matthews, 1969). Some smooth muscle cells extend their cytoplasmic processes through the IEL into the nerve bundle (Gardner and Matthews, 1969).

Decrease in calibre of the vessels is accompanied by an increase in the number of unmyelinated nerves. The distance between the axon and the smooth muscle cell's basement membrane decreases from several hundred or thousand Å in large arteries (Zelander et al., 1962; Ehinger et al., 1966; Gardner and Matthews, 1969) to 45 Å in the smallest ones (Rhodin, 1967).

VASA VASORUM

The nutrition of the arterial wall takes place through the lumen; some of the large vessels and the aorta are nourished also through the vasa vasorum (Winternitz, 1954; Woerner, 1959). Animals of less than 5–6 kg body weight, i.e. having less than 26 medial lamellar units, have no vasa vasorum in the aortic media (Wolinsky and Glagov, 1967), only in the adventitia (Schlichter et al., 1949; Adams, 1964). In large mammals including man, final vascularization develops only with the establishment of the vascular wall structure. In these species, the vasa vasorum arise chiefly in the aortic branches, form a vascular plexus in the adventitia and another in the external third of the media (Clarke, 1965a, b, c, d; Wolinsky and Glagov, 1967; Putte, 1969). The electron-microscopic structure of the vasa vasorum corresponds to that of the capillaries (Parker, 1958; Shimamoto, 1969a).

LYMPH VESSELS

Only a few authors have reported studies of arterial lymphatic drainage by means of a contrast medium (Hoggan and Hoggan, 1883; Lee, 1922; Papamiltiades, 1952; Setti, 1965). Electron-microscopic observations have as yet been made only on the lymph drainage of the mesenteric vessels and aorta of normal rats maintained on an atherogenic diet (Borst et al., 1969; Jellinek et al., 1970).

On concluding this summary of details of the normal structure, it should be noted that differences from the normal have been observed in all species studied (Wilens and Sproul, 1938; Morehead and Little, 1945; Simms and Berg, 1957; Karrer, 1960a; Jones and Zook, 1965; Stehbens, 1965b; Schenk et al., 1966; Gupta et al., 1969; Likar et al., 1969).

CYTOLOGY

ENDOTHELIUM

The inner surface of the arterial wall is covered by endothelial cells. These form a flat layer in vessels fixed under pressure, bulging forward only near the nuclei. In collapsed vessels, the entire endothelial cell bulges into the lumen and its cross-section is cuboidal. According to quite recent observations by scanning electron microscopy, 'the endothelial cells form folds running along the blood stream like rifling (or spiral) in the barrel of a gun'. The endothelial cells are equipped with two types of intercellular bridge. The first starts from an endo-thelial cell near the top of the endothelial fold and connects obliquely with the neighbouring fold, and the other starts near the bottom of the endothelial fold and connects vertically with the neighbouring fold (Shimamoto et al., 1969a, b; Sunaga et al., 1969a, b). The endothelial cells are surrounded by a trilaminar cytoplasmic membrane; recently a mucopolysaccharide covering over the luminar surface has been demonstrated by special methods (Luft, 1965; Takagi et al., 1967a; Groniowski et al., 1969) (Plate II/3). The capillary endothelium thins out in several places to form pores 600–700 Å wide (Moore and Ruska, 1957; Fawcett, 1959; Movat and Fernando, 1964a, b, c). The extracellular and intra-cellular spaces probably do not communicate directly even through the pores, as these are closed by a thin membrane diaphragm with a central thickening (knob) (Kobayashi, 1968a, b; Friederics, 1969). In places the arterial endothelium extends a foot-process into the lumen (Pease and Paule, 1960; Matthews and Gardner, 1966). A similar foot-process has been observed in the small arterioles, in which it extends through the fenestrae of the IEL into the media (Moore and Ruska, 1957; Fawcett, 1959; Rhodin, 1967). The proximal sides of two endothelial cells are as a rule parallel to one another, and are separated by a 100–250 Å wide gap; this intercellular gap is supposedly filled by a substance of mucopolysaccha-ride nature (Fawcett and Wittenberg, 1962; Luft, 1965a, b; Groniowski et al., 1969). In newborn rats, the capillary junctions are wide and permeable to various substances (Suter and Majno, 1965). These junctions may infrequently become distended also in older rats (Tranzer, 1967). Opinions have been divergent con-cerning trans-junctional flow in the arteries or aorta. Certain authors (Florey, 1966) believe that the capillary junctions correspond both functionally and morphologically with the structures observed at the junctions of epithelial cells (Farquhar and Palade, 1963), thus the permeating substances cannot pass beyond the initial portion; Shimamoto (1969b), in contrast, observed the passage of col-loidal substances through the aortic endothelial cell junctions, and believes that these structures bear primary responsibility for the transport of material across the vessel wall. The cytoplasm of endothelial cells possesses the usual cell organelles. Vesicles 5–70 μ in diameter are surrounded by a single-layered membrane and localized along the luminal and basal surfaces of the cell; they probably play a role in intracellular transport. Such vesicles have been observed in both arterial and capillary endothelium. Delicate filaments 50–70 Å in diameter have been found in the endothelium of various arteries; these are thought to play a role in the recently observed contractility of the endothelium (Majno, 1968; Constantinides and Robinson 1969a, b, c). Relatively little studied endothelial structures are the membrane-surrounded microtubuli (Weibel and Palade, 1964; Sun and Ghidoni, 1969). The capillary endothelium lies on a basement membrane 500–600 Å wide and is composed of delicate filaments embedded in a homogeneous matrix, as shown by electron micrographs. A longitudinal fragmentation of the basement membrane occurs in the small arteries, it appears discontinuous in the larger muscular vessels and is entirely absent from the aorta of various species. (For more details see Altschul, 1954; Florey, 1966, French, 1966.)

SMOOTH MUSCLE CELL

The shape of the smooth muscle cell depends largely on the technique employed for fixation of the artery. The sarcolemma of the muscle cell is composed of a 70–80 Å wide cytoplasmic membrane (unit membrane), and a basement membrane which lies on its external surface. The fine structure of the basement membrane is the same as that described in connection with the endothelium. The aortic smooth muscle cells of rodents have a less distinct basement membrane (Keech, 1960; Pease and Paule, 1960b; Karrer, 1961; Ham, 1962). The sarcolemma shows in places densely staining areas which probably serve as an anchorage for myofilaments. Many micropinocytotic vesicles, 450 Å (Gardner and Matthews, 1969) to 800 Å (Cliff, 1967) wide, are located along the cytoplasmic membrane. The presence of the so-called intercellular bridges, inferred from light-microscopic examinations, could not be confirmed electron microscopically, but a membrane-to-membrane contact between the smooth muscle cells of small arteries could be seen in many places. At the point of contact smooth muscle cells lose their basement membranes and often also the external lamellae of the two unit membranes merge with one another; this phenomenon is called nexus (Dewey and Barr, 1962). The aortic smooth muscle cells of the newborn rat are still in nexus (Cliff, 1967), but later connective tissue separates them in the rat and in other species as well. The thin myofilaments are characteristic components of smooth muscle cells of the mammalian artery. Their thickness varies between 30 Å (Pease and Molinari, 1960) and 100 Å (Gardner and Matthews, 1969) and they are connected with the dense bodies of the cytoplasmic membrane. The other intercellular components of smooth muscle cells are identical with those of other cells.

Apart from a few exceptions, the media of the mammalian vascular wall contains exclusively smooth muscle cells (Karrer, 1960a; Hess and Stäubli, 1963a, b; Simpson and Harms, 1968). Medial smooth muscle cells constitute the cellular elements of the intimal proliferation (IP) in pathological processes (Hess and Stäubli, 1963a, b; Geer 1965a; Veress et al., 1969c) and substitute for the deteriorated endothelial cells (Ts'ao, 1968). In addition, they play a decisive role in the production of extracellular substances, collagen, elastin and basement membrane, similar to that of the smooth muscle cell population of other areas (Ladányi and Lelkes, 1968). Thus the vascular smooth muscle elements possess essentially the properties of the primordial mesenchymal cells, being capable of responding to altered circumstances by change of shape and functions (Wissler, 1967; Kádár et al., 1969b). (For more details see Somlyó and Somlyó, 1968; Hamoir, 1969; Shoenberg, 1969.)

FIBROBLAST

This is an elongated cell and its cytoplasm emits several thin processes, usually from opposite sides (Movat and Fernando, 1962; Ben-Ishay et al., 1968). Fibroblasts have no basement membrane; their chief function is the synthesis of adventitial collagenous elements (Takagi and Kawase, 1967; Takagi, 1969a, b).

Apart from the components listed above, many unknown factors are present in the vessel wall. The structural relations of the individual vascular segments vary widely even in areas close by. The basic vascular structure and its characteristic components are essentially the same throughout, but the combination and proportions of the latter play a decisive role in vascular wall function and thus also in the morphological appearance of lesions. The fact that vessels identical in calibre show structural variation according to the organ supplied indicates a vascular adaptation to organic function; it follows that vascular response to an identical injury will vary with the organ on a structural basis.

The transitory morphology of certain adjacent or nearby vascular areas often renders the correct judgement of normal or altered structure difficult.

Vascular innervation is still poorly understood at both histological and ultra-structural levels. In this context, innervation means not only the morphologically definable nerve structures, but also the functionally connected stimulus-conducting substances. Investigations into the nature of the latter humoral factors have as yet revealed nothing but our ignorance of their response to hormones, drugs, etc. As long as these gaps in knowledge continue, functional morphology will remain the most reliable approach to the understanding of vascular diseases and their related lesions.

*

The mammalian artery is characterized by a three-layered structure, composed of the same basic components in all mammals. Species and individual variations within the frame of the general structure are, nevertheless, great, and structural details alter also with growth and aging.

CHAPTER 2

AORTIC RESPONSE TO VARIOUS EFFECTS

INTRODUCTION

Thickening of the intima of large vessels, so-called intimal proliferation (IP), is a very typical change in chronic vascular diseases. The IP or its variations always constitutes the basic change of arteriosclerotic vascular impairment. Certain lesions associated with hypertensive vascular disease or the final stage of vascular inflammations also appear in the form of an IP. Organized thrombi are replaced by IP. The establishment of IP characterizes not only the progression of a vascular disease, but also vascular regeneration. The inner surface of vascular grafts is overgrown by several layers of proliferating cells, the so-called neointima.

Intimal proliferation develops not only in human vascular diseases, but also appears as a spontaneous lesion in vessels of various animals, above all in association with arteriosclerosis (ASC). Changes resembling the IP developing in human ASC have been observed among others in monkey (McGill et al., 1963; Middleton et al., 1964; Gresham et al., 1965), swine (Gottlieb and Lalich, 1954; Jennings et al., 1961; French et al., 1963; Campbell, 1965; McCombs et al., 1969), parrot (Finlayson et al., 1962), pigeon (Prichard et al., 1964; Cooke and Smith, 1968), cat (Lindsay and Chaikoff, 1955), dog (Svekerud et al., 1962) and cattle (Knieriem, 1967).

Intimal proliferation soon became a subject of research, because understanding of its development, in addition to clarifying in part the pathomechanism of vascular diseases might throw a light on certain important biological processes such as fibre formation. The experimental observation that IPs of essentially similar nature can be induced by various factors supports the now fairly widely accepted concept that the aetiology of ASC is complex.

Intimal proliferation could be induced experimentally by ligation of the vessel (Jores, 1898; Buck, 1961; Dauid et al., 1963; Hackensellner and Töpelmann, 1965a; Hackensellner et al., 1965, and others), by painting of the vessel wall with silver nitrate (Fabris, 1901; Sminkova, 1903), formaline (Fox et al., 1963), hydrochloric acid or alkali (Szemenyei et al., 1961, 1968; Kádár et al., 1965, 1969a, b; Veress et al., 1969c), by stricture of the vessel (Efskind, 1941), cold or warm treatment (Jaffe et al., 1929; Solovev, 1929, 1930; Kelly et al., 1952; Cox et al., 1963; Taylor et al., 1963), injury to the intima (Prior et al., 1956; Poole et al., 1958; Gutstein et al., 1963; Björkerud, 1969a, b), subcutaneous implantation of vessel (Solovev, 1932), inflation of a balloon catheter placed in the vascular lumen (Baumgarten and Studer, 1963), nerve stimulation (Gutstein et al., 1962; Thorban, 1961); by treatment with beta-aminopropionitril (Paik and Lalich, 1970), vitamin D (Hass et al., 1958; Eisenstein and Zervlois, 1963, 1964; Constantinides, 1965), adrenalin and thyroxin (Lorenzen, 1963), methoxamine (Herbertson and Kellaway, 1960) or methylcellulose (Stehbens and Silver, 1966). Development of IP was observed after X-ray irradiation (Dobrovolskaya-Zavadskaya, 1924; Mogilnitzky and Podljaschuk, 1929; Sheehan, 1944; Sheehan and Davis, 1959; Berdjis, 1960; Gold, 1962; Yarygin and Nikolajev, 1961; Lindsay et al., 1962; Kirkpatrick, 1967) in experimental hypertension (McGee and Ashworth, 1963; Spiro et al., 1965; Esterly et al., 1968; Veress et al., 1969a), in pyridoxin depletion (Rinehart and Greenberg, 1951) and after an atherogenic diet (Buck, 1958, 1961; Constantinides, 1961; Constantinides et al. 1960; Parker, 1960; Still and O'Neal, 1962; Thomas et al., 1963; Suzuki et al., 1964; Geer, 1965a, b; Imai et al., 1966; Scott et al., 1967a, b).

The IPs induced by different methods have, in addition to certain common basic characteristics, some distinguishing features. Simple and complex IPs can be distinguished by the number and quality of the constituent elements of the cell proliferation. The simple IP consists of endothelial and smooth muscle cells and contains about as many elastic and collagenous fibres as the normal vessel wall, or somewhat less. The complex IP either contains additional cell elements (connective tissue cells, macrophages, foam cells, monocytes, lymphocytes), or its intercellular substance is abnormally bulky, whether it contains elastic or collagenous fibres, or both. A simple IP develops among others in the process of regeneration, involution or atherogenic diet. But the simple proliferation may become complex if degenerative phenomena set in, as shown in combined or prolonged experiments (Anitschkow, 1933; Huezer, 1944–1945; Schlichter et al., 1949; DeSuto-Nagy and Waters, 1951; Cox et al., 1963; Taylor et al., 1963; Hass et al., 1966; Still et al., 1967; Constantinides, 1968; Wexler, 1968; Veress et al., 1969a–d).

A clue to the understanding of intricate processes is the scrutiny of the simple ones. The various kinds of simple IP were therefore studied in detail, because the phenomena taking place in them form the basis of the degenerative, or progressive regenerative processes, by which the complex arteriosclerotic lesions develop.

DEVELOPMENT AND STRUCTURE OF REGENERATIVE IP

COURSE OF AORTIC REGENERATION

In studying the course of regeneration experimentally, realistic results are obtained if a given segment of the aorta of normally managed healthy animals is so damaged that only the cellular elements deteriorate, but fibres persist, even if in a degenerated state. The persisting laminas serve as a guiding frame for the regenerating elements; this can be regarded as a kind of autotransplantation. Cell deterioration without fibre damage can be most easily achieved by painting the vessel wall with a caustic liquid. In this laboratory, the 10–20 mm long infrarenal portion of the rat abdominal aorta was painted on the adventitial surface with two brush strokes of 5 per cent hydrochloric acid, after exposure of the vessel by abdominal incision under ether anaesthesia. The nuclei of the damaged cells lost stain affinity immediately after painting (Plate LXI/1), the smooth muscle cells lost their phosphotungstic acid binding ability and anisotropy, and the cellular enzyme reactions ceased. The ATPase activity of the endothelial cells and the acid phosphatase and non-specific esterase activities of the medial smooth muscle cells were no longer demonstrable (Plate LXI/2); also the positive alkaline phosphatase reaction of the network situated at the borderline between the rat media and adventitia (LXI/3) disappeared (Lojda, 1962; Gardner, 1963; Gardner and Laing, 1965; Sótonyi et al., 1965; Hüttner et al., 1967a). The elastic fibre system differed markedly from that of the undamaged vessel portion. Normally, the elastic fibres are undulating and 1–2 μ thick in the rat aorta; on painting with hydrochloric acid they become straight, longer and thinner (0.3–1 μ). This morphological change does not, however, imply a major structural disorganization; the altered fibres continued to show anisotropy in polarization micrographs (Plate IX/32, 33) and they behaved in phenol and anilin reactions like normal fibres.

Neither the intima nor the media showed further change one day after painting with acid, but a marked cell increase was noted in the adventitia at the border zone between damaged and intact vessel wall. The cells showed a distinct non-specific esterase activity (Plate LXI/2), the intercellular AMP increased and the borderline alkaline phosphatase activity rose, as compared to normal (Plate LXI/3). Two days after painting, mononuclear cells with round nuclei appeared above the bare IEL (Plate LXI/4) and on the second to the fifth day endothelial cells, more active enzymatically than the controls, migrated from the intact vascular areas to the damaged segment (Plate LXI/5). Simultaneously, smooth muscle cells at the border between the intact and damaged part of the media began to divide and showed an increased non-specific esterase activity (Plate LXI/5); they then became mobilized and migrated to the straightened elastic fibres in the deteriorated internal third of the vessel wall. Twelve days after painting, the entire damaged segment was lined by a single cell row, which rendered the intima complete again. Between the 14th and 18th day, elongated cells with cytoplasmic processes began to appear between the damaged IEL and the lining cell row. This resulted in the formation of a stratified IP which made up the new vessel wall (Plates VIII/30; LXI/6–9); the latter was complete by the 30th–50th day. A considerable amount of AMP substances appeared intercellularly, as in the adventitia (Plate LXI/9). No regeneration of the original media took place, but its elastic fibres persisted (Plate LXI/7, 10). The place of the deteriorated smooth muscle cells was occupied by thick, compact, collagenous fibres, and a few fibrocytes appeared in the outer and middle thirds of the media (Plates III/4; LXI/7, 9). Simultaneously with the cicatrization of the media, cells decreased, but fibres increased in number in the adventitia (Plates III/5; LXI/7, 9) and by the 90th day the alkaline phosphatase active net appeared, although in a rudimentary form, at the borderline between the two vascular wall layers (Plate LXI/12).

The inferiority of the regenerative IP in general, and of the newly formed media in particular, is signified by the fact that degenerative phenomena developed in them after a certain period of time. Hundred and fifty-two days after painting, the proliferate showed sudanophilia, and after 261 days extensive calcification and increase of hyaline connective tissue were noted (Plate III/6).

As to the cell population of the IP formed in the course of vascular regeneration, conflicting observations have been made. Fabris (1901), Sminkova (1903) and Lange (1924) saw connective tissue elements. Kirkpatrick (1967) found mesenchymal cells in the proliferate of the auricular artery of rabbits kept on a normal diet after X-ray irradiation. Szemenyei et al. (1968), Buck (1963) and Kádár et al. (1965a) observed smooth muscle cells in the regenerative IP. Evidence of the true nature of the cellular composition of IP was finally obtained by electron-microscopic examinations.

ANALYSIS OF THE CELLULAR COMPONENTS OF IP

ULTRASTRUCTURE OF THE LINING CELLS OF IP

Initially, endothelial cells are present above the impaired IEL, and later these constitute the surface row of the multilayered IP. The cytoplasmic membrane of the endothelial cells is a regular, on the average 96 Å thick unit membrane, which maintains its trilamellar structure throughout (Plate IV/7, 8). No zonula occludens has been observed between the cells; they adhere to one another by the glove-like interdigitations typical of endothelial cells (Plate V/12). The gaps between the junctions are filled by a delicate granular substance, having the same density as the ground substance. If fixation is perfect, a similar layer, 80–100 Å thick, is seen on the luminal surface of the cytoplasmic membrane; this is the 'external coat', which has been observed on several kinds of cell surfaces (Bennett, 1963; Fawcett, 1965) and is rich in AMP (Luft, 1965a, b). In proliferates older than 30 days, 400–800 Å wide osmiophilic clumps lie on the cytoplasmic membrane of the endothelial cells (Plates IV/9, 10; V/17); similar structures were observed by Parker (1960), who regarded them as lipoprotein molecules. According to Courtice and Garlick (1962), the lipoprotein molecules circulate in the blood in the form of granules 200–700 Å in diameter. It seems, therefore, very probable that the clumps we had seen were lipoprotein molecules.

Both on the luminal and external sides of the cytoplasmic membrane there are many pinocytotic vesicles (Plates IV/7, 8, 10; V/15), 700–900 Å in diameter. Some of them are patent, others are closed toward the lumen by an amorphous zone, similar in density to the external coat, as observed also by Luft (1964a). A uniform, single-layered closing membrane is seen on only few vesicles and the central thickening or knob described by Kobayashi (1968b) and Rhodin (1962b) cannot be seen. Some vesicles opened into the intercellular junctions (Plate IV/11). All vesicles localizing along the luminal surface are single, but many of those along the external surface are confluent, multiple or even cluster-like (Plate V/13). Vesicles at both surfaces contain a granular, medium electron-dense material.

Two types of endothelial cells can be distinguished on the basis of the density of the hyaloplasm (Plate V/13, 17). Cells of one type are dark and compact, those of the other type are light and looser in structure. Of the cell organelles, the smooth endoplasmic reticulum prevails in the dark cells and the rough endoplasmic reticulum is more marked in the light ones. The ductuli, cisterna-like in places, contain low electron-dense granules 60–70 Å in diameter, as observed also by Weibel and Palade (1964). The Golgi apparatus of the dark cells consists of many tubules and vesicles (Plate IV/8). According to Karrer (1960b), Dauid et al. (1963) and Schoefl (1964), young immature endothelial cells are characterized by the presence of several membrane systems. This supports the view that newly formed endothelial cells help to form the proliferate. The mitochondria are generally small, with a dense matrix, and aggregate as a rule around the nuclei. Free ribosomes are more numerous in the light cells. In addition to the above organelles, the cytoplasm contains vesicles surrounded by a unit membrane, a few lysosomes and 50–70 Å thick filaments. The latter correspond either with contractile elements (French et al., 1963), or with supporting structures forming part of the cytoskeleton (Rhodin, 1962b). Most cells have an oblong spindle-shaped nucleus, with the chromatin aggregating along the nuclear membrane (Plate IV/7).

At the basal surfaces of the endothelial cells there is in places a 200–350 Å thick discontinuous basement membrane (Plate V/15); a 100–200 Å wide electron-dense layer separates it from the cytoplasmic membrane (Plate IV/7, 8). Its outer surface shows no sharp demarcation, being in places continuous with the intercellular fibrous elements of the proliferate.

The endothelial cells of the IP contain, in addition to the above cytoplasmic structures, neutral lipid droplets surrounded by a unit membrane (Plate V/14). This correlates well with the observation that young or not completely differentiated cells are more permeable to lipids than the mature older cells of the intact vessel wall (Constantinides, 1965). A greater lipid susceptibility of young regenerative cells as compared to mature ones has also been reported (Hass et al., 1961; Constantinides and Lawder, 1963; Cox et al., 1963; Taylor et al., 1963).

ORIGIN OF ENDOTHELIAL CELLS OF IP

According to Altschul (1954), the new endothelial cell row arises by the division of pre-existing intact mature cells; these migrate to the damaged segment to initiate regeneration. Dividing endothelial cells were first observed by Zahn (1884) in the rabbit carotid artery; later Efskind (1941) saw them in a regenerative process of rabbit aorta. Gottlob and Zinner (1962) observed multinucleated endothelial cells. Poole and Florey (1958, Poole et al., 1959) demonstrated endothelial cell division in regenerating rabbit aorta by means of a membrane preparation. Although we failed to obtain electron-microscopic evidence of such divisions in our material, we have been able to confirm it indirectly. It is known that embryonic cells as well as young or premitotic cells have a lighter electron-lucent hyaloplasm than mature ones, owing to their higher water contents. We believe that the pale cells with relatively few organelles which we saw among the endothelial cell populations of the impaired vascular segments corresponded with the premitotic, newly formed cells. The lipid accumulating capacity and rich membrane systems of the latter (Karrer, 1960a, b; Constantinides, 1963, 1965; Dauid et al., 1963; Schoefl, 1964), as well as the absence of highly differentiated cell linking systems are also in support of this interpretation.

The activated endothelial cells migrate to the deteriorated media or the exposed IEL (Plate LXI/2, 5, 6) and form a confluent layer in 10–12 days. This is in good accordance with the observation that the migration rate of the regenerating endothelium is 0.1–0.15 mm daily (McKenzie and Drewenthal, 1960). The migration rate is apparently higher, 3 mm daily, in the case of transplantation (Ghidoni et al., 1968).

Additional cell elements playing a role in vascular regeneration are the mononuclear cells originating from the blood. They appear over the damaged IEL (Plate LXI/4) already after 2 days, to judge from light- and electron micrographs (Plate V/16). This confirms the observations of Stump et al. (1963) and O'Neal et al. (1964) who saw mononuclear cells and endothelial and smooth muscle cells differentiating from mononuclear blood cells in dacron tubes placed in the aortic lumen of pigs or dogs.

Apparently, most of the endothelial cell population of the regenerative IP originate from intact cells of the adjacent unimpaired vascular segment, and the rest arise by differentiation from mononuclear cells of the blood.

STRUCTURE OF CELL COMPONENTS OF THE PROLIFERATE

The precise nature of cells appearing between the newly formed endothelial cell row and the original damaged IEL cannot easily be identified by light microscopy. They are elongated cells with cytoplasmic processes, hence they might as well represent smooth muscle cells as fibroblasts. They stain red with azan (Plate LXI/7), brownish-black with Mallory (Plate LXI/6) and yellow with van Gieson's technique. These staining properties are indicative of smooth muscle cells. Evidence was obtained by polarization microscopy (Romhányi, 1962, 1966). In specimens mounted in Canada balsam, certain cell and fibre components of the proliferation showed a positive birefringence (Plate IX/32, 33). After an aniline reaction, which eliminates the anisotropy of collagenous and elastic fibres, the elongated cells continued to show a positive birefringence, like the smooth muscle cells of the normal media (Plate IX/32, 33). Anisotropy is due to the many myofibrils which pass along the cell's longitudinal axis; connective tissue cells and macrophages do not possess such elements and are, therefore, isotropic. Thus polarization microscopy has unequivocally attested that the cellular components of the proliferation are smooth muscle cells and this was subsequently confirmed by electron microscopy.

Rhodin (1962a, b) has established six main characteristics of smooth muscle cells as follows:

1. they are associated with a basement membrane;
2. pinocytotic vesicles are connected with the cytoplasmic membrane;
3. the hyaloplasm is filled by myofilaments lying along the cell's longitudinal axis;
4. highly electron-dense bodies, as a rule triangular or spindle-shaped, are present in the cytoplasm, and along the cytoplasmic membrane. These so-called 'attachment bodies' serve to fix the myofilaments;
5. the other cell organelles lie centrally around the nucleus in a cap-like manner;
6. the nucleus is an elongated ellipsoid in shape.

The ultrastructural characteristics of the cellular components of the regenerative IP corresponded in every respect to the above criteria (Plates VI/19–23; VII/24), but differed slightly in certain features from common smooth muscle cells. Their Golgi apparatus and rough endoplasmic reticulum were extraordinarily well developed (Plates VI/19; VII/24); the canaliculi of the latter distended in places in a sac- or cisterna-like manner and contained a medium electron-dense, granular substance (Plate XXI/91). Some cells contained more numerous organelles and fewer myofilaments than the rest. The basement membrane was 250–400 Å thick and consisted of granular and filamentous elements; in places it formed two or three layers along the cytoplasmic membranes (Plates VI/20–23; XXII/95–99). Some cells were associated with rudimentary, discontinuous fragments of a presumably newly formed basement membrane (Plate VII/25), localizing below the detached original one. On the basis of these characteristics, the cellular components of the regenerative proliferation are regarded as modified smooth muscle cells, similarly to the muscular elements of arteriosclerotic lesions (Thomas et al., 1963; Parker and Odland, 1966a). In addition to relaxation and contraction, these modified cells play an important role in fibrillogenesis (for details, see p. 42).

The greater activity of the modified smooth muscle has been confirmed by enzyme histochemical studies (Hüttner et al., 1967a). They show a considerably greater non-specific esterase activity than the normal medial smooth muscle cells (Plate LXI/5, 6); this activity, however, returns to normal after the proliferation has fully developed (Plate LXI/8).

Certain changes in old proliferations can be regarded as a transition to the complex arteriosclerotic IP. For example, three months after vascular surgery myelin figures appeared in the smooth muscle cells. Electron micrographs suggest a tendency of the cells to eliminate these degeneration products; first they became demarcated, then they were extruded from the cells (Plate VII/26). The extra- and intracellularly localizing myelin figures, as well as lipid droplets (Plate VII/27) appearing inside the endothelial cells and in the intercellular space, are responsible for the sudanophilia of aged lesions. The accumulation of lipid, reported by others (Geer et al., 1961; Haust and More, 1963; Parker et al., 1963; Balis et al., 1964; Geer, 1965b) in smooth muscle cells of proliferations induced by an atherogenic diet did not appear in our normally fed experimental animals. Nagy and Szemenyei (1965) observed, however, that switch to a cholesterol diet in the postoperative period resulted in an early accumulation of cholesterol in the endothelial and smooth muscle cells of the newly formed IP (Plate LXI/13, 14). On administration of calcium, sclerotic deposits arose in the IP, but they did not appear in the normal segment (Plate LXI/15). This kind of sclerotization was accelerated by vitamin D_2 treatment.

ORIGIN OF SMOOTH MUSCLE CELLS

Smooth muscle cells can in principle arise from four sources:

1. endothelial cells;
2. subintimally localizing multipotent mesenchymal cells;
3. mononuclear cell elements of the circulating blood;
4. smooth muscle cells of the media.

Altschul (1954) regards the endothelial cells as multipotent elements with a capacity for multiple differentiation and thinks it probable that the cell elements of the proliferation originate from endothelial cells.

Baumgarten (1876) was the first to observe the presence of subintimally localized cells ('angioblasts') from which all layers of the vessel wall can develop. Recently Seifert (1962, 1963a, b) and Rodbard et al. (1962) have considered the existence of such intermediary multipotent cell forms and Rodbard and his co-workers believe that their differentiation to endothelial, smooth muscle or connective tissue cells is determined by the dynamic function of the vessels.

Since in our experiments the cell elements of the impaired aortic segment were completely destroyed, pre-existing subintimal cells as a source of the proliferation can be excluded. Similar cells from the adjacent intact segment can also be disregarded as a source, because they formed only a single row of endothelium over the damaged vascular wall portion, and no undifferentiated cells could be demonstrated under this layer by either light- or electron microscopy.

Stump et al. (1963) and O'Neal et al. (1964) mention in their previously cited publications the differentiation of smooth muscle cells from corpuscular elements of the circulating blood. We observed the attachment of blood monocytes to the lesion only in the earliest phase of regeneration and think that such elements play a role exclusively in endothelial cell formation. The fact that transitional types between blood corpuscular elements and smooth muscle cells have never been observed militates against the validity of such hypotheses.

The most widely accepted source of the cell elements of IP is the media of the unimpaired vascular segment; its smooth muscle cells undergo proliferation and migrate into the subendothelial space of the impaired segment, as confirmed by experimental evidence. The medial origin of smooth muscle cell components has been demonstrated by Buck (1961) in involutional IP, by Thomas et al. (1963), Still (1964), Balis et al. (1964) and Scott et al. (1967a, b) in IP induced by an atherogenic diet and by Szemenyei et al. (1968) in regenerative IP of muscular arteries. Medial smooth muscle cells of the border zone between normal and impaired vascular tissue showed a considerable increase of enzyme activity and dividing cell forms appeared already during the first days of regeneration (Plate LXI/5). Subsequently, the cells migrated toward the impaired area and appeared between the degenerated elastic lamellae of the vascular wall's interior third. From there they proceeded to the subendothelial space (Plate VII/28, 29) between the fragments of the broken IEL or through the distended stomae. The smooth muscle cells did not lose their mobility, to judge from the presence of smooth muscle cell protrusions in the newly formed IEL stoma of a 90-day old proliferation (Plate VIII/31); according to Hoff (1968), such protrusions signify a cell migration. It seems fairly certain from the above considerations that the muscle cell elements of the regenerative IP originate from smooth muscle cells of the unimpaired vascular media and they reach the damaged area by migration, to form a multilayered proliferation between the damaged IEL and the row of newly formed endothelial cells.

THE INTERCELLULAR SUBSTANCE OF IP

Light- and electron-microscopic examinations of the intercellular substance of experimental IP were performed to follow up the course of elastic fibre formation under pathologically altered conditions. As the ultrastructure of experimental

3

aortic IP was found to resemble that of early arteriosclerotic change, elastic fibre genesis in the regenerative IP was regarded as conclusive of the mechanism of similar processes under pathologic conditions of a different nature (ASC, organization of vascular graft). Recently, many literary reports have dealt with the formation or ultrastructure of elastic fibres in the extracellular space of various tissues or in the wall of elastic arteries and aorta (Lansing et al., 1952; Movat et al., 1959; Pease and Paule, 1960; Karrer, 1960b; Fernando and Movat, 1963; Haust et al., 1965a; Haust and More, 1966; Bartman, 1968). Despite great interest in elastic fibre genesis, the morphological steps of elastin formation are still poorly understood compared with those of collagenous fibre formation. On the basis of our light- and electron-microscopic studies of the extracellular space of experimental IP, the process of elastic fibre formation can be outlined as follows: First a single row of endothelial cells grows over the damaged area, then a proliferation, composed of several layers of smooth muscle cells, appears between the straightened IEL and the endothelial layer. Fibres staining positively with resorcin-fuchsin arise between the cells of the proliferation and a coherent IEL develops one year later (Plate LXI/10,11).

Initially, a delicate, granular, phosphotungstic acid positive substance appears between the newly formed, single endothelial cell row and the straightened IEL. Later the IP becomes stratified and a delicate fibrillar substance is seen in polarized light, after aniline reaction (Plate VII/32, 33). Electron microscopically, medium electron-dense aggregates, 800–2000 Å in diameter, with 70 Å wide, electron-dense elastic granules at their margins, are seen between the smooth muscle cells on counterstaining with uranyl acetate (Plate XI/42, 44). At a higher magnification, elastic granules are seen also inside some aggregates. In places the elastic granules are arranged in a row, forming filament-like structures (Plates IX/35, 37; XI/42); these are 70 Å wide and have a periodicity of 140 Å. We propose to denote these structures elastic fibrils. In some areas the elastic granules clump together; these appear in cross-section as tubular structures with an electron-lucent centre averaging 110 Å in diameter (Plate IX/35). They are in fact pseudo-tubuli, as the tubular appearance of their cross-section arises by the circular arrangement of the granules, i.e. elastic fibrils.

Apart from the above structure there were also delicate filaments on the average 30–40 Å in diameter, not showing a periodicity; these appeared either in close association with, or independently of, the elastic granules or aggregates (Plate IX/34–37). Elastic clumps in the diameter range of 400–2000 Å showed a marked affinity to phosphotungstic acid (PTA); but stain-binding capacity tended to diminish together with the electron density after coalescence to larger clumps or fibres (Plates X/38–41; XI/43–46). PTA-affinity persisted at the marginal areas of the larger elastic aggregates, because they were surrounded by elementary granules and fibrils (Plates IX/35–37; X/38–41). After 3 months, the IP contained almost fully mature elastic fibres, and a newly formed elastic lamella appeared below the row of endothelial cells. Maturity was signified by a high degree of electron lucence on counterstaining with uranyl acetate, and by the absence of PTA-binding capacity in the body of the elastic structures; only a very narrow marginal zone remained PTA-positive (Plates X/41; XI/46). Structures corresponding to the above elementary elastic units were seen also inside the basement membrane associated with the smooth muscle cell components of the IP. The basement membrane was 200–500 Å wide on the average, and granular and filamentous structures could be identified in it at a higher magnification (Plates XX/93; XXII/94). The basement membrane appeared not only in association with smooth muscle cells, but also independently of them in a multilayered form with the contours of cytoplasmic membranes still impressed (Plate XXII/95–99). Whether associated with smooth muscle cells or not, the basement membranes contained myofilaments, 30–40 Å in diameter, and arranged in a nest-like manner. When our findings are correlated with observations and speculations by others, information about elastic fibre formation may be summarized as follows:

Many authors agree that the morphological unit of the elastic substance is a fibril or filament of electron-microscopic order, composed of either granular, or vesicular subunits (Pease and Molinari, 1960; Pease and Paule, 1960; Takagi et al., 1968; Keech, 1960; Bierring and Kabayashi, 1963; Schwarz, 1964; Greenlee et al., 1966; Ghidoni et al., 1968; Kádár et al., 1967, 1969a–d; Chase, 1969). Rannie (1963) supposes that the so-called oxytalan fibres, which are visible under the light microscope after special staining, might be the precursors of the elastic fibrils.

We explain elastic fibre formation as follows:

Two basic elements can be distinguished in the extracellular matrix. One is a fairly electron-lucent filament, 30–40 Å in diameter, not showing a periodicity. This element has been regularly observed in the extracellular space of the IP and consists probably of AMP as suggested also by Gardner (1965) and Fahrenbach et al. (1965). The other basic element is the homogeneous electron-dense particle, 70 Å in diameter, termed an elastic granule. Such granules combine, probably with the help of AMP filaments, to form elastic fibrils, which are 70 Å in diameter and show a periodicity of 140 Å. The role of the AMP microfilaments in elastic fibril formation has not yet been fully confirmed, but it seems likely that they support the combining granules as a guiding framework.

Elastic fibrils arranged in rows appear as vesicle-like structures in cross-section. The fusion of elastic granules and fibrils results in the formation of larger elastic clump, 400–2000 Å in diameter, and these join to form elastic fibres or elastic lamellae, according to the functional requirements of the vessel wall.

The chemical composition of the above elements is better known than their structural relations. The most important investigations were carried out by Bedford and Katritsky (1963), Partridge et al. (1963), Partridge (1966) and Miller et al. (1964). Elastin contains a specific amino acid, desmosin or isodesmosin, not to be found in any other protein. Desmosin arises from 4 molecules of lysine through the oxidative deamination of three of them. This proelastin substance contains globular molecules which link with one another by free amino acid radicals on the surface of the paired lysin molecules. The globular molecules are of an alkaline nature, which is probably determined by the two free amino groups on the surface. We think that the protein molecules which contain the globular desmosin and isodesmosin should be sought in the elastic granules. Partridge holds a similar view (Personal communication), because he saw similar structures on electron-microscopic examination of hydrolysed elastin; the fact that his and our structures differed in size may have been due to a loss of water during hydrolysis. It seems likely that the elastic fibrils constituting the fibres do not pass parallel to the latter's longitudinal axis, but rather form a spiral, as has been inferred from Romhányi's (1965) analysis by polarized light microscope; a spiral structure would explain also the typical picture, shown by polarized optics, consisting of one central isotropic line and two lateral anisotropic ones. The fibrils arising from the combination of elastic granules probably become embedded in the AMP substance to form the larger elastic fibres.

An important structural aspect of elastic fibrils and fibres is their relation to the various AMPs. A related problem is the variation of the PTA-binding ability of elastic elements according to their degree of maturity. The high PTA-affinity of the developing elastic fibrils may be due to the presence of excess lysin, the free amino acid groups of which do not participate in the desmosin cross-linkages. In the course of clumping and subsequent fibril and fibre formation from the elastic elements, lysin and its free amino groups tend to diminish and PTA-binding is limited to the marginal parts of the developing elastic structures. Lysine not yet embedded in AMP is present at the marginal zones as long as elastic elements are still in the process of development. A direct binding of PTA by AMP has also been reported (Takagi, 1967a, b; Bartman, 1968; Pease and Molinari, 1960a). In our opinion, PTA-affinity is not so much a property of AMP as of those elastic fibrils and granules which possess free amino groups. It has been demonstrated that mature fibres still showing a PTA-affinity at the marginal zones are surrounded by a coat rich in AMP (Banga et al., 1965; Banga, 1966).

The distribution of AMPs in the vascular wall and their relation to the elastic fibres will be discussed later.

The role of the elastic element-like structures of the basement membrane in elastic fibre formation can be explained as follows: Filaments 30–50 Å in diameter and granules 60–80 Å in diameter localizing in the basement membrane are very similar to certain extracellular ultrastructural elements not associated with a basement membrane. The fusion of these elementary units into elastic fibrils or fibres is likely to take place outside the basement membrane. The fundamental similarity of basement membrane and ground substance has been observed by several authors. Jarmolich et al. (1968) reported the increase of AMP and appearance of typical fibrils and dense granules in vascular smooth muscle cell explants. Rodgers et al. (1967) observed that in small arteries a basement membrane structure fulfilled the function of the elastic lamella. Movat and Fernando (1963b) observed a basement membrane structure and ground substance in the elastic membrane. Our findings support Paule's hypothesis (1963) that the basement membrane of smooth muscle cells plays an important role in elastin formation and also that its AMP components are involved in this process.

In our experimental model, detached portions of the basement membrane of smooth muscle cells greatly resembled the extracellular substance present in other areas of the IP. After a gradual detachment, the basement membrane reached the extracellular area in which the fusion of elastic granules and fibrils into clumps and fibres, respectively, was taking place. The basement membranes still associated with smooth muscle cells appeared as a rule discontinuous, suggesting an asynchronism of detachment and resynthesis. An intensive resynthesis was indicated by the increased metabolic activity of the smooth muscle cells; this was signified by a considerable distension of the endoplasmic reticulum and by the appearance of a large amount of delicately granular material in the distended organelles. This process of elastic fibre genesis resembled in every respect the ultrastructural details of human and experimental arteriosclerotic lesions (Rhodin and Dalhamm, 1955; Constantinides, et al., 1958; Constantinides, 1965) (see Chapter 3).

The elementary units of elastic fibres arising in the IP were the elastic granules, 70 Å in diameter, and the elastic microfibrils formed by the coalescence of these granules and fine AMP filaments; the latter showed in places a periodicity of 140 Å. These units and extracellular AMP fused to form the PTA-binding elastic clumps, and the latter coalesced to give rise to the elastic fibre. This lost its PTA-binding capacity when mature. The synthesis of the elementary units, and of the AMP also, seemed to be connected with the presence of smooth muscle cells.

ELASTIC FIBRE GENESIS IN EMBRYONIC VESSELS

Elastic fibre genesis has been shown to play an important role in the establishment of regenerative, involutional and transplantation IP. In aortic IP, elastic fibre genesis appears to be connected with the smooth muscle cells of the vascular wall. To clarify the precise role of the smooth muscle cells and AMPs, normal embryonic fibre genesis was studied as the most suitable model. In this monograph, only the normal aortic elastogenesis is discussed in detail.

Most investigators have studied elastic fibre genesis in a given period of embryonic development. Examinations have chiefly been carried out on newborn or embryonic rats, rabbit and chicks. Bartman (1968) studied the aortic ultrastructure of newborn rats, Bierring and Kabayashi (1963) that of newborn rabbits. Fahrenbach et al. (1965) examined the nuchal ligament of a calf foetus for elastic fibre structure, and described the elementary elastic unit of this system as a filament, 130 Å in diameter. He observed that filament formation, i.e. elastogenesis, is accompanied by a distinct cellular activity. Ross and Sandberg (1967) inferred from electron-microscopic examinations of embryonic rat tendon that one elementary unit of the elastic fibre is the so-called tubular fibril, 100 Å in diameter, and another unit is the so-called central semi-amorphous substance. They concluded that the first unit is present during early elastogenesis, while the second characterizes the mature elastic fibres and correspond therefore to the elastin itself. The tubular fibrils are composed of a kind of fibrous protein (connective tissue fibre) rather than elastin or collagen.

From their examination of chick embryo explants, Lelkes and Karmazsin (1965) regarded the intercellular substance arising under the influence of pulsation as an elastic substance or AMP. Karrer (1960b) and Takagi et al. (1967a, b) studied the ultrastructure of the embryonic chicken aorta in great detail and described the cell forms of the aortic wall and the morphology of the intercellular substance.

Examinations in this laboratory have shown that elastic fibre genesis takes essentially the same course in the embryonic rat aorta as in the IP. In the early stage, elastic clumps showing a marked affinity to PTA and uranyl acetate appeared below the endothelial cell layer and between the smooth muscle cells (Plates XII/49, 50; XIII/53, 54). Elastic granules, fibrils and microfilaments were seen at the margins of the clumps and also independently of them (Plate XII/47–49). The collagenous fibres appeared very early between the elastic ones, and this was probably the only notable structural difference from the extracellular fibre genesis of the IP.

A close connection between the basement membrane of smooth muscle cells and the developing elastic elements was observed also in embryonic fibre genesis. This seemed to commence at the luminal side of the inner medial portion and gradually involved the middle and outer layers of the media and the adventitia. While mature elastic fibres had already developed in the medial portion adjoining the endothelium (Plates XII/52; XIII/55, 56), to judge from the loss of PTA-binding capacity, elastic clumps, granules and fibrils with a strong PTA-affinity were still present in the outer layer of the media and in the adventitia.

During the development of the embryonic rat aorta, multipotent mesenchymal cells are transformed into vascular smooth muscle cells. The latter, which can be regarded as modified smooth muscle cells, have a special fibre-producing function and, in addition, play a role in the synthesis of elementary elastin units and ground substance. The elastic granules, synthesized in all probability by the smooth muscle cells, form elastic fibrils in the extracellular space, these again form elastic clumps, which become embedded in AMPs to give rise to elastic fibres or lamellae, according to the functional requirements of the vascular wall. This process corresponds in every respect to the course of elastogenesis in the IP.

Further studies in this laboratory concerned the ultrastructure of the thoracic aorta of the developing chick embryo. The span of embryonic life is 21 days for both chickens and rats; our light- and electron-microscopic examinations of the various aortic segments were conducted between the 6th and the 21st days of embryonic development.

Light microscopy showed a demonstrable amount of orcein-positive elastic substance at as early as 8 days. This appeared in the middle layer of the media, but was not yet present in the inner and outer layers. Elastic clumps and fibres were seen in the aortic wall peripheral to the orcein-positive area (Plate XIV/57, 58). Later the orcein-positive aggregates approached the endothelial cells and after 17 days they localized immediately below the endothelial layer. The alcian-blue, PAS-positive substance showed a reverse tendency; initially it was present in large amounts in the inner and middle thirds of the media, later it tended to diminish with the progression of the process.

The shapes of the cell components changed in the course of fibre genesis. Prior to the appearance of the early elastic elements, the cells could only be defined by light microscopy as being oval or round, with relatively large nuclei and a few cytoplasmic processes. At 8 days, elongated cell forms were already seen in the middle layer of the media, and by the time the elastic fibres had begun to develop, these smooth muscle cell-like forms appeared also in the areas adjoining the endothelium (Plate XIV/57, 58, 59).

Electron-microscopic examinations of the developing embryonic chick aorta revealed the following extracellular structures:

At 6 days, no PTA-positive substance was yet present between the cell components of the media (Plate XV/63), but small elastic aggregates were seen at 8 days (Plate XV/64). At 9 days, elastic granules, averaging 80–110 Å in diameter, appeared at the marginal parts of the PTA-positive elastic clumps. In places the granules were arranged in a thread-like manner, forming microfibrils similar in diameter and with a periodicity of 140–160 Å. In other places the granules were arranged in an annular or tubular manner, as in the IP; these structures might have corresponded with cross-sections of aggregated fibrils. The microfibrils were closely associated with the elastic clumps, lying at their margins (Plate XV/65–67). Elastic fibres developing at the external part of the media began to lose PTA-binding capacity (Plate XV/68) after 9 days, and completely mature fibres with exclusively marginal PTA-affinity were already seen after 14 days (Plate XVIII/78). Both light- and electron-microscopic observations suggest that elastic fibre genesis proceeds towards the vascular lumen and reaches the extracellular area below the endothelial cell row by the 17th day.

Counterstaining with uranyl acetate revealed the presence of a delicate fibrillar substance between the cells at as early as 6 days, when the extracellular area was still PTA-negative. This phenomenon is known from the literature as characteristic of early elastic substance.

The nature of the cells was studied after counterstaining with uranyl acetate and lead citrate.

As already noted, initially the cells are round or oval, with processes and ample subcellular structures (Plate XVI/69–71). After 8 days they become elongated, myofilaments appear in them and attachment bodies develop close to the cell surface. The cell organelles aggregate around the nucleus. At this stage, the cells correspond in every respect to smooth muscle cells and acquire a basement membrane (Plate XVI/72, 73). Increased cellular activity is manifested by the distension of the cisternae of the endoplasmic reticulum and the appearance of a delicate granular substance in the cisternae. Many free ribosomes and many vesicles, surrounded by a unit membrane, appear in the hyaloplasm (Plate XVI/71). Some vesicles contain a substance of lipid density, others are filled by an electron-lucent material.

The process of elastic fibre genesis in the embryonic chick aorta can be summarized as follows: The first electron-microscopically recognizable structural units are the so-called elastic granules. Then microfibrils arise and aggregate to form elastic clumps which are characterized by a strong affinity to PTA. The fusion of the elastic clumps gives rise to elastic fibres and elastic lamellae, which lose PTA-affinity except at the marginal zones, where elastic clumps and fibrils are present.

A decreased capacity to bind PTA signifies the maturation of the elastic structures. Elastic material appears early in embryonic life, first at the outer part of the media, then progressing gradually up to the endothelium. A corresponding sequential synthesis can be seen during the maturation of arterial cells. These have initially an undefinable structure, then become more and more similar to adult smooth muscle cells. They have specialized functions, being capable of the complete or partial synthesis of the basic elements of elastin and probably also of ground substance, a function of which the primitive mesenchymal cells appear incapable.

EXAMINATIONS BY DIGESTION WITH ELASTASE

Elastase (serine proteinase), isolated by Baló and Bangha (1949b), is the only known enzyme that can hydrolyse elastin. Experiments with elastase have been widely performed to obtain more information on elastic fibre structure. Lansing et al.

(1952) added elastin to a suspension of elastic fibres and Keech (1960) injected it *in vivo* into the thoracic aorta prior to embedding for electron-microscopic examination. Yokota (1957) applied elastase to embedded specimens of calf nuchal ligament, after removal of methacrylate from the ultra-thin sections, while Waisman (1968) applied it to the tissue block before embedding. Ross and Bornstein (1969) digested fibres from the nuchal ligament with collagenase and the residues with elastase. These authors agree that the elastic substance, i.e. the elastic fibre, has two main components, a microfibrillar structure and an amorphous material. The latter, which appears late in embryonic life and characterizes the mature fibres of the nuchal ligament, is the elastin-digestible substance.

In this laboratory, elastase was applied to Durcupan-embedded aortic specimens from chick embryos of various ages, in order to study enzyme action on the elastic structures in various stages of maturation. Digestibility by elastase was found to be the property of mature elastic clumps and fibres, since none of the early PTA-binding elastic structures was decomposed by the enzyme (Plate XV/64–67). Apparently, sensitivity to elastase increases with the decline of PTA-affinity (Plate XVII/74, 75). Elastase appears to act specifically on mature clumps, fibres, and lamellae, as it never digested microfibrils, elastic fibrils, collagenous fibres or intracellular structures (Plates XVII/76; XVIII/79). It digested, however, the contents of the membrane-surrounded vesicles which appear in aortic cells of the chick embryo after 6 days. Partial or complete digestion of the vesicles commenced after 8 days (Plate XVII/77). Mature elastic fibres with a low PTA-binding capacity were almost completely decomposed (Plate XVII/78), while the PTA-positive immature clumps remained intact (Plate XVIII/79). The fully developed IEL of the newly-hatched chick binds PTA only at the margins (Plate XVIII/80); at this stage of maturity the elastic fibre is completely digestible by elastase (Plate XIV/61, 62), while collagenous fibres, microfibrils and intracellular structures (myofilaments, etc.) resist enzymatic action (Plate XVIII/81). The action of elastase is thus highly specific, and it follows that the intracellular vesicles sensitive to this enzyme resemble in composition the mature elastic elements. Elastase digestion had similar results in experimental IP of rat aorta. The mature, fully developed IEL and the elongated elastic fibres of the damaged vascular wall area were sensitive to the enzyme, whereas the immature, delicate elastic fibrils resisted its digestive action (Plate LXI/16, 17). This insensitivity is apparently due to the protein nature of the fibrils; the enzyme cannot link with this type of substrate. It remains to be clarified by further examination whether the substrate is an AMP, a lipoprotein, or a protein-polysaccharide or elastin-AMP complex.

The specimens used to demonstrate elastic elements were subsequently treated by special techniques to visualize the AMPs for electron-microscopic examination. Fixing solutions containing ruthenium red (glutaraldehyde and osmium tetroxide) have a strong affinity to highly polymerized AMPs (Luft, 1964b). Ruthenium red links selectively with the AMPs, above all with heparin and chondroitin sulphate, and has a lesser affinity to certain acid substituents (aliphatic polymers) and acid polypeptides. It does not bind to neutral polysaccharides, proteins and aliphatic compounds. It stains selectively the cartilaginous matrix, the myotendinous junctions and the surfaces of the intestinal microvilli, i.e. all sites where AMPs are present (Luft, 1966). Its affinity to the cementing substance of collagenous fibres (Luft, 1964b) has been shown to be due to the latter's high AMP content (Myers et al., 1969). The AMP-containing structures appear in various forms: as an amorphous coat surrounding the collagenous fibres, as a transversal belt or as delicate lateral filaments linked with one another by fibrils. These structures are usually composed of chondroitin sulphate and a hyaluronic acid–protein complex. On staining the cartilaginous matrix with ruthenium red Luft (1965a, b) observed two basic AMP structures, a fibre 100–180 Å in diameter and a granule, 100–140 Å in diameter. According to Luft (1965b), the cartilaginous matrix is composed of dense spherical particles, linked with one another by delicate filaments, on the average 50 Å thick. A net-like structure constituted by granules and fibres of varying thickness corresponds to the protein polysaccharide macromolecule, which has a specific affinity to ruthenium red. The specific binding of ruthenium red by highly polymerized AMPs was demonstrated by Siew and Wagner (1968).

Aortic specimens from chick embryos of various ages were fixed in ruthenium red containing glutaraldehyde and osmium tetroxide for electron-microscopic examination of the localization of AMPs. Net-like aggregates of ruthenium-red positive granules and thick and thin fibrils were seen between the smooth muscle cells, in close association with the marginal parts of the smaller extracellular elastic clumps. After the fusion of these clumps, the ruthenium red-positive aggregates appeared at the surface and a few granules or fibrils remained inside the elastic clump or fibre. The ruthenium red-positive substance also occurred independently of elastic structures in the extracellular space (Plates XIX/83; XX/86, 87), and in the coat surrounding the collagenous fibres.

The ground substance contains a considerable amount of AMP in the early phase of embryonic development. In the intercellular space scarcely any ruthenium red-positive substance is present prior to the appearance of PTA-positive elastic structures, i.e. after 6 days of embryonic life (Plate XIX/82). After 8 days, however, the entire extracellular space of the media is filled with AMP up to the subendothelium (Plate XIX/83). Later when the developing elastic clumps and fibres replace the ground substance, the extracellular AMP tends to diminish (Plate XIX/84, 85), and ruthenium red-positive meshworks are seen primarily at the surfaces of elastic and collagenous fibres (Plate XX/86, 87). The ruthenium-red positive AMPs are not digested by elastase and thus they persist after the enzymatic decomposition of the clump or fibre with which they are associated. In certain cases also the AMPs incorporated into the elastic fibre resist elastase action and persist in a honeycomb-like arrangement after the elastic substance has vanished (Plate XX/88, 89). Extended enzyme action, however, decomposes the incorporated AMPs, probably because their protein bonds are sensitive to elastase. The mesh of ruthenium red-positive spheres and threads might correspond to protein-polysaccharide macromolecules. The fine threads probably correspond to the AMP filaments seen in preparations counterstained with PTA and uranyl acetate, and the microfibrils are probably the elastic microfibrils observed by Ross and Bornstein (1970) and also by us, in embryonic rat aorta and in experimental aortic IP. The finding that the proportions of extracellular AMPs and elastic fibres are reverse, suggests that the former become incorporated into the elastic structures. We believe that elastic fibre genesis takes place in an essentially similar manner in chick embryo aorta, rat embryo aorta and in IP induced by

41

vascular damage, and that the formation of elastic substance is associated with the vascular smooth muscle cells.

In summary, the digestibility of aortic elastic tissue by elastase appears to increase with the latter's maturation during embryonic development or in the course of IP. Sensitivity to elastase is inversely related to the PTA-affinity of the developing elastic tissue. Early elastic elements (granules, microfibrils, developing clumps and immature fibres) bind PTA readily and resist the action of elastase, while mature elements (clumps, elastic fibres or elastic lamellae) gradually lose affinity to PTA and simultaneously become susceptible to elastase.

The AMP components of the vascular wall, i.e. the ruthenium red-positive network of spheres and threads in the intercellular space of the chick embryo aorta appear in increasing amount from media to endothelium in the early stage of embryonic development between 6 and 8 days. The amount of AMP decreases parallel to the development of elastic clumps and fibres between the smooth muscle cells. The elastic clumps and fibres are surrounded by the ruthenium red-positive material. After the fusion of clumps into fibres, AMP becomes incorporated into the latter. The AMPs associated with elastic fibres are less susceptible to elastase action than the amorphous-appearing basic substance.

FUNCTION OF SMOOTH MUSCLE CELLS AND THEIR ROLE IN FIBRILLOGENESIS

Our examinations indicate that the precursor of the elastic fibres is synthesized in the IP by the latter's cellular components, i.e. by vascular smooth muscle cells which can be regarded as mesenchymal cells specialized for a fibre-producing function. This process seems to be analogous to tropocollagen synthesis by fibroblasts. The desmosin and isodesmosin produced by smooth muscle cells require additional components to make up the elastic substance, i.e. the elastic fibre. The probable additional components are, on the one hand, the extracellular AMP filaments which help to form microfibrils from elastic granules, on the other hand the amorphous AMP substance which serves as a matrix for the embedding of elastic clumps during the process of elastic fibre formation. The functional requirements of the vessel wall induce the transformation of multipotent mesenchymal cells and vascular smooth muscle cells into modified smooth muscle cells specialized for fibre synthesis. The modified cells are capable of a partial, or perhaps complete, synthesis of the elementary units of elastin and probably also of the ground substance, as inferred from examinations of elastogenesis in experimental IP and embryonic chick and rat aorta.

In discussing elastic fibre formation in vascular smooth muscle cells, one cannot avoid dealing with the much disputed problem of whether or not cells specialized for elastic fiber synthesis, the so-called elastoblasts, do in fact exist.

In a paper written in 1928, Krompecher supported the elastoblast theory, but recently (Personal communication) he has agreed with the opinion of others that probably no elastoblasts exist in the vascular wall. The vascular smooth muscle cells are, however, in all probability capable of synthesizing either a precursor or certain components of the elastic fibre. According to Krompecher's interpretation, no elastoblast, but a specialized cell function does in fact operate in elastic fibre genesis. This function, attributed to vascular smooth muscle cells, requires the presence of pulsation to come into display. On examining heart and aortic explants from chick embryo, Lelkes and Karmazsin (1965) observed that elastic membrane formation took place exclusively in the presence of pulsation. Krompecher (1966) regards pulsation as the specific stimulus of elastic membrane formation, and elastin production as the response of the undifferentiated mesenchymal cells to the intermittent mechanical stimulus. Ladányi and Lelkes (1968) arrived at a similar conclusion from examinations of ligated rat ureter; cells of the pulsating tunica were involved in elastic fibre formation above the ligature. They regard this cell function as a qualitative adaptation, resulting in the activation of the primordial fibro-elastoblastic capacity by the mechanical stimulus.

As already noted, parallel to the appearance of elastic substance in the developing chick embryo aorta, transformation of undifferentiated mesenchymal cells to forms corresponding in every ultrastructural detail with smooth muscle cells, proceeds inwardly from the outer part of the wall. In addition to the static morphological observations, functional implications can be derived from electron micrographs. Intensive cellular activity is indicated by the extraordinary distension of the endoplasmic reticulum, the presence of a fibrillar, granular substance in the dilated ductules, and the presence of many ribosomes (Plate XXI/90–92) and of vesicular structures showing dissimilar density on counterstaining with uranyl acetate.

In summary, studies on chick embryo aorta serve as additional proof for the observation that the presence of smooth muscle cells is indispensable for the appearance of elastic fibres or clumps.

STRUCTURE OF INACTIVITY (INVOLUTIONAL) PROLIFERATION OF THE INTIMA

Constriction of the vessel by a simple or double ligature was already employed in the past century for study of the pathomechanism of arteriosclerotic vascular lesions. The considerable, or complete depression of blood flow by ligation results in a functionally inactive state of the vessel. The IP developing in response to inactivity has been named inactivity (involutional) proliferation on the analogy of post-partum vascular occlusion in the uterus.

Investigation of lesions developing in response to inactivity was pioneered by Baumgarten (1876) who analysed the organization of thrombi formed after simple ligation. Double ligature was used first by Böttcher (1888). Since then many authors have studied the development of IP after simple or double ligation (Auerbach, 1877; Senftleben, 1879; Burdach, 1885; Pick, 1885; Beneke, 1890; Pekelharing, 1890; Sokoloff, 1893; Jores, 1898; Meckel, 1903; Schaeffer and Radosh, 1924; Malyschev, 1929; Efskind, 1941; Mehrotra, 1953; Williams, 1956; Schmidt-Diedrichs and Courtice, 1963; Hackensellner et al., 1965; Kunz et al., 1967a, b; Zollinger, 1967; Jurukova and Rohr, 1968; Wexler, 1968; Hoff and Gottlob, 1969; Hassler, 1970).

Electron-microscopic examination of inactivity IP was first reported by Buck (1961), who employed double ligature on rabbit carotid aorta. The multilayered IP developing in the damaged segment occluded the vascular lumen. It contained macrophages and modified smooth muscle cells. Buck called the latter myointimal cells and believed that they originated from the media, while the macrophages derived from the blood stream. Hackensellner et al. (1965) reported similar investigations, but they saw only smooth muscle cells originating from the media in the proliferation below the endothelial coat. On investigating the early phase of the lesion, Hoff (1968) observed that changes of mitochondria and endoplasmic reticulum appeared already 1–5 minutes after ligation; subsequently, large, oedematous, electron-dense vesicles appeared in the endothelial cells and subendothelial oedema developed. They attributed these changes to anoxic permeability disturbances and/or to the release of vasoactive substance from the vascular segment impaired by ligation. Still (1967) described subendothelial plasma deposition and appearance of macrophages as early ultrastructural changes in the segment above a simple ligature. Hoff and Gottlob (1969) demonstrated the accumulation of lipoproteins in endothelial and smooth muscle cell components of the IP forming between two ligatures in a rabbit vessel. Using a double ligation of rat abdominal aorta, Kunz et al. (1967a) arrived at the same conclusion as Hackensellner et al. (1965) on rabbit aorta. Kunz et al. (1967b) were the first to test drug influence on the development of IP. Hydrocortisone delayed the formation of the lesion and there was a corresponding decrease of ^{3}H thymidine index and ^{3}H proline and ^{35}S sulphate incorporation.

Using a double ligature in this laboratory, the rat aorta was not completely occluded, only constricted, and the two ligatures were placed at 5 mm distance from one another. The structure of the IP developing in the ligated segment corresponded in every respect to the regenerative IP (Plates XXIII/100; LXI/18, 19). The medial smooth muscle cells migrated into the subendothelial space across the stoma of the IEL. Contrary to Still (1967), we observed neither macrophages nor lymphocytes. The modified smooth muscle cells of the inactivity IP played the same role in elastic fibre formation as in other types of proliferation (Plates XXIII/103; XXIV/104, 105). After 95 days, myelin figures (Plate XXIV/105–107) appeared in the cells and intercellular space, as with regenerative IP. The two kinds of proliferation differed only in the time required for development. The inactivity proliferation took a shorter time to establish, probably because the media did not deteriorate, so that the smooth muscle cells could soon become activated after the trauma, and also because their route of migration was shorter.

The question arises, what factor or mechanism might be responsible for the initiation of smooth muscle cell migration. This is probably the most important aspect of the vascular reaction, yet one still poorly understood. The tendency towards regeneration after complete vascular wall destruction might in itself offer a sufficient explanation. But no convincing explanation has as yet been found for smooth muscle cell mobilization in connection with changes resulting from aortic constriction or an atherogenic diet. This problem will be discussed in more detail when dealing with the development of IP in response to an atherogenic diet.

INTIMAL PROLIFERATION IN TRANSPLANTED GRAFTS (NEO-INTIMA)

DEVELOPMENT AND STRUCTURE OF THE NEO-INTIMA

Voorhees et al. (1952) were the first to introduce permeable grafts into vascular surgery, and they studied the structure of the tissue overgoing the inner surface of the graft (neo-intima). Similar examinations were soon reported by Blakemore and Voorhees (1954), and since then both the surgical and pathological aspects of the problem have been investigated in great detail (Szilagyi et al., 1954, 1963, 1964, 1965; Deterling and Bhonslay, 1955; Creech et al., 1957; Martinez et al., 1957; Petry and Heberer, 1957; Szöllősy et al., 1958; Meijne, 1959; McKenzie and Drewenthal, 1960; Bartos et al., 1961, 1965a, b; Florey et al., 1961, 1962; Jellinek et al., 1961a, b, 1963; Wosolowski et al., 1961; Wosolowski, 1962; Wosolowski and Dennis, 1963; Wosolowski et al., 1963; Jordan et al., 1962; Dauid et al., 1963; Stump et al., 1963; Voorhees, 1963; Voorhees and Wosolowski, 1963; DeBakey et al., 1964; O'Neal et al., 1964; Warren et al., 1965; Halpert and O'Neal, 1966; Jennings et al., 1966; Bartos and Szöllősy, 1967; Ghani and Still, 1967; Still et al., 1967; Bartos, 1968; Ghidoni et al., 1968; Kádár et al., 1969c; Veress et al., 1970). The development and structure of the neo-intima, the degenerative processes taking place in it and the origin of its cell components are discussed here on the basis of the literature and our own observations on the aortic reactions of dogs to graft implantation.

A fibrin film, containing various numbers of leukocytes and red blood cells, deposits first on the inner surface of the graft. The surface of the film is as a rule smooth, but sometimes turbulent blood flow imparts to it a ribbed appearance (Voorhees, 1963). A secondary thrombosis is rare; usually small clumps of platelets or red cells deposit on the surface of the fibrin film and slowly become organized (Jellinek et al., 1963). The neutrophilic leukocytes disappear from the fibrin mass by the end of the first week, and macrophages, histiocytes and foreign-body giant cells appear, with abundant cytoplasm indicating vigorous phagocytic activity (Ghidoni et al., 1968).

Simultaneously, degenerative processes (smooth muscle cell necrosis, deterioration of elastic membrane) take place in the proximal and distal aortic portions adjoining the graft, but also a regenerative tendency can be observed. Endothelial cells and smooth muscle cells become active and migrate to the surface of the graft and into the fibrin film. The observed rate of endothelial cell migration varies between 0.15 mm per day (McKenzie et al., 1960) and 3 mm per day (Ghidoni et al., 1968); it is in any case faster than that of the cell components of the neo-intima which replaces the fibrin film. Thus a coherent endothelial cell layer grows over the inner surface of the graft within 2–3 weeks; at this time fibrin or macrophages are still present below the newly formed endothelium.

According to Voorhees (1963), the final neo-intima migrates to the vascular prosthesis like a pannus. Its rate of progress does not exceed 1.5 mm daily (Ghidoni et al., 1968). Voorhees et al. (1952) saw fibroblasts in the pannus, but other authors dealing with the neo-intima (Karrer, 1960a; Hess et al., 1963a, b; Simpson et al. 1968) reported that the overwhelming majority of the proliferative cells were modified smooth muscle cells (Plate LXI/20). Probably Voorhees and Wosolowski

(1963) mistook the latter for fibroblasts for lack of special muscle stains. Anyhow, Voorhees (1963) reported later that smooth muscle cells were present in the neo-intima of a vascular prosthesis implanted for 8 years.

The development of the neo-intima is complete after 3 months; its surface is covered by endothelium and subjacent are many smooth muscle cells (Plate LXI/20) and some fibroblasts and fibrocytes (Plate XXV/108–111). A variable amount of collagenous fibres is present between the cells (Plate XXVI/112, 113) (the older the preparation, the more numerous), and delicate elastic fibres lie chiefly at the surface or near the host aorta (Plate LXI/21). In the literature the presence or absence of elastic fibres is controversial. Voorhees and his co-workers failed to observe them in 1952 and neither Petry and Heberer (1957), nor Ghidoni et al.(1968) saw elastic elements in the neo-intima, while their presence was reported by Florey et al. (1961), Dauid et al. (1963), Voorhees (1963), Jellinek et al. (1963), Bartos (1968), Kádár et al. (1969c), Veress et al. (1970). The number of these fibres, however, tends to decrease with the time elapsing after implanta tion (Bartos, 1968).

Simultaneously with the processes taking place at the inner surface of the graft, a tissue proliferation consisting of connective tissue cells, histiocytes and capillaries develops in the adventitial region, and connects with the neo-intima between the units of the graft.

Thus on full organization of the graft, three layers can be distinguished:

1. Neo-intima, consisting of an endothelial layer, and a subjacent population of many smooth muscle cells and a few fibroblasts, with elastic and collagenous fibres in the intercellular spaces. Kerényi (Personal communication) observed that in human subclavial-femoral bypass prostheses, neo-intima developed only to a level 5–8 mm away from the host vessel and that the fibrin film still lined the intermediate area after one and a half years.

2. Neomedia, formed by the graft itself, with granulation tissue filling its pores.

3. Neo-adventitia, consisting of proliferative tissue, which contains elastic fibres and, depending on its age, also capillaries (Halpert and O'Neal, 1966; Bartos, 1968).

ORIGIN OF CELL COMPONENTS OF NEO-INTIMA

Three sources have been considered as the possible origin of neo-intimal cell components:

1. blood stream;
2. host aorta;
3. neo-adventitia.

Observations have been reported in support of all three possibilities.

Stump et al. (1963) and O'Neal et al. (1964) placed small dacron tubes in the blood stream, attaching them to the vessel wall by means of a thin thread. Since no cells were found on the threads, a vascular wall origin of the cell population on the tubes was excluded, and it was therefore postulated that monocytes from the blood stream became differentiated into endothelial cells or smooth muscle cells inside the tubes. Halpert and O'Neal (1966) and Ghani and Still (1967) also believe that the cell components of the vascular graft neo-intima derive from the blood stream.

The recent investigations of O'Neal and his research group have tended more to support the hypothesis of Florey et al. (1961), Dauid et al. (1963), Ghidoni et al. (1967), and Ghidoni et al. (1968). The eventual contribution of the adventitia was excluded by the use of impermeable prostheses, and as neither leukocytes nor monocytes appeared in the initial fibrin film, and no transitory forms were seen among the modified smooth muscle cell components of the neo-intima, a possible role of blood cells in neo-intima formation was rejected. This could easily be done because the authors were able to follow up the entire migration process of endothelial and smooth muscle cell elements from the adjoining areas of the host aorta. From these findings the definitive conclusion was drawn that neo-intimal cell constituents originated from the host aorta.

Voorhees et al. (1963), Dauid et al. (1963) and Jellinek et al. (1963) have stressed the role of adventitial cells growing into the pores of the graft and they believe that either the capillaries growing into that tissue or immature connective tissue cells serve as the sources of neo-intimal cell elements. This might be true if porous prostheses are used, but with impermeable grafts these sources are insignificant.

According to present knowledge, the host aorta seems to be the most probable source of the neo-intimal cell components, and the contribution of the blood stream and adventitia is in all probability unimportant.

DEGENERATIVE CHANGES IN TRANSPLANTATIONAL IP

Degenerative processes of the neo-intima play a decisive role in the fate of the patient and of the graft as well. Wosolowski (1962) described in his monograph a cartilaginous islet formation, and Voorhees (1963) observed hyalinization, appearance of bone tissue and chronic inflammation. Hyalinization of the neo-intima was also reported by Bartos and Szöllősy (1967). Authors dealing with the factors eventually involved in degenerative processes have arrived at controversial conclusions. Wosolowski et al. (1961) and Bartos and Szöllősy (1967) have attributed the primary role to porosity, while Szilagyi et al. (1964) have disputed this.

To obtain more information on the problem, the structure of the neo-intima was examined electron microscopically in both a compact (4 ml per cm^2 per min per mm Hg) and a porous (29 ml per cm^2 per min per mm Hg) graft, each implanted for 4 years. Bartos has kindly collaborated in these studies. The neo-intima of the porous graft contained beneath the endothelial lining a row of smooth muscle cells embedded between thick collagenous fibres, and also fibroblasts (Plates XXV/108–111; XXVI/112). Cell degeneration was indicated by the extracellular presence of lipid droplets, myelin figures and dense bodies, congregating around cell processes (Plate XXVI/113). Also elastic fibres were seen in the intercellular space, in areas adjoining the lumen and the host aorta.

The neo-intima of the compact prosthesis showed microscopically the appearance of a hyaline cartilage (Silberberg et al., 1966; Silva and Hart, 1967; Meachim and Roy, 1967; Roy, 1968; Silva 1969), composed of regular cartilaginous cells and intercellular substance (Plate XXVI/114, 115).

These findings support the views of Wosolowski et al. (1961) and Bartos and Szöllősy (1967), and suggest that graft pore size plays a role in the degenerative process. The more compact the graft, the fewer neo-adventitial capillaries can pass through its pores to supply the deep neo-intimal layers distant from the lumen. A chronic hypoxia develops in the poorly supplied area and a bradytrophic hyaline, cartilaginous or osseous tissue arises as a result of adaptation. These tissues render the prosthesis rigid and insufficient and are indeed of a lower functional value (in respect of graft function) than a proliferation rich in elastic fibre and smooth muscle elements.

It is concluded that the transplantational IP (neo-intima) arising on the inner surface of vascular grafts resembles structurally the regeneration and inactivity IPs and that its cell components originate chiefly from the host aorta. A decisive difference between the two is the scarcity of elastic elements in the graft neo-intima. The porosity of the graft plays a fundamental role in the nature of the degenerative changes taking place in transplantational IP.

CHANGES OF LARGE VESSELS IN EXPERIMENTAL HYPERTENSION

SURVEY OF THE LITERATURE

Data in the literature (see Introduction) and our own observations (see p. 27), have shown that the aortic changes elicited by different factors have some common characteristics. The development of IP is the primary response of the aorta to various injuries. This suggests that there is a fundamental difference in the reactions of small and large arteries. In fact, neither a subendothelial nor a media fibrinoid has been observed either in human aorta or in experimental aortic change.

Hypertension affects the vessels in all segments of the arterial system. Yet hypertensive lesions of large vessels have been relatively little studied compared to the number of reports on arteriosclerotic lesions. Investigators of the human aorta take two different views, depending on the type and location of the primary changes. According to the first school of thought, the aorta responds to hypertension by IP. Fishberg (1925) and Dietrich (1930) believe the earliest reaction to be the multiplication of the intimal layers with, in addition to cell proliferation, a concomitant marked increase of elastic fibres. According to Fishberg's newer interpretation (1954), hypertension only accelerates the development of arteriosclerotic lesions. Vascular reaction by IP has also been observed by Lange (1924) and Smirnova-Zamkova (1951), but they regard the proliferation as a secondary change, developing in response to the impairment of adventitial vessels. Thus while Fishberg (1925) and Dietrich (1930) have regarded the intima as the primary site of attack of hypertension also in the large vessels, Lange (1924) and Smirnova-Zamkova (1951) have interpreted IP as a secondary change to adventitial vessels.

Ashworth and Haynes (1948) and Zlateva (1960) also hold the latter view, but their findings do not correspond with those of Lange (1924) and Smirnova-Zamkova (1951). Ashworth et al. observed hyperplasia and hyalinization of smooth muscle cells of the vasa vasorum and Zlateva describes in addition a fibrinoid necrosis of the vasa vasorum and smooth muscle cell hyperplasia in the media as the earliest aortic changes. The necrotic areas of the walls of the vasa vasorum later undergo a fibrotic or hyaline transformation, and vasa vasorum lesions result in degeneration and necrosis of the smooth muscle cells of the media, owing to the reduction of oxygen supply.

The early stage of the experimental hypertensive change of large vessels was examined by Still (1967) on rat aorta. He constricted the aorta by ligation and examined its proximal segment by electron microscopy. The first change was the widening of the subendothelium, accompanied by the accumulation of a granular, fibrillar substance. Simultaneously, the endothelial cells became vacuolized and the contents of the vacuoles resembled the granular, fibrillar substance. Subsequently, monocytes and lymphocytes migrated into the vessel wall across the endothelium and deposited to form an IP (Pollák, 1969). McGill et al. (1961) examined monkey aorta with hypertension of 19–29 months duration. The animals were fed on a normal diet and had no lipaemia. The gross and microscopic damage of the aorta corresponded to that of arteriosclerotic lesions. The IPs formed were either fibrotic, containing many connective tissue fibres and few smooth muscle and connective tissue cells, or consisted of foamy cells characteristic of atheroma and smooth muscle cells. In both types of lesions, the intercellular space contained a considerable amount of metachromatic substance and delicate elastic fibres. The two main differences from human arteriosclerotic lesions were (i) a greater amount of mucinous extracellular substance and (ii) fewer collagenous and elastic fibres in the fibrous plaques. Salgado (1970) has observed medial smooth muscle cell degeneration as the early aortic change in DOCA-hypertension. Rabbits rendered hypertensive and maintained on a normal diet developed arteriosclerotic lesions in the aorta (Dill and Isenhour, 1942) and similar changes could be induced by an atherogenic diet (Wilens, 1943; Bronte-Stewart and Heptinstall, 1954; Heptinstall and Porter, 1957; Fischer et al., 1958). Campbell (1954) and Moses (1954) examined the effect of experimental hypertension and high cholesterol diet on dogs. Whether the serum lipid level was normal (Wakerlin et al., 1957), or elevated (Moses, 1954; Wakerlin et al., 1957), the arteriosclerotic lesions of the aorta were rendered more severe by the hypertensive state. Similar observations have been made on rats by Wissler et al. (1954), Deming et al. (1957, 1958), Renaud and Allard (1963), Eadles et al. (1965) and Koletsky et al. (1968).

MORPHOLOGY OF LARGE VESSEL CHANGES IN EXPERIMENTAL MALIGNANT HYPERTENSION

Most experimental hypertensive lesions described in the literature developed in consequence of a slowly progressive, essentially benign hypertensive state. Still (1967) produced in experiments a malignant hypertension but mechanically and examined only acute cases. If irrespective of mural structure and calibre, the

4

vessels are regarded as parts of a uniform organ system, the uniformity of their responses to certain injuries might well be postulated; presumably the structural differences, and the severity and duration of the inducing factors do not alter but merely modify the fundamental response.

Based on the hypothesis of 'uniform response' it was postulated that given influences of an appropriate severity and duration would elicit similar changes in the aorta and large muscular-type vessels as in small arteries. Painting with a caustic substance destroyed the aortic wall and was strongly aphysiologic, therefore to determine whether structural differences between vessels fundamentally alter the response or only modify it, the experimental malignant hypertension model elaborated by Lőrincz and Gorácz (1954) was chosen (Veress et al., 1969a). The operative procedure proposed by Lőrincz and Gorácz is described in detail in the Appendix.

One week after the operation, malignant hypertensive changes developed in the small arteries of the rats, whereas in the large vessels the first lesions appeared only about one month later.

The initial change was, as usual, necrosis of the vascular smooth muscle cells; this could be clearly visualized by staining with PTA (Plate LXI/22). The lesions, however, were initiated by a change of permeability, as judged by the appearance of vacuoles in endothelial cells and subendothelium (Plate LXII/26) and a subsequent intra-subendothelial diffusion of plasma (Plate LXII/28, 29), clearly visible after staining with PTA or azan, or in polarized light (Plate XXVII/117). The subintimal fibrinoid deposition occasionally extended over one-third of the width of the vessel wall. At this stage, smooth muscle cell necrosis and subendothelial fibrinoid were simultaneously present (Plate LXII/23, 27). A periarterial inflammatory cell reaction might additionally develop, as in the small arteries (Plate LXII/23). Single muscle cells between the elastic fibres might fuse with one another during the development of the subendothelial fibrinoid, but large vessel lesions never assumed the homogeneous appearance found in small vessel changes (see p. 26.).

In large vessels, the subendothelial fibrinoid becomes transformed in two ways: one is signified by a black-to-yellow colour transition on M-staining and flame-red-to-blue transition on azan staining (Plate LXII/30), the other is the phagocytosis of the fibrinoid by macrophages, foamy RES cells and smooth muscle cells (Plates XXVII/116; LXII/25); the phagocytic cells contain lipid-like substances (Plate LXII/24).

Changes of the various types of vessels at the same stage of hypertension can be compared in Plate LXII/31. While in the small artery the lesion has already become transformed to scar tissue, the musculoelastic femoral artery still contains some subendothelial fibrinoid, but predominantly IP, and in the aorta there is only subendothelial fibrinoid and as yet no IP. Thus the progress of the change is largely influenced by the vessel wall structure.

A widening of the subendothelial space can be observed electron microscopically already on the second day of hypertension (Plate XXVII/118), with basement-membrane-like granular, filamentous substance and medium electron-dense granules reminiscent of plasma. Increase of endothelial cell activity is indicated by a hypertrophy of the Golgi-apparatus (Plate XXVII/118). Polymeric fibrin appeared in the vascular wall already at this stage (Plate XXVII/120). Bundles of fibrin and degenerative membrane formations were seen 19 days after the operation (Plate XXVII/119), but crystal-like fibrin bodies did not appear until the 41st day (Plate XXVIII/121), in contrast to the small arteries where they developed by the end of the first week (see p. 70). Simultaneously with the deposition of plasma substances in the vessel wall, corpuscular elements of the blood entered the subendothelial space. This process started on the second post-operative day (Plate XXVIII/122). Apart from plasma substances, the main components of the 65-day-old proliferation were smooth muscle cells, which synthesized elastic fibres in the same manner as in other types of proliferation, as shown by the presence of elastic clumps between the rows of smooth muscle cells constituting the proliferation (Plate XXVIII/123, 124).

Serial experiments have clearly shown that structurally different vessels respond to the same damage in the same way: first endothelial permeability increases, then plasma is deposited in the subendothelial space, fibrinoid develops and smooth muscle cell necrosis takes place. Intimal proliferation develops only secondarily, partly through phagocytosis of the fibrinoid, partly through mobilization and migration of smooth muscle cells.

Apart from the fundamental identity of the primary response, the modifying effect of the structural differences also comes into display.

1. The most conspicuous modifications have been observed in connection with the elastic elements. In small arteries, in which the IEL represents a single continuous elastic structure, necrotic medial smooth muscle cells and inflowing plasma together formed a media fibrinoid (see Chapter 9). No such lesion developed, however, in the large muscular and elastic vessels. In these arteries, including the aorta, only single smooth muscle cell necrosis was seen, or—in muscular-type large arteries—the coalescence of a few necrotic muscle cells between two elastic lamellae (Plate LXII/23, 27). It appeared that the strong elastic lamellae prevented the inflow of a larger amount of plasma. This had a double effect: on the one hand, the small amount of plasma deposition in the media impaired the nutritional conditions of the smooth muscle cells to a lesser extent than in the small arteries, in which the smooth muscle cells were practically 'drowned' by the copious inflow of plasma. On the other hand, the presence of elastic lamellae reduced the possibility of the admixture of smooth muscle cells with one another and with the plasma, because they isolated the cells from one another, thus preventing the development of a fibrinoid over the entire width of the media. The minor extent of plasma flow through the walls of the large vessels was indicated by the observation that, while perivascular granulation was marked around the small vessels, it was slighter around the large ones and did not appear at all around the aorta (Plate LXII/27, 31). The radial pattern of plasma diffusion in the perivascular area of small vessels was clearly visible in fluorescence micrographs (Hüttner et al., 1966a). The development of granulation was probably related to the extravasation of plasma into the perivascular space. Thus the absence of granulation around the aorta could be attributed to two causes: (i) plasma extravasation was insignificant owing to the barrier effect of the elastic fibres; (ii) the barrier function of the elastic lamellae prevented the progression of vascular wall destruction to such a degree that the development of a massive fibrotic granulation would be required to prevent rupture.

2. The time required for the development of the lesion differs for each type of vascular structure. While in the small arteries the IP had already constricted the lumen and the subendothelial and the perivascular granulation had progressed to fibrous tissue, the large muscular vessels showed only a minor degree of plasma deposition and single muscle cell necroses. A corresponding delay in changes was observed in the aorta as compared to large arteries (Plate LXII/31). The temporal delay in changes seems to be due not so much to the quantity of elastic elements as to the dissimilar degrees of permeability of small and large vessels. Damage of the endothelial cell or of that component primarily responsible for permeability (coat surface, pinocytosis, basement membrane, etc.) seems to take place earlier in small than in large vessels (see Chapter 10); and vice versa, the endothelial cells of large vessels are probably more resistant to the permeability-increasing effect of malignant hypertension. If there were no such differences, subendothelial plasma deposition would probably take place simultaneously in all vascular areas. Anyhow, the known morphological differences between endothelial cells of vessels of different calibres cannot fully account for this phenomenon (see Chapter 1).

CHARACTERISTICS OF HYPERTENSIVE REPARATIVE IP

The various types of simple IP have been considered in the sections 'Development and structure of regenerative IP' (p. 27.), 'Structure of inactivity (involutional) proliferation of the intima' (p. 43.) and 'Intimal proliferation in transplanted grafts' (p. 45). The main cellular components of simple IP were found to be smooth muscle cells, migrating from the media of adjoining vessel portions into the space between the endothelium and original IEL or to the inner surface of the vascular graft. In regenerative and inactivity IPs, the trend of cell migration was inward, while in the transplantational IP it is horizontal. Most migrating cell elements were common components of the normal vessel wall. In hypertensive regenerative IP, a modification and extension of the range of cellular components could be observed. This type of IP differed not only from simple IP, but also from complex arteriosclerotic IP, representing a transitional type between the two.

In the first stage of the development of simple IP, a subendothelial space was either absent owing to the destruction of the endothelium, or it widened slightly, if at all, in consequence of a minor plasma deposition.

In malignant hypertension, in contrast, the development of the IP is preceded by massive vascular damage and by the development of a so-called subendothelial fibrinoid from the large amount of plasma depositing in the subendothelial space. The fibrinoid is composed of highly oriented fibrin formations and fibrin crystals (Kerényi et al., 1966a; Hüttner et al., 1968). The disappearance of the subendo-thelial fibrinoid requires cellular activity, whether it takes place by phagocytosis or by hyaline transformation (see Chapter 7). This fact can in itself account for the dissimilar characteristics of the reparative IP. While the cell components of simple IPs migrate inwardly, or horizontally, some cells of the reparative IP take an opposite route of migration, proceeding outward from the lumen. This applies, of course, only to the few cells—phagocytes, lymphocytes—moving into the subendothelial space. Ingestion of the fibrinoid requires the phagocytic activity of macrophages derived from the blood stream and approaching the subendothelial fibrinoid across the endothelial junctions. This explains the observation that in the initial phase of the organization of the fibrinoid, the macrophages with their round nuclei occupy first the luminal third of the lesion under which the fibrinoid is still preserved. The involvement of phagocytic activity in the organization process has been confirmed by electron micrographs of small vessels (see Chapter 7). As organization progresses, residues of the fibrinoid are seen in the form of minor clumps localizing immediately above the IEL, deep in the proliferation. Unlike the macrophages, the smooth muscle cell components of the proliferation migrate inwardly, from the media into the subendothelial space. Although according to Hüttner (Personal communication) the smooth muscle cells of the media show ultrastructural signs of an increase in activity already in an early stage, they do not appear in greater numbers in the subendothelial space until the chronic stage. Intensive elastic fibre genesis commences simultaneously with the subendothelial establishment of the smooth muscle cells (Plate XXVIII/123, 124).

Thus the first stage of the formation of large vessel IP in malignant hypertension mobilizes a lesser number of smooth muscle cells, connective tissue cells, fibroblasts and fibrocytes than of macrophages. Hence not only the trend of cell migration, but also the cell composition appears modified compared to simple IP. These differences, nevertheless, vanish during the further progression of the lesion, because degenerative changes and macrophages may also appear in simple IP, and smooth muscle cells and elastic fibres increase in number in the regenerative IP, while the initially numerous macrophages diminish.

The pathomechanism of the IP associated with benign hypertension differs from that of the reparative IP. In the former process, plasma deposition and the consequent fibrinoid formation are minor, and the mechanism of the change resembles primarily that of a simple involutional IP. A slight plasma deposition does not provoke a mass migration of macrophages into the vessel wall, but the smooth muscle cells become mobilized, probably by the intramural plasma diffusion and migrate into the subendothelial space to form the proliferation.

To summarize, the early changes found in large vessel lesions of experimental malignant hypertension (increase of permeability, subendothelial plasma deposition and fibrinoid formation, smooth muscle cell necrosis) are fundamentally the same as in the small vessels. This supports the hypothesis that vascular reaction to a given injury is uniform throughout the entire system, and the difference of vascular structure only modifies, but does not alter the response. Modification comes into play either as a temporal difference in the appearance of the changes (related to a dissimilar permeability of endothelium), or as the absence of the development of a media fibrinoid or perivascular granulation (barrier role of elastic fibres).

CHAPTER 3

DEVELOPMENT AND ULTRASTRUCTURE OF ARTERIOSCLEROTIC LESIONS

INTRODUCTION

'Totally new concepts were not spawned' conclude Ghidoni and O'Neal in their study on human arteriosclerosis, written in 1967. In fact a survey of earlier publications will soon convince the reader that despite persevering research work, no notable progress has been made in this field during recent decades.

Of the hypotheses advanced to explain the origin of ASC, the so-called filtration theory has been most widely accepted.

Virchow stated in 1856 that in the initial phase of arteriosclerosis, a mucinous substance from the blood plasma gains access to the intima, and connective tissue cells appear in turn in the subendothelial space. He observed the presence of delicate elastic fibres in the mucinous substance. Both Virchow and Aschoff (1924) thought that the appearance of lipids was a secondary phenomenon. The present interpretation of Virchow's hypothesis is that the primary phenomenon of atheroma development is the increase of endothelial permeability, allowing the accumulation of a fluid rich in AMP in the subendothelial space (Bredt, 1961; Doerr, 1963; Shimamoto, 1963; Nakashima, 1967; Avtandilov, 1970), and this is followed by cell proliferation (formation of IP from smooth muscle cells) and finally by degenerative processes (appearance of lipid, foam cell lesions, etc). Also Gerő et al. (1961b) have shown that lipoprotein originating from the blood plasma links with the AMPs previously accumulated in the vessel wall and that the complex thus formed deposits to form the atheromatous plaque.

The primary lipid filtration theory was originally advanced by Marchand in 1904, and confirmed by Anitschkow in 1913 on the basis of his fundamental experiment in which rabbits fed cholesterol developed lesions reminiscent of human ASC. According to the lipid filtration theory, disturbances of the physiological transport across the vessel wall give rise to intramural lipid depositions and these initiate the development of IP.

Rokitansky suggested in 1852 that the arteriosclerotic plaques resulted from the organization of mural thrombi. This thrombogenic theory was revived by Duguid (1949) and several other workers (Morgan, 1956; More and Haust, 1961; Mustard, 1967; Likar et al., 1968; Kagan et al. 1968). Recent observations (Walton and Williamson, 1968), however, suggest that the role of mural thrombi is only secondary to filtration changes.

Entrance of blood lipophages into the vessel wall (Leary, 1941) has also been considered the primary factor in eliciting ASC. Several investigators (Rannie, 1963; Poole et al., 1958; Simon et al., 1961; Still and O'Neal, 1961) have confirmed this theory, but according to present knowledge, lipophages play only a secondary role, like the *in loco* lipid synthesis, which also has a strong experimental support (Geer et al., 1961; Adams and Bayliss, 1963; Parker et al., 1963; Balis et al.,

1964). According to Baló (1958), the deterioration of elastic fibres is the decisive factor in the development of ASC, and in this connection Baló and Banga (1949a) examined the role of the elastase enzyme and its inhibitor, which they discovered in 1949. Acid treatment destroyed the inhibitor and elastase acted freely on the elastic elements of the vessel wall. This seems to confirm the acidotic theory of ASC, according to which the condition is elicited by the shift of the blood pH toward the acid region (Banga et al., 1954; Alekseyeva, 1959).

It can be seen even from this short and incomplete survey that the basic theories of ASC development and the structure of the lesions have been known for decades. The question is therefore justly posed, what morphological knowledge has been contributed, if any, by the persistent investigations of the recent ten years. Knowledge has indeed accumulated mainly in three areas: (i) more details have become known and certain earlier concepts have been proved or disproved; (ii) an important theory has been advanced concerning the role of auto-immune processes in the pathomechanism of ASC (Robert et al., 1963; Szigeti, 1964; Gerő, 1969; Robert and Robut, 1969). Anestyadi and Zota (1970) believe that the elastin plays the role of an antigen; (iii) the most important change occurred probably in the basic concept of aetiology, because ASC has increasingly been regarded as a multicausal disease (Constantinides, 1965).

The general acceptance of a complex aetiology may fundamentally alter the trends of ASC research. Once multiple causation is accepted, investigations will be centred on the pathomechanism and on the factors influencing it in a positive or negative direction. The knowledge of these factors is for the establishment of successful therapy and prevention of ASC.

ULTRASTRUCTURE OF ARTERIOSCLEROTIC LESIONS

Comparison of the ultrastructures of human and experimental arteriosclerotic lesions reveals a fundamental similarity, in certain respects even an identity of pathomechanism and components.

Geer et al. (1961) were the first to examine human lesions by electron microscope, and subsequently, several authors reported similar observations on the aorta or coronary arteries (Haust et al., 1962; Laitinen, 1963; McGill et al., 1963; McGill and Geer, 1963; Watts 1963; Geer and Guidry, 1964; Daoud et al., 1964a, b; Balis et al., 1964; Still and Mariott, 1964; Geer, 1965a; Haust and More, 1966; Marshall et al., 1966; Scott et al., 1966; Weller, 1966; Ghidoni et al., 1967; Paegle, 1969).

The following authors examined by electron microscope spontaneous or experimentally induced arteriosclerotic lesions in the following animal species: rabbit: Buck (1958, 1962); Parker (1960); Parker et al. (1963); Still (1963); Congin and Baccino (1964); Still (1964); Still and Mariott (1964); Still and Prosser (1964); Imai et al. (1966); Parker and Odland (1966a, b); Iwanaga et al. (1969); Shimamoto et al. (1969a, b); Björkerud (1969a, b); rat: Simon et al. (1961); Still and O'Neal (1962); Hess and Stäubli (1963a, b); Thomas et al. (1963); Scott et al. (1964); Marshall and O'Neal (1966); Suzuki and O'Neal (1967); dog: Westlake et al. (1963); Suzuki et al. (1964); Geer (1965b); cock: Berki et al. (1969) parrot: Hess and Stäubli (1969); turkey: Simpson and Harms (1966, 1968);

55

white pigeon: Cooke and Smith (1968); monkey: Scott et al. (1967a, b); Geer et al. (1968); McCombs et al. (1969); swine: French et al. (1963); Campbell (1965); Daoud et al. (1968); Thomas et al. (1968); cattle: Knieriem (1967).

Daoud et al. (1964b) distinguished two developmental forms of the arteriosclerotic plaque, a lipid-less early pre-atheroma and a lipid-containing necrotizing atheroma, and suggested that, while the former consisted exclusively of smooth muscle cells, the latter also contained foam cells and showed degenerative phenomena. Hess and Stäubli (1969) distinguished three fundamental lesions: fibromuscular proliferation, fatty streak and fibrous plaque.

In accordance with the classification described in connection with the development of the experimental IP, we believe that the arteriosclerotic IP (plaque) develops in two steps, of which the second has two forms. The first step is the early simple IP, which corresponds essentially with the pre-atheromatous or fibromuscular lesion. Terminologically, the name 'pre-atheroma' (Daoud et al., 1964b) seems to be correct, because it expresses clearly that lipid deposition may occur in the early phase of the lesion, but degenerative phenomena are not yet present and the proportion of cellular components is roughly the same as in the normal vessel wall. The second step is the development of a complex IP (arteriosclerotic plaque); this has two forms depending on the predominance of degenerative changes or a pathological increase of fibrous elements: the first is the classical atheroma, characteristically referred to in the English literature as 'fatty streak' and the second is the fibrous plaque. This agrees with the interpretation of Hess and Stäubli (1969), but we would lay more emphasis on the sharp distinction of the two steps, because we believe that the fate of the arteriosclerotic lesion is in fact decided in the simple IP. Depending on the size of the simple plaque and the nature of the processes taking place in it, an atheroma is either liable to ulceration, or to the development of a smooth-surfaced fibrous plaque. On the other hand, the study of the simple IP (pre-atheroma) is the only possible approach to the knowledge of the early phase of ASC.

STRUCTURE OF THE PRE-ATHEROMA

The pre-atheromatous phase of the IP is characterized by the presence of several rows of modified smooth muscle cells below the endothelium, with newly formed elastic and collagenous fibres in the intercellular spaces. The original IEL is either preserved or becomes enlarged or fragmented, while the proportion of the cellular and fibrous elements is the same as in the normal vessel wall.

The development and structure of the pre-atheroma as well as the fine structural characteristics of its components have been described in the chapter on experimental IP (see p. 27), thus under this heading references are made only to certain details.

A certain modification of the 'pure' pre-atheroma has been observed under the influence of an atherogenic diet or a high blood lipid level. The reason for discussing the diet-induced modified lesion under the heading of 'pure' pre-atheroma is that the proportion of its components is roughly the same as in the normal vessel wall. Modifications of the individual components of the pre-atheroma under the influence of an atherogenic diet are described below.

In both human and diet-induced lesions, the earliest changes have been observed in endothelial cells and subendothelial space. According to Florentin et al. (1969), after 3 days of atherogenic diet the endothelial cells already show an increased incorporation of ^{3}H thymidine, signifying a rise of the DNA-synthesis, while the smooth muscle cells show no sign of activation. Using the scanning technique, Shimamoto et al. (1969a, b) described the swelling of endothelial cells and destruction of their intercellular bridges as an early lesion.

Parker (1960) saw dense bodies, resembling caps or clumps, on the luminal surface of the endothelial cells. Clumps of a similar appearance were present in the pinocytotic vesicles, in the distended cisternae of the endoplasmic reticulum, and in the subendothelial space. Parker regards these bodies as lipoproteins, entering the vessel wall via cytopempsis (More and Haust, 1957). Similar observations have been reported by Buck (1958).

Parker and Odland (1966b) report that vacuoles appeared in the aortic endothelial cells of the rabbit after 2 weeks of an atherogenic diet. Hess and Stäubli (1963a) observed the same phenomenon in rats during the third week. In electron micrographs, some vacuoles appeared empty, some contained drops of neutral lipids surrounded by a unit membrane (Thomas et al., 1963; McGill and Geer, 1963; Simpson and Harms, 1968; Hess and Stäubli, 1969). Still (1964) observed a hypertrophy of the Golgi apparatus with appearance of lipid droplets, as well as a simultaneous increase and distension of the rough endoplasmic reticulum. Still and Mariott (1964) believe that the Golgi region of the endothelial cells plays a role in intracellular lipid synthesis. Increase of the mitochondria and the darkening of their matrix (Hess and Stäubli, 1963a) as well as the increase of free ribosomes (Parker and Odland, 1966a, b) also indicate greater activity of the endothelial cells. Several workers, however, particularly those concerned with human lesions (Balis et al., 1964; Geer, 1965a), found no endothelial cell change.

In this laboratory, a medium electron-dense layer has been observed on the luminal side of the unit membranes of pinocytotic vesicles in aortic endothelial cells of rats maintained on Loustalot's (1960) atherogenic diet for three weeks (Plate XXIX/128). Neutral lipid droplets surrounded by a unit membrane were seen in the cytoplasm (Plate XXIX/127) at the phase of the initial slight distension of the subendothelial space. The free ribosomes increased in number and formed many rosette-like patterns (Plate XXIX/126); the ductules of the endoplasmic reticulum similarly increased. We also observed a greater than medium electron density of the mitochondrial matrix (Plate XXIX/125, 126) and many empty vesicles in the cytoplasm (Plate XXIX/126, 128). In places double ring-like structures, with outer and inner diameters of 900 Å and 700 Å, respectively, were present in the cells (Plate XXIX/126). A widening of the intercellular space was reported by Parker and Odland (1966a, b), but their electron micrographs seem to show processes of endothelial cells and a tangential section of the subendothelial space. We were able to follow up the process whereby the intercellular junctions opened to allow the entrance of membrane-surrounded chylomicrons into the vessel wall (Plate XXX/130).

Extracellular Space. Buck (1962), Still and O'Neal (1962), Thomas et al. (1963), Daoud et al. (1964*a*, *b*), Geer (1965*b*), Parker and Odland (1966*b*), Ghidoni and O'Neal (1967) and Hess and Stäubli (1969) observed a widening of the subendothelial space already in the early phase of the atherogenic diet, with accumulation of a delicate granular or fibrillar substance resembling the electron-microscopic image of blood plasma. All authors agree that this substance originates from the blood; Gresham et al. (1962) regard it as a protein, Still and O'Neal (1962) as a plasma substance, French et al. (1963) as a mucoprotein and Hess and Stäubli (1963*a*, *b*) as a lipoprotein.

Geer (1965*b*) saw extracellular lipid inclusions, but Hess and Stäubli (1969) believe that no extracellular lipid is present in the pre-atheroma. Balis et al. (1964) and Still and Mariott (1964), however, observed a small amount of lipids in early human arteriosclerotic lesions. Geer (1965*b*) believes that the extracellular lipid originates from the blood; this has been supported by demonstration of lipids in the vessel wall by various techniques (see p. 62).

Also fibrin appears in early and late arteriosclerotic lesions; it is identified either by its characteristic 230 Å periodicity (Haust et al., 1965; Marshall et al., 1966; Ghidoni and O'Neal, 1967) or by its specific antibody-binding capacity (Haust et al., 1964, 1965; Koo and Wissler, 1965; Walton and Williamson, 1968).

After 3 weeks of an atherogenic diet, we observed a widening of the subendothelial space, due to the accumulation of a granular, filamentous substance (Plate XXIX/127). Structures which might have corresponded to lipids from the blood were already present in the lesion at that time (Plate XXIX/127). It is known that phospholipids are highly osmiophilic owing to their unsaturated bonds. Their hydrophilic and hydrophobic groups cause them to form a membrane-like or myelin sheath like structure in aqueous media (e.g. in the extracellular space) (Stoeckenius, 1959; Romhányi, 1962, 1966).

We failed to demonstrate fibrin in the subendothelial space.

Role of Cell Components (Smooth Muscle Cells) of the Pre-atheroma in Atherogenesis. After the widening of the subendothelial space, cells appear in it, which have been identified electron microscopically as 'modified' smooth muscle cells in both human and experimental lesions (Parker, 1960; Geer et al., 1961; Haust et al., 1962; Thomas et al., 1963; Ghidoni and O'Neal, 1967; Hess and Stäubli, 1969). The ultrastructural characteristics of these cells resemble those of the cell components of the regenerative IP (Plate XXXI/136), except that in the former, lipid inclusions, surrounded by single, double or no membrane (Plate XXXI/137) are already apparent in the early stage of the change (Geer et al. 1961; McGill and Geer, 1963; Balis et al., 1964; Geer et al., 1968). Since the smooth muscle cells show no sign of a phagocytic activity at this stage, Geer et al. (1961), Newman et al. (1961) and Geer (1965*a*) explain the phenomenon by an *in loco* lipid synthesis. Modification of the smooth muscle cells is indicated by the presence of many cell organelles in a very active functional state and by a simultaneous decrease of the contractile structures. For this reason the modified cells occasionally resemble fibroblasts (Scott et al., 1967*b*). Increased cellular activity is centred chiefly on fibre genesis. The basement membrane accompanying the smooth muscle cells is sometimes double, sometimes discontinuous, probably as a result of detachment (Geer et al., 1961; Parker and Odland, 1966a, b; Imai et al., 1966). The distended ergastoplasmic ducts of the smooth muscle cells contain a granular substance which resembles the elementary units of extracellularly localizing elastic or collagenous fibres. Thus, since the fundamental observations of Haust et al. (1960) have been published, all morphologists engaged in the study of arteriosclerotic lesions have accepted the role of smooth muscle cells in fibrillogenesis, and Jarmolich et al. (1968) confirmed it by autoradiographic examination of cultured aortic smooth muscle cells.

According to Thomas et al. (1963), the smooth muscle cell components of the pre-atheroma originate either from the endothelium, the media or from circulating monocytes. The view presently held by most authors is that all cell components originate from the media and they reach the subendothelial space via migration through the stomas and discontinuous fragments of the IEL (French et al., 1963; Daoud et al., 1964a; Geer, 1965a, b; Parker and Odland, 1966a, Simpson and Harms, 1968; Wissler, 1968; Hess and Stäubli, 1969). We observed similar phenomena in aortic specimens from rats killed during the 6th week of an atherogenic diet (Plate XXXI/133, 134).

The factor responsible for the initiation of smooth muscle cell migration remains to be identified. According to Constantinides (1965), two mechanisms are able to elicit ASC in animal experiments: (i) a high degree of lipaemia, or (ii) vessel wall impairment plus a slight degree of lipaemia. In the latter case, cell necrosis appears to elicit cell proliferation, as a compensating mechanism in the process of regeneration. But as regeneration can never restore the original vessel wall, an arteriosclerotic plaque develops at the site of the lesion.

It seems less easy to explain the cause of smooth muscle cell mobilization if the pre-atheroma is induced by atherogenic diet alone, without a vascular injury. In the latter case, namely, the interaction between cell destruction and regeneration provides a reasonable explanation of this phenomenon. Thomas et al. (1963), who identified vascular smooth muscle cells as components of the initial lesion, did not identify the factor responsible for the cell migration, neither did many other authors in similar reports. Wissler and Kao (1962), however, speculated that certain lipids may affect the medial smooth muscle cells of cebus monkeys in two different ways, i.e. either they stimulate the cells and initiate their proliferation, or damage them and thereby elicit a cell necrosis. An indirect proof of this hypothesis is the observation that smooth muscle cell mobilization takes place after the first intimal changes have already become established (Bálint et al., in press), i.e. when lipids appear in the media (Hess and Stäubli, 1963a, b). In addition to the direct effect of lipids, either the change elicited in the ground substance by plasma deposition or the hypoxia induced by the accumulation of plasma and lipids might be responsible for the activation and migration of the smooth muscle cells.

The further development of the pre-atheroma can proceed in two directions depending on the nature of the predominant smooth muscle cell processes, and the level and duration of lipaemia. Predominance of the fibrillogenetic function of smooth muscle cells results in the development of a fibrous plaque, and predominance of lipid synthesis and/or uptake results in the development of an atheroma.

Transformation of a simple pre-atheroma to an atheroma is indicated by the appearance of cell forms other than smooth muscle cells (macrophages, connective

59

tissue cells, lymphocytes) in the IP (Still, 1963; Balis et al., 1964; Still and Prosser, 1964; Geer, 1965b).

THE ARTERIOSCLEROTIC PLAQUE

As already noted in the Introduction, two forms of arteriosclerotic vascular lesions (ASC plaques) can be distinguished depending on the nature of the predominant change. The ultrastructural characteristics of the two forms, atheroma and fibrous plaque, are discussed in the following sections.

STRUCTURE OF THE ATHEROMA

The endothelial cells of the atheromatous change contain lipid droplets, and the multilayered IP subjacent to the endothelium contains, in addition to smooth muscle cells, many foam cells (Plate XXXI/137). In the intercellular spaces there are newly formed elastic and collagenous fibres (Plate XXXI/135–138) and many lipid droplets and myelin figures (Plate XXX/132). The foam cells and the penetration of lipids into the vessel wall are discussed here in detail; for discussion of the other components of the atheroma, the reader is referred to the reports and reviews cited in the Introduction.

STRUCTURE AND ORIGIN OF THE FOAM CELLS

The main electron-microscopic characteristic of the foam cell is the presence of homogeneous or reticular lipid droplets, surrounded or not surrounded by a membrane, and occasionally of myelin figures and ceroid pigment in the cytoplasm. The ultrastructural characteristics of foam cell components of the ASC plaque were first observed by Poole et al. (1958) in experimental lesions and by Geer et al. (1961) in human lesions.

Foam cells of the atheroma can arise in four different ways:

1. blood lipophages penetrate into the vascular wall;
2. blood monocytes phagocytose lipids from the atheroma;
3. endothelial cells are formed or pre-existing subendothelial cells;
4. smooth muscle cells transform to foam cells via degeneration or an active lipid synthesis *in loco*.

Poole et al. (1958) were the first to publish electron micrographs in which lipophages were seen to adhere to the surface of endothelial cells, and similar cell forms were seen within the vascular wall below the endothelium. Subsequently, Still and O'Neal (1962), Still (1963), Still and Mariott (1964) and Marshall and O'Neal (1966) concluded from their observations that lipid-containing macrophages enter the vessel wall. This supported the lipophage theory of Leary (1941). Rannie. (1963) believe that the lipophages gain access to the vessel wall passively rather than by active migration, in that a row of endothelial cells migrates to them after they have become attached to the intima. Sinapius (1968) holds a similar view.

In contrast, Haust and More (1963), McGill et al. (1963), Dauid et al (1963), Balis et al. (1964), Geer (1965a, b), Parker and Odland (1966a, b) and Hess and Stäubli (1969) have doubted the importance of lipophage invasion on the ground that they have never observed such a process. Constantinides (1965) regards the distended gaps between endothelial cells in which processes of lipophages are extending as post-mortem changes and considers the possibility that the cells might migrate from the vessel wall into the blood rather than vice versa.

On the basis of experiments on rats, we have taken a definite position in respect of lipophage migration into the vessel wall. The electron micrographs permit a follow-up of the subsequent steps of the movement of lipophages towards the subendothelial space. The lipid-carrying macrophages adhere first to endothelial cells (Plate XXXI/138), then extend pseudopodia into the intercellular junctions and, pushing them apart, they migrate into the widened subendothelial space (Plate XXXII/140, 141). Occasionally, two or three lipophages join to enter the vessel wall simultaneously, lifting the processes of endothelial cells in the course of migration.

The hypothesis that the lipophages actively penetrate the vessel wall is supported by the observation that no foam cells were seen subendothelially, in the stomas of the IEL or in the media.

Still and Mariott (1964), Balis et al. (1964) and Geer (1965a, b) observed that lymphocytes or monocytes appearing in the atheroma were able to phagocytose the lipids which enter the extracellular space of the lesion from the blood and can transform to foam cells. Balis et al. (1964) have established the features differentiating macrophages from myogenic foam cells. They state that foam cells transformed from macrophages have neither a basement membrane nor cytoplasmic myofilaments, and thus no trace of filament can be seen around the lipid droplets; signs of phagocytosis are, however, present. Geer and Guidry (1964) observed in addition that foam cells transformed from macrophages have circular mitochondria and a clear hyaloplasm.

Poole et al. (1958) and Friedman et al. (1966) presented experimental evidence that endothelial cells can transform to foam cells. On examining human coronary arteries, Sinapius (1968) found that the endothelial cells phagocytose the lipid layer or lipid droplets attaching to their surface and then transform to foam cells. Duff and McMillan (1951) thought that foam cells arise from pre-existing subendothelial cells.

The most generally accepted theory of foam cell formation has been the transformation of smooth muscle cells. Many transitional forms between modified smooth muscle cell and foam cell have been observed (Geer et al., 1961; Laitinen, 1963; Watts, 1963; Still and Mariott, 1964; Balis et al., 1964; Geer 1965a, b; Imai et al., 1966; Ghidoni et al. 1967; Cooke and Smith, 1968). According to the criteria established by Balis et al. (1964), the myogenic foam cells possess a basement membrane and myofilaments (although the latter may be rudimentary) and their cytoplasmic lipid droplets are always surrounded by a filamentous structure.

As the smooth muscle cells show no signs of phagocytosis (Geer et al. 1961; Newman et al., 1961; Geer, 1965b), but their metabolic activity is high (Parker et al., 1963; Balis et al., 1964) and they possess all enzymes necessary for lipid synthesis (Werthessen et al., 1954; Zilversmit et al., 1961; Dayton, 1961; Whereat, 1961; Stein and Stein, 1962; Adams and Bayliss, 1963), the *in loco* lipid synthesis seems to be the primary factor of myogenic foam cell formation.

To summarize these observations on the origin of foam cells, findings by others and ourselves have shown that they arise in part from the modified smooth muscle cells of the atheroma (myogenic foam cells), and in part from lipid-loaded lipophages migrating into the lesion from the blood stream, or from monocytes which phagocytose the extracellular lipids of the atheroma. With extreme lipid deposition, the foam cells fall apart and the lipid figures stored in them are released into the extracellular space.

SOURCE OF LIPIDS LOCALIZING IN THE ATHEROMA

The atheroma is characterized by the presence of a large quantity of lipids, localizing either intracellularly in the foam cells or in the extracellular space. After an atherogenic diet for 6 weeks, lipid membrane formations fill almost the entire subendothelial space (Plate XXX/132). The 'empty' spaces between the membranes might represent dissolved saturated or non-polar lipids, which cannot be seen in common electron-microscopic preparations (Thomas and O'Neal, 1960). Lipids from the blood stream can enter the vessel wall in three ways:

1. via cytopempsis across the endothelium;
2. across intercellular junctions in the form of a chylomicron;
3. via transport by lipophages.

Passage of lipids across endothelial cells is probably analogous to lipid transport across intestinal epithelial cells. The lipoprotein-lipase enzyme acting on the surface of endothelial cells (Holle, 1967) breaks the neutral lipids into fatty acids and glycerol, which diffuse through the cytoplasmic membrane and cell body and reach the subendothelial space via 'reverse' pinocytosis. The partial re-synthesis of lipids from fatty acids and glycerol on the ergastoplasm or Golgi apparatus might correspond with one process of mural lipid synthesis (Werthessen et al., 1954; Zilversmit et al., 1961; Dayton, 1961; Whereat, 1961; Loomeijer and Van der Veen, 1962; Stein and Stein, 1962); while the other process would be a similar synthesis in smooth muscle cells. The presence of lipid droplets in the ergastoplasm (Geer, 1965b) and Golgi apparatus (Still and Mariott, 1964) can be interpreted as the morphological sign of endothelial lipid-synthesizing capacity. This process seems to be responsible for the marked accumulation of lipids in endothelial cells (Plates XXIX/127, XXXI/137). The simultaneously observed ring-like intracytoplasmic structures (Plate XXIX/126) might represent phospholipids which pass across the cell membrane by direct diffusion and form membrane systems in the hyaloplasm.

We observed that the intercellular junctions opened and membrane-encased chylomicrons gained access to the subendothial space (Plate XXX/129) between the processes of endothelial cells (Plate XXX/130). No similar observations have been made by others, although Hess and Stäubli (1969) suggested that this phenomenon might take place.

Lipid transport by lipophages has been described in connection with the nature and function of the latter cells.

It should be noted that only part of the characteristic extracellular lipid content of the atheroma might result from filtration of blood plasma through the endothelial cells or between them; a substantial part could well originate from lipid release by degenerated foam cells or synthesis and subsequent release of lipids by smooth muscle cells, as postulated by Geer et al. (1961).

STRUCTURE OF THE FIBROUS PLAQUE

This type of advanced arteriosclerotic lesion is characterized by the predominance of fibrous elements in the extracellular space. Three forms can be distinguished according to the quality or quantity of the fibres: musculo-elastic, fibromuscular or fibrous change. The first two forms contain relatively numerous smooth muscle cells, whereas in the third form cellular components are scarce. A varying amount of lipid inclusions may be present between the fibres; these are either derived from the lumen by filtration or originate from disintegrated foam cells (Geer et al., 1961; Constantinides, 1965), some of which persist in the fibrous plaque. According to McGill et al. (1963), the formation of a fibrous plaque from foam cells is preconditioned by the release of lipids into the extracellular space. The ground substance between the smooth muscle cells has a granular and filamentous structure and it contains elastic granules and elastic clumps of different degrees of maturity (Plate XXXI/135, 136, 138).

Ghidoni et. al (1967) observed in the fibrous plaque fibrin of a regular periodicity, bodies reminiscent of 'amyloid starlets' and accumulated fine filaments, 40–100 Å thick, of as yet unidentified nature. The immunomorphological studies of Haust et al. (1964, 1965b) suggest that part of these filaments also correspond to fibrin.

The further fate of the arteriosclerotic lesion is in part determined by local factors, in part by the general condition of the organism as a whole. The atheroma may undergo hyalinization, chalk deposition (Paegle, 1969) or further disintegration and secondary thrombosis; or the formation of a vascularized proliferative tissue may become associated with these processes (Constantinides, 1965; Bredt, 1969).

COMPARISON OF AORTIC RESPONSES

The preceding chapters dealt with the analysis of the different types of aortic reaction under different conditions. These analyses aimed at the recognition of the fundamental morphological changes which underlie the aortic lesions. The different models used in the various experimental schemes were set up with the aim of obtaining more information by variation of the experimental approach and thus facilitating the understanding of certain intricate processes. The investigations disclosed the characteristic properties of the changes. Although mural plasma deposition occurs regularly in the early phase of both hypertensive and arteriosclerotic lesions, still the IP should be regarded as the most general and fundamental reaction type. The fundamental structural elements of vascular lesions have become known by analysis of the simple IP and this had enabled a systematic study to be made of the processes taking place in the complex proliferation.

All three types of simple IP (regenerative, inactivity, transplantational) are characterized by a proliferation composed of several rows of smooth muscle cells originating from the media. A vigorous fibre synthesis takes place in the proliferation, during which elastic lamellae may also be formed. The component parts of the elastic lamellae are the same in the simple and complex proliferations, and also the morphological steps of the maturation process are identical.

Degenerative phenomena occurring in the lesion with aging (lipid deposition, cartilage formation, chalk deposition) gradually render it similar to advanced complex arteriosclerotic changes. The latter are characterized by the presence of degeneration products in both endothelial and smooth muscle cell components and by the appearance of cell elements other than smooth muscle cells. Intercellularly, collagenous fibres predominate over elastic ones in the aged lesions.

Early arteriosclerotic changes elicited by a high blood lipid level differ from the above-described lesions in certain respects. The main characteristic is an accumulation of lipids in the affected area, resulting from permeability change, lipophage invasion, and fat degeneration of endothelial and smooth muscle cells. But in a more advanced stage, proliferative structural elements become predominant also in this type of lesion and at this stage it is already hard to differentiate the 'fat by streak' from an aged, simple IP.

The reparative IP developing in the course of hypertension represents a transitional form between simple and complex proliferations. In the early phase of this change, plasma deposition and fibrinoid formation occur in consequence of permeability increase. Intramural plasma diffusion of the same type, but of a lesser degree, occurs also in the initial stage of inactivity (involutional) IP and in arteriosclerotic lesions. At a later stage, either macrophages and smooth cells appear in the subendothelial fibrinoid to form a proliferation, or the fibrinoid undergoes a hyaline transformation, as in the small vessels.

At the present state of knowledge, research is centred on three main lines of investigation which generally correspond with the subsequent phases of the pathomechanism of vascular lesions:

1. Alteration of the endothelial cell, or more strictly speaking, of its AMP-rich coat surface, which might be regarded as the first step of the process of ASC.

2. The nature and mechanism of action of the factor(s) responsible for smooth muscle cell mobilization and the metabolic processes of the smooth muscle cells.

3. Shift of the proportions of extracellular components and the factors influencing these, i.e. the predominance of collagenous fibres over elastic elements in aged lesions and the intercellular accumulation of degeneration products.

The clarification of the morphological and biochemical aspects of these problems will, it is hoped, promote not only the therapeutic treatment, but also the prevention of vascular diseases in general and of ASC in particular.

CHAPTER 4

STUDIES OF LARGE MUSCULAR VESSELS

The preceding chapter dealt with the impairment, reaction types and regenerative changes of the large elastic vessels, with special regard to the pathologic phenomena elicited by vascular impairment. Similar investigations have been carried out on muscular-type large vessels, using the same model of impairment by painting with acid. A total of 31 rabbits of both sexes, 2–3 years old and weighing on an average 4–5 kg, were used. A 3 cm long portion of the adventitia of the femoral artery was painted *in vivo* with 33 per cent or 8 per cent hydrochloric acid, to vary not only the duration, but also the degree of exposure. After treatment, the rabbits were killed in succession at predetermined intervals from 5 minutes to 352 days. Undamaged arterial segments served as control. In addition to the usual staining techniques, some formalin-fixed specimens were stained with Carere-Coombs' Siena-orange technique, to demonstrate smooth muscle cells which stain specifically yellow owing to the reaction of their potassium contents.

The endothelial cells became necrotic within a few minutes after painting, and began to separate from the IEL which contracted in an undulating manner. The medial smooth muscle cells became vacuolated, their nuclei hyperchromatic and a few leukocytes appeared in the adventitia (Plate LXII/34). After 20 minutes, muscle cell damage became more pronounced; the cells showed an increased affinity to the M-stain, assuming a black colour (Plate LXII/35). After a few hours, cell necrosis became apparent over the entire width of the damaged vascular segment and after 24 hours no more cells were present; the affected vessel portion became homogeneous and more straitened than the adjoining viable portion (Plate LXII/36). By the time the cellular elements of the vessel wall disappeared, the IEL stretched, its undulation diminished and the vessel wall reduced to one half of its original width (Plate LXII/37).

Staining with azan still revealed smooth muscle cell necrosis at the borderline between affected and intact vascular tissue; finally the vessel wall became narrow and acellular and collagenous fibres appeared in it (Plate LXII/38). After about one week, the muscle cells localizing at the border between changed and preserved vascular areas began to divide and the newly formed cells migrated toward the surface across the stomas of the IEL, to form an IP (Plate LXII/39). A delicate meshwork of elastic fibres appeared first at the demarcation between affected and intact vascular wall segments, then gradually also in the intima (Plate LXII/40).

Depending on the degree of the damage, a multilayered IP forms a new vessel wall at the luminal surface; certain cell components of the IP appeared to be smooth muscle cells (Plate LXII/41), because they stained red with azan, black with M-stain and yellow with Siena-orange stain and showed a positive birefringence in polarized light after anilin reaction. Simultaneously, a broad adventitia, rich in collagenous fibres, was newly formed above the original, collapsed adventitia. Patches of collagen were seen also between the proliferating cells (Plate LXII/41).

Staining of the IP with specific elastic fibre stains reveals a marked increase of the elastic elements; in places they form a multilamellar layer and may even constitute a new elastic membrane (Plate LXII/42).

Regeneration after painting with acid was essentially the same in large muscular vessels as in large elastic vessels. The former, however, showed a marked narrowing of the wall during the acute stage of the change; this might be explained by the absence of elastic fibres. Proliferation phenomena during the reparative stage were similar to those observed in aortic lesions. Elastic fibre genesis matched, or even exceeded that observed in elastic vessels; this is probably due to an inducer effect of the pulsation of the markedly narrowed wall. The thinned wall synthesizes multiple lamellar elastic elements to reinforce its structure. This is the reason why the regeneration of the muscular-type vessel wall results in elastic or elastofibrotic rather than muscular reparation and this accounts for the decrease of smooth muscle cells in the lesion after 100–120 days.

The above observations clearly indicate that identical vascular injury elicits an identical response, irrespective of the muscular or elastic type of the vessel, and also initiates the same kind of regenerative processes, which result finally in a musculo-elastic-fibrotic change of the vessel wall.

The same conclusion could be drawn from the study of experimental hypertensive lesions of large muscular-type vessels. As described on p. 26, the hypertensive changes of large muscular arteries (femoral artery) were in every respect similar to those encountered after painting with acid (Plate LXI/22). The smooth muscle cells showed initially an increased affinity to PTA, then single smooth muscle cell necroses appeared, i.e. the microscopic picture was the same as shown in Plate LXII/35. The absence of the subendothelial fibrinoid after the acute stage of hypertension was clearly due to the lack of blood pressure rise. The cell components of the chronic proliferation were, however, the same as those encountered during the regenerative phase of vascular hypertension (Plate LXII/25, 41).

In the chronic stage, the IP was as thick as the vessel wall or thicker and contained many delicate undulating elastic fibres and a newly formed IEM, which imparted an elastic character to the changed segment of the muscular vessel. The presence of elastic fibres in the IP has been observed by several authors (Jellinek et al., 1958; Kellaway et al., 1962; de Faria, 1965a), but Courtice et al. (1963) and Schmidt-Diedrichs and Courtice (1963) consider that this depends on the actual state of the IEM: if it is intact, predominantly elastic fibres are formed, whereas if it becomes fragmented, predominantly collagenous fibres (fibrous tissue) arise.

Experimental production of vascular damage by ligation of the vessel was already practised in the past century (Raab, 1879; Pick, 1885; Pekelharing, 1890; Sokoloff, 1893; Jores, 1898), and has been employed ever since. Ligature of the carotid artery has generally been preferred, because it rarely endangers survival, and several authors have complemented it with further procedures. While Lange (1924), Mehrotra (1953), Buck (1958), Schmidt-Diedrichs and Courtice (1963) and Hackensellner et al. (1965) have contented themselves with a simple circular suture or a double ligature, Courtice et al. (1963) injected saline of 60 °C temperature into the ligated vessel portion and fed the animals a high cholesterol diet. Hoff and Gottlob (1969) treated the animals with Intralipid in addition to the ligature, and Wexler (1968) used multiparous rats with pre-existing ASC for vascular ligature. Záhoř et al. (1967) fed the animals cholesterol only, while others applied other injuries to elicit regeneration. Makoff (1899) employed a vascular compression, Andriewitsch (1901) used a thermocauter, Jaffe et al. (1929) used electricity, and Sminkova (1903) employed painting with turpentine and silver nitrate. Mairano and Giugiano (1954) placed a suture and injected a fibrinolytic pancreatic enzyme into the femoral artery of dogs. Csillag et al. (1955) and Jellinek et al. (1958) exposed the vessel to gastric acid. Husni and Manion (1967) implanted a piece of wire into the femoral artery of dogs and this resulted in thrombosis and hypertension. Björkerud (1969a, b) elicited endothelial damage by inserting a catheter containing diamond crystals, into the femoral artery of the rabbit. Rosnowski (1968) produced compression of the vessel by means of plastics cuffs. Gage et al. (1967) froze the femoral artery by means of liquid nitrogen flow in a tube. Garbarsch et al. (1969) elicited vascular change by creating hypoxia. Altschul and Paul-Boemler (1963) observed endothelial damage after contraction of the ear vessels as a result of puncture. Rowley (1963) elicited permeability disturbance and mural damage by local injection of thorotrast. The vasoconstrictor action of adrenalin has also been utilized; Hayes (1967) employed it together with deep freezing or heat exposure on auricular arteries of rabbits and Cavallero and Tutolla (1964) combined its use with an orthostatic collapse. Mustard (1967) employed ADP infusion to elicit platelet aggregation and intimal damage. Thoma (1883) produced an IP by alteration of the mechanical conditions of blood flow. Cappelli et al. (1968a, b) observed the effect of the P-factor on the arterial wall in tissue explants. Patek et al. (1963a) described arteriosclerotic lesions in parabiotic animals after blocking of the RES and cholesterol feeding.

The results of these model experiments on large muscular-type vessels may be summarized by saying that the various causative factors gave rise to identical morphological and structural changes which fairly corresponded with the arteriosclerotic lesions produced by other authors under different conditions. It appears that the morphological changes taking place in the course of vascular regeneration may serve ultimately as a basis of arteriosclerotic lesions.

CHAPTER 5

MORPHOLOGICAL CHANGES OF SMALL MUSCULAR-TYPE VESSELS AND ARTERIOLES UNDER THE INFLUENCE OF VARIOUS INJURIES

The various types of lesions in large elastic and muscular-type vessels have been discussed in the preceding chapters. This chapter deals with pathologic changes in those vessels which still have a distinct elastic membrane and, for comparison, with those which possess few or no elastic elements (arterioles). Although the ultrastructural relations of small vessels have not yet been fully clarified, the presence or absence of elastic fibres seems to be the decisive factor in their response to damage. The pathomorphology of the lesion depends largely on this factor over and above the degree and duration of the damage. To obtain more information on this factor, the temporal course of the changes was followed up under different experimental conditions.

Experimental hypertension was chosen as the basic model. Hypertension was induced by the method of Lőrincz and Gorácz, as in the experiments on large vessels. Painting with acid elicited similar changes to those found in large vessels. Noradrenalin treatment, not used for the large vessels, was also applied. The fourth model was hypersensitization by means of horse serum.

All four experimental models, each representing a different type of injury, elicited identical tissue reactions with the same rate and sequence of pathomechanical events but differing in the degree of severity. It appears that in the small vessels, muscle cell necrosis and subsequent plasma deposition are the decisive changes, influenced only by the presence or absence of elastic elements. Reparative changes of the small vessels, which will be discussed in a separate chapter, appeared as proliferative phenomena resembling in every respect those observed in large vessel regeneration.

LESIONS OF MUSCULAR-TYPE SMALL VESSELS IN ACUTE EXPERIMENTAL HYPERTENSION

ACUTE HYPERTENSIVE LESIONS OF SMALL VESSELS AS A MODEL OF VASCULAR DAMAGE

Hypertensive vascular damage involves not only the risk of an acute disturbance of blood supply but usually serves also as a basis of later sclerotic lesions (McGill et al., 1961; Duncan, 1963; Gutstein et al., 1962, 1963; Loth, 1965; Texon, 1967; Packham et al., 1967; Still et al. 1967; Hoff et al., 1969; Björkerud, 1969a, b; Silver et al., 1969). The multifactorial theory of ASC was advanced by Constantinides in 1965. However, the sclerotic changes are not conclusive as to the nature either of the initial lesion, or of the original injury, because they depend on the degree rather than on the quality of impairment (Jellinek et al., 1965b, 1967b, c). Hypertensive and other injuries of the muscular-type small vessels and arterioles may be segregated as a separate group on the basis of the structural uniformity of this vessel system. The knowledge of the pathomechanism of small vessel lesions is very important, because such changes develop in various kinds of diseases other than hypertension (periarteritis nodosa, Wegener's granulomatosis, vascular changes associated with lupus erythematodes, etc.). Thus the hypertensive lesions of small vessels can be regarded as a model not only of hypertensive vascular disease, but to a certain extent also of other conditions.

Hypertension research and the study of the effects of hypotensive drugs on man have verified the more than fifty-year-old theory that the two forms of hypertensive changes in muscular-type small vessels, arteriolosclerosis and arteriolonecrosis, represent essentially two degrees of a basic response to the same fundamental damage (Löhlein, 1917; Herxheimer, 1923; Jores, 1924). The factors involved in the initial stages of lesions associated with benign hypertension and of necrotizing vasculitis associated with malignant hypertension are the same, except that the change is less extensive and develops in a less explosive manner, if the process is benign (Jellinek et al., 1967b). Our investigations were, therefore, based on the working hypothesis that acute lesions are more conclusive than chronic ones in respect of initial and essential changes.

The rat was chosen as experimental animal because it is physiologically hypertensive, and renal hypertension was chosen as the experimental disease, because it can be adjusted to different degrees (Lőrincz and Gorácz, 1954; Campbell et al., 1963; Rojo-Ortega et al., 1968) and alters only indirectly the water and electrolyte equilibrium (Katz et al., 1962; Schmidt, 1962). Although there is no close relationship between the severity of acute vascular damages and the extent of blood pressure rise (Campbell et al., 1963), necrotizing arteritis has been regarded as equivalent to malignant renal hypertension in the rat (Churg, 1963b; Opie et al., 1970).

ACUTE HYPERTENSIVE LESION OF THE INTIMA

The earliest hypertensive change of small vessels is the appearance of a PAS-positive subendothelial oedema (Zollinger, 1959; Gardner, 1963). Electronmicroscopic and physiological studies have disclosed the role and functions of endothelial cells in basement membrane formation (Laitinen, 1963), in the synthesis of histamine, the production of renin activators, and the conditions of normal and pathologic permeability (Movat et al., 1963a; Nowak et al., 1969) and have identified the materials which promote clotting (Weibel et al., 1964; Fuchs et al., 1966; Burri et al., 1968). In the initial stage of hypertensions, the number of microvilli increases, owing probably to a local hypoxia. The mitochondria become denser and the Golgi apparatus and rough endoplasmic reticulum hypertrophy (Plate XXXIV/154, 155). These phenomena indicate, in addition to a disturbance of cell metabolism, an increased synthesis of basement membrane components (Kunz et al., 1968). As the bulk of plasma substances diffuse from the lumen (Wiener et al., 1969) into the vessel wall via patent endothelial junctions (Cotran,

1967), the basement membrane acts as a barrier and ultrafilter and as such plays a decisive role in vascular permeability (Hager, 1961; Majno et al., 1961). We observed that in the early stage of hypertension the subendothelial space always appears broadened subjacent to the endothelial junctions, and contains an increased amount of a floccular, loosely layered subendothelial substance which shows the same density as the basement membrane. This substance either originates from the blood plasma, or represents increased ground substance synthesis by the endothelial cells (Plate XXXIV/156, 157).

The ultrastructure of the endothelial cells responds extremely rapidly to changes of environmental pH and osmolarity (Constantinides et al., 1969a, b), to vasoactive amines (Burri et al., 1968; Constantinides et al., 1969) and toxins (Stearner et al., 1969). The cytoplasmic filaments of these cells (Mollo et al., 1965; Cecio, 1967; Puchtler et al., 1969) may even promote active constriction (Anderson, 1963; Bensch et al., 1964; Majno, 1968).

DEVELOPMENT, FORMS AND COMPONENTS OF THE VASCULAR FIBRINOID

Fibrinoid degeneration, as a characteristic change of hypertensive vascular disease, has been studied by many authors (Schürmann et al., 1933; Muirhead et al., 1951a–d; Endes et al., 1952; Montgomery et al., 1953; Zollinger, 1959; Still et al., 1959; Ohta et al., 1959; Gumenyuk, 1960; Gorácz, 1963; Churg, 1963a, b; Gardner, 1963; Kojimahara, 1967; Hüttner et al., 1966a, 1968). Several workers (Schürmann et al., 1933; Šoustek, 1956; Lendrum, 1963; Kerényi et al., 1966a, b; Hüttner et al., 1966a, 1968) have attributed its formation to increased vascular permeability and fibrin precipitation. The presence of fibrin among extravasated plasma proteins (dyshoria) has been evidenced by immunofluorescence tests (Fennel et al., 1961; Paronetto, 1965; Walton, 1968), and the characteristic ultrastructure of fibrin has been identified electron microscopically (Geer et al., 1958; Spiro et al., 1965; Wiener et al., 1965; Ooneda et al., 1965; Hüttner et al., 1968; Wiener et al., 1969). Apart from fibrin, other plasma proteins also gain access to the vessel wall and together with the degenerating cellular and fibrous elements they help to form the change known as fibrinoid necrosis (Adams et al., 1966; Lendrum et al., 1967). The diffusion of these substances into the vessel wall is impossible unless the blood–arterial wall barrier becomes damaged. Damage can arise from the following causes: (i) impairment of the endothelium by hypoxia due to a circulatory disorder, muscle spasm or other cause (Kjeldsen et al., 1968, 1969); (ii) disorder of mural electrolytes (Gardner et al., 1964); (iii) direct action of hypertension with the endothelium preserved; (iv) circulating vasoactive substances with constrictor- or permeability-enhancing effects (Koletsky et al., 1964; Murakami et al., 1964; Nikulin et al., 1965a); (v) antigen–antibody reaction (Kühl, 1956) (vi) auto-immunization against endogenous substances (White et al., 1964; Paronetto, 1965); (vii) increase of fibrinolytic activity (Onoyama et al., 1969) and (viii) alteration of plasma proteins (Grundmann et al., 1961).

Kojimahara (1967) believes that hypertension and haemodynamic factors play the decisive role in focal plasma protein deposition (dyshoria) and changes of the media, whereas Gardner (1962), Cain et al. (1963), Bednar (1965) and ourselves attribute it to a durable recurrent or intermittent long-standing vascular spasm, i.e. to an alternation of dilatation and spastic constriction (Kóczé et al., 1970). Unlike Duguid et al. (1952), Downing et al. (1963), Ashford et al. (1967) and Stout (1969), we have never observed a primary thrombosis on the endothelial surface.

Histochemically, the fibrinoid is eosinophilic; it is PAS-positive, stains red with azan and black with M-stain and appears as a birefringent, non-metachromatic homogeneous substance. Two main forms of fibrinoid can be distinguished on the basis of localization, fine structure and mechanism of development in muscular-type small vessels:

1. Subendothelial fibrinoid arises exclusively from plasma substances admixed with the subendothelial basement membrane (Plate LXIII/52–57). The characteristic histochemical and polarization optical properties (Jobst, 1954) of the subendothelial fibrinoid are due chiefly to the presence of fibrin, to judge from a quantitative polarization optical analysis (Hüttner et al., 1966a) and from electronmicroscopic examinations (Plates XXXV/158–160; XXXVI/161–164). The establishment of the subendothelial fibrinoid serves as a proof of the important barrier role of the IEL in the prevention of deep vascular damages (Fischer, 1965; Lang, 1965; Jellinek et al., 1965b; Lang et al., 1966; Adams et al., 1966).

2. The media fibrinoid arises from the admixture of necrotic medial smooth muscle cells with plasma proteins entering the vessel wall through the pores of the IEL (Hassler, 1962; Kretzschmann, 1963; Lang et al., 1966); pore size depends on the age and functional state of the IEL. Fibrin plays a less important role in the formation and histochemical properties of the media fibrinoid than of the subendothelial fibrinoid, and also the birefringence of the former is rather of the smooth muscle cell type (Hüttner et al., 1966a; Kerényi et al., 1966a; Veress et al., 1966a; Jellinek, 1967b) (Plate XXXVII/165, 166).

The adventitial fibrinoid consists chiefly of fibrin, like the subendothelial fibrinoid. It does not, however, arise by an independent mechanism; it is formed by plasma flowing across the deteriorated vessel wall, fibrin deposition, and necrotic muscular and fibrous elements of the wall.

ACUTE HYPERTENSIVE DAMAGE OF SMOOTH MUSCLE CELLS OF THE MEDIA

The other basic change that appears simultaneously with the development of the vascular fibrinoid is the necrosis of the smooth muscle cells. As vascular muscle cells originate from multifunctional mesenchymal elements (Wissler, 1967, 1968), their responses differ in many respects from those of s mooth muscle cells in other organs (Rhodin, 1962a; Kasai et al., 1964; Ehrreich et al., 1968; Esterly et al., 1968; Weiss, 1968; Somlyo et al., 1968). In addition to contraction activity, which is a general muscle cell property, vascular smooth 'muscle cells are capable of synthesizing ground substance and precursors of elastic and collagenous fibres (Haut et al., 1960; Pease and Molinari, 1960a; Karrer, 1961; Biava, 1962; Biava et al., 1962; Szabó, 1962; Seifert, 1962, 1963b; French et al., 1963; Costa et al., 1964; Haust et al., 1965a). Vascular muscle cells are very sensitive to environmental ionic changes (Ryden et al., 1967; Phelan et al., 1968; Scott et al., 1968). Local modification of the anion milieu can be elicited by vascular spasm resulting from the activity of the renin-angiotensin systems which bears primary responsibility for acute renal hypertension (Gardner, 1962, 1964; Gardner et al., 1963; Garrett et al., 1967; Hiraoka et al., 1968; Schoeffeniels, 1969; Kalliomäki et al., 1969). On bilateral nephrectomy in renal hypertension, blood pressure can be adjusted simply by the control of salt intake (Keynan et al., 1969). Thus hypertension alters the sensitivity of muscle cells to drugs and vasoactive substances (Honore et al., 1962; Gardner et al., 1964; Carettero et al., 1967; Konold et al., 1968; Kanishawa et al., 1969). The activity of the renin-angiotensin system depends on various organic and general factors (Wolff et al., 1962; Zimmerman, 1962; Endes, 1963; Masson, 1967; Biron et al., 1969).

Muscle cell necrosis is initiated partly by the ionic changes resulting from a lasting vasospasm, partly by hypoxia resulting from the intramural diffusion of plasma (DeFaria, 1961; Moss et al., 1968). Necrobiosis or necrosis of the muscle cells results in the reduction of the synthesis of elastic and collagenous precursors (Biava, 1962; David et al., 1963); the consequent weakening of the fibrous vascular wall elements promotes intramural plasma protein deposition (dyshoria). In addition, the release of endogenous histamine from the hypoxic prenecrotic cells can further enhance the dyshoria (Nikulin et al., 1964).

CHAPTER 6

EXPERIMENTAL OBSERVATIONS

INVESTIGATIONS BY LIGHT MICROSCOPY

Small vessel lesions were studied in experimental renal hypertension of albino rats, induced by a bilateral compression of the renal cortex (Lőrincz and Gorácz, 1954). The first light-microscopic change was the swelling and clumping (Altschul, 1957) of endothelial cells. Simultaneously, the smooth muscle cells of the media became swollen and vacuolized, and disseminated necroses appeared in the outer muscular layer of the media (Plate LXIII/45–49). The prenecrotic phase of the muscle cells could be traced by autoradiography prior to the visibility of microscopic changes (Plate LXII/43, 44). The water content of the swollen hypertensive arterial wall rose markedly compared to normotensive subjects (Tobian et al., 1969). The oedematous swelling of the wall constricted the lumen, diminished, distension by pulsation and the peripheral resistance tended to rise. Necrosis involved the inner muscular layers as early as in 3–6 days and, in the meantime, the intensive intramural diffusion of plasma proteins (dyshoria) resulted in fibrinoid formation which first appeared confluent (Plate LXIII/47–50), then became circumferential (Plate LXIII/51). In the newly formed fibrinoid, single necrotic muscle cells could still be distinguished by M-stain (Veress et al., 1966a; Jellinek et al., 1967c). The preserved mural structures naturally influence the localization of the fibrinoid and substances present at the site of the change may modify the lesion when they admix with the plasma substances (Altmann et al., 1962). The priority of intramural plasma diffusion or muscle cell necrosis remains to be determined by further studies, but the two basic phenomena are clearly related to one another. The focal appearance of muscle cell necroses in the outer cell row of the media suggests that the cells which receive a direct nerve supply are damaged first (Barajas, 1964; Devine, 1967; Devine et al., 1968a, b), probably by a lasting vasospasm (Bednar, 1965). The supposition of a relationship between innervation and necrotic change is corroborated by the fact that the outer cell layer of the media is better provided with oxygen than the middle layers. If a metabolic factor were responsible, it would damage the middle area (Moss et al., 1968). The vascular spasm is responsible for part of the microscopic endothelial changes (Altschul et al., 1963).

Examinations of intramural plasma diffusion by tracer substances and immunohistochemical methods have shown that it starts very early (Vazquez et al., 1958; Giese, 1961, 1964; Olsen, 1968; Nagy et al., 1968; Jellinek et al., 1969) and floods and distends the media already in the initial stage. Seven to nine days after the establishment of the circumferential fibrinoid necrosis and plasma extravasation, a perivascular granulation develops, and replaces the necrotic media.

MECHANISM OF DEVELOPMENT OF THE SUBENDOTHELIAL FIBRINOID

A subendothelial fibrinoid (Plate LXIII/52–57), accompanied by medial damage of various degrees, develops chiefly in those muscular small vessels which possess a strong IEL (Jellinek et al., 1965b; Kerényi et al., 1966a, b). If the IEL is weak, the fibrotic granulation tissue which replaces the media often prevents further intramural diffusion of plasma, thus furnishing the conditions required for the development of a subendothelial fibrinoid.

ELECTRON-MICROSCOPIC STRUCTURE AND FIBRIN FORMATIONS OF THE SUBENDOTHELIAL FIBRINOID

The following fibrin formations were identified in experimentally induced vascular fibrinoid of mesenteric and coronary arteries of albino rats, depending on the age and localization of the lesions:

1. Loose, lightly contoured fibrillar fibrin, usually lacking a transversal periodicity (Plate XXXV/158). This formation could be identified in all layers of the vessel wall during fibrinoid transformation, especially after 5–7 days when, if the typical axial periodicity was seen at all, it was in the range of either 160–170 Å or 200–220 Å (Plate XXXV/159). Fibrin formations of this kind have been observed in impaired vessels, inflamed tissues, in thrombi, in the early neo-intima of vascular grafts, in thrombocytes and myxoma cells (Vassali et al., 1963, 1964; Hirano et al., 1965; Prose et al., 1965; Nam et al., 1965; Haust et al., 1967; Kerényi et al., 1971a). Köppel (1967) has postulated that the two different periodicity ranges of the fibrin bundles result from two possible orders of the regular dodecahedron-shaped fibrin molecules. Bundles without periodicity correspond to an incompletely polymerized fibrin, i.e. to the initial stage of fibrin deposition.

2. Compact, sharply demarcated crystalline fibrin formations, hexagonal, clustered or clumped. The appearance of this formation in the subendothelial fibrinoid and less often in the media fibrinoid parallels the progression of hypertension (Plates XXXV/160; XXXVI/161, 162). Periodicity, 160–170 Å or 200–220 Å, is most distinctly seen in the clustered (bundled) order. In polygonal forms, 2–3 linear structures lie at angles of 60°; these have a periodicity of 90–115 Å. The latter could be observed in some bundles which showed a typical axial periodicity, usually with an angle of 60° (Plate XXXVI/161, 162). Wiener et al. (1965) and Ben-Ishay et al. (1966) observed this fibrin formation in hypertensive lesions of vessels and glomeruli. Similar formations were seen in the subendothelial space of renal arteries (Esterly et al., 1963) and in fibrinous necrotizing vasculopathy induced by proton irradiation (Andres, 1963). Wiener et al. (1965) determined the periodicity of the fibrin formation as 230 Å and saw in it stripes at a periodicity of 115 Å. Clumps and bundles of fibrin are seen in a photomicrograph of a human atheromatous plaque published by Haust et al. (1967), but their structure is indefinite, owing probably to the autolysis of the autopsy material. The

polygonal fibrin bodies which show a linear periodicity of 90–115 Å probably correspond with the cross-sections of the sharply contoured bundles.

3. Crystal-like bodies with a broad periodicity occur exclusively in the sub-endothelial fibrinoid and increase in amount with the progression of hypertension (Plate XXXVI/163), until finally they fill almost the entire subendothelial space (Plate XXXVI/164). Their shape is the same as that of the polygonal fibrin described under 2, but a periodicity of 600–1500 Å is superimposed on the basic 90–115 Å periodicity. The role of these fibrin formations will be discussed in connection with chronic vascular changes. Their occurrence in mesentric arteries of rats with renal hypertension (Kerényi et al., 1966b) and in coronary arteries (Hüttner et al., 1968) has already been reported. Formerly, they were believed to be connected with perivascular collagenous structures showing a periodic striation (Wetzstein et al., 1963; Pillai, 1964). Andres (1963) observed similar bodies after chronic radiation damage of the vessel wall, but he did not specify their fibrin nature. Ooneda (1965) saw fibrin clumps of similar structure in the subendothelial fibrinoid of mesenteric vessels, but in addition to the broad basic periodicity he observed another periodicity of 230 Å; we failed to identify the latter in our material.

The broad periodicity of the crystalline form probably appears in connection with the incorporation of globular plasma proteins into the crystal (Ohta et al., 1959), but the effect of pulsation may also play a role. Broad periodicity could be excluded as a summational phenomenon, since rotation of the ultra-thin section 40° around an imaginary axis parallel to one line of the striation did not change the value of periodicity. Pulsation in itself does not impart a broad periodicity to the fibrin structures. In experimental fibrinous pleuritis and pericarditis as well as in the fibrinous neo-intima of human arterial grafts, only loose fibrillar fibrin forms develop despite exposure to pulsation (Kerényi et al., 1971a). The accumulation of the more mature and structurally more organized formations of fibrin in the subendothelial space, their scarcity in the media, and the fact that the adventitia contains only loose fibrillar fibrin can be explained by the observation of Onoyama et al. (1969), that each vascular wall layer has a different fibrinolytic activity, being weakest in the endothelium and strongest in the adventitia. The probable role of fibrin-stabilizing substances may also be considered (Bleyl, 1967).

The electron-microscopic definition of the fibrinoid has not yet been determined. According to Vassalli et al. (1963, 1964) and Choi et al. (1968), the fibrinoid is less electron dense than fibrin itself, and shows a granular incomplete polymerization or a partial structural decomposition. Most authors, however, use 'fibrinoid' as a collective term in the light-microscopic sense, to denote substances having fibrin as the main component, which admixed with other plasma proteins, connective tissue fibres and necrotic cells, assume a homogeneous eosinophilic appearance (Gitlin et al., 1957; Movat et al., 1957; Chrug, 1963a; Lendrum, 1963). The contributors of this monograph (Hüttner et al., 1966a, 1968; Jellinek et al., 1966a; Jellinek, 1967) also use the term 'fibrinoid' in this wider sense and accordingly denote all fibrin formations described here as such.

ELECTRON-MICROSCOPIC STUDY OF THE MEDIA FIBRINOID AND OF NECROTIC MUSCLE CELL CHANGES

Electron microscopy of the media fibrinoid has shown that in addition to loose fibrillar fibrin and occasional sharply demarcated, crystal-like fibrin formations, smooth muscle cells showing different degrees of a necrobiotic change are present in the plasma-inundated vessel wall (Plate XXXVII/166). The most frequent muscle cell change is the necrotic oedema described by Korb (1965). The cytoplasm

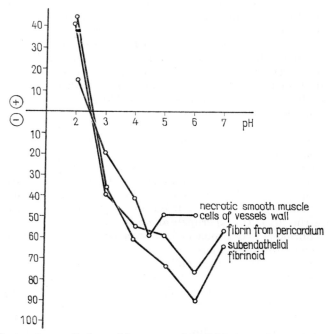

Fig. 1. Anisotropic methylene blue–potassium bichromate precipitation staining reaction as a function of pH. Curve for necrotic smooth muscle cells differs greatly from curves for subendothelial fibrinoid and fibrin from pericardium; the latter two run almost parallel and the muscle cell curve deviates from both (Romhányi's method)

of the muscle cells becomes clear, glycogen disappears; the myofilaments first separate, then undergo a lysis and the mitochondria show various forms of degeneration (Plates XXXVII/166–168; XLII/184). After these damages, which result primarily from hypoxia, the muscle cells are obviously incapable of any mechanical activity (Shibata et al., 1967). A tubulo-vesicular hyperplasia of the smooth endoplasmic reticulum ensues and the Golgi apparatus becomes distended. These changes seem to suggest an increased intake of water (Gardner, 1963; Hatt et al., 1966; Kent, 1967, 1969) and are not specific (Ashford et al., 1966). Other muscle cells show a clumping of the myofilaments with shrinkage of the entire cell body

(Takebayashi, 1970) and increasing osmiophilia (Plate XLII/184). A quantitative analysis suggests that the latter form of muscle cell necrosis might be responsible for the increased disseminated birefringence of the media (Fig. 1; Plate XXXVIII/171*f*) in the initial stage of the fibrinoid change (Jellinek et al., 1965*b*; Kerényi et al., 1966*a*; Veress et al., 1966*a*; Hüttner et al., 1968).

A small amount of fibrin from the fibrinoid, above all from the media fibrinoid, may potentiate the contraction-inducing actions of angiotensin, adrenalin, nor-adrenalin, or histamine, and may modify the further reactions of the vascular wall (Buluk et al., 1969). The adventitial fibroblasts are already swollen after 3 days of hypertension. The rough endoplasmic reticulum increases markedly in the cytoplasm (Plate XXXVIII/169), signifying the preparation of the cells for a greater fibre precursor synthesis to cope with the increased strain. The light microscopic manifestation of this phenomenon is the abrupt increase of alkaline phosphatase activity in the adventitia (as discussed later).

LOCALIZATION OF ACUTE HYPERTENSIVE DAMAGE IN SMALL VESSELS

The localization of malignant hypertensive lesions in vessels has suggested the decisive role of vasodilation (Gorácz, 1963). By administering vasodilators several times daily, Kóczé et al. (1970) were able to elicit a vascular muscle cell necrosis followed by intramural plasma diffusion (Plate XXXVIII/171*g*). Similar implications have been made in human pathology (Meyer, 1964). Uchida et al. (1969) have, nevertheless, presented convincing evidence in support of a reverse relationship between the distribution of the intrinsic myogenic tone and the lo-calization of hypertensive lesions in rat vessels. The mesenteric vessels, which are the main localization of hypertensive lesions, have no myogenic tone themselves; thus they are the ideal site of unhampered development of innervation disorders. The focal character of the changes in the exposed areas is probably due to the dissimilar sensitivity or nerve receptors (Godfraind et al., 1968). The nerve plexus accompanying the vessel (Bednař et al., 1965) is a means of central and local calibre regulation and, as such, influences local tension, blood flow and int-ramural flow. As already noted, prolonged states of vasospasm play a decisive role in the establishment of vascular wall lesions.

HISTOCHEMISTRY OF ACUTE VASCULAR LESIONS

HISTOCHEMICAL EXAMINATIONS FOR PROTEIN, CARBOHYDRATE AND LIPID

The histochemical study of protein, lipid and carbohydrate components of muscu-lar-type small vessels is relatively less informative than enzyme-histochemical investigation. In the early phase of the vascular change, the Feulgen-positive nuclear substances (Plate LXIII/46) of the rapidly necrotizing smooth muscle cells can be identified in the media fibrinoid (Kerényi et al., 1966). Apart from M-staining and PAS-reaction, the fibrinoid can be visualized by the rose indole reaction involving the tryptophane component of fibrin. This amino acid is present in the fibrin at a concentration of 3.3 g%, i.e. at a higher proportion than in any other kind of protein (Skjørten, 1968). The fibrinoid and the necrotic smooth muscle cells can be readily demonstrated by the fluorescent staining technique of Haitinger (Plate LXIII/48). Differentiation by polarization microscopy is always helpful if the fibrillar proteins form a supramolecular micellar structure; in this case it can distinguish the fibrin, necrotic smooth muscle cell (Fig. 1; Plate XXXVII/171e, f) and collagenous fibre components of the fibrinoid, as described by Jobst (1954). A quantitative polarization optical analysis of the entire vessel wall has been performed by Hüttner et al. (1966a) and Jellinek (1967)

The vascular smooth muscle cells metabolize lipids actively (Nakatani et al., 1967a, b) and play a key role in the development of the atheroma. The pertinent studies have, however, dealt chiefly with chronic lesions of large vessels, either with respect to their biochemistry (Whereat, 1966, 1967; Constantinides, 1968a), or in connection with the appearance of ceroid pigments (Gedigk et al., 1959, 1964). Lipid histochemical studies conducted during the acute stage of experimental malignant hypertension (Veress et al., 1969b) have disclosed a definite difference between the two kinds of vascular fibrinoid: while the subendothelial fibrinoid never showed a sudanophilia, either the damaged smooth muscle cells of the media, or the intercellular space between them, always contained a considerable quantity of lipids (Plate LXIV/73). In the advanced stage of the change, lipid droplets were present chiefly in macrophages appearing in the subendothelial space, and the sudanophilia of the media tended to diminish.

As to carbohydrates, the glycogen content of the vascular muscle cells varies with the species (Reale, 1965; Biava et al., 1966; Imai et al., 1966; Luciano et al., 1968). The glycogen content and the activity of the vessel are related (Laszt, 1964). The glycogen is synthesized and utilized by the cells of the vessel wall and noradrenalin enhances its synthesis (Wertheimer et al., 1961).

Increased basement membrane synthesis can be followed by PAS-reaction. The quantitative and polymeric changes of AMPs in small vessel lesions histochemically are demonstrable scarcely if at all (Kunz et al., 1965), in the acute lesion for this reason they have usually been investigated in connection with chronic small vessel changes.

ENZYME HISTOCHEMICAL STUDIES

Reviews of the vascular wall enzyme systems have naturally been centred on arteriosclerotic lesion rather than on acute vascular damage (Zemplényi, 1962, 1968; Berlepsch, 1964; Lojda, 1965; Kahn et al., 1967). The variation in enzyme activity of the hypertensive and normal vascular wall with age and sex can probably account for age- and sex-related differences in the frequency of occurrence of ASC (Kirck et al., 1955a, 1967; Kirck, 1962, 1964; Oka et al., 1968).

Although the vessel wall is regarded as a bradytrophic ('show') tissue, its metabolic activity is high (Rudolph, 1964). Vessels less than 150 μ in diameter use roughly twice as much oxygen *in vitro* than larger ones, 250–400 μ in diameter, as calculated for dry material content (Howard et al., 1965). Oxygen consumption increases in parallel with the intensity of contraction induced by vasoactive amines (Kosan et al., 1966).

The conventional enzyme-histochemical methods do not indicate early vascular changes, but quantitative assays show a marked alteration of activity prior to the appearance of morphological lesions (Gardner et al., 1965). Increase of glucose-6-phosphatase and alkaline phosphatase activity precedes vascular changes. Inferences as to activity changes in the individual vascular wall layers based on this information, however, remain speculative. The most informative enzyme-histochemical reaction, although not specific, is the activity increase of adenosine monophosphatase during the prenecrotic phase (Oka et al., 1965, 1967). In small vessels this reaction becomes positive later in postnatal life than it does in the aorta, but it is less common than the ATPase reaction and a more sensitive indicator of necrobiosis (Oka et al., 1967; Stefanescu-Gavat et al., 1967). The activity of DPNH diaphorase often changes parallel to the adenosine monophosphatase reaction.

Non-specific esterase, some of which localizes in the lysosomes (Hess et al., 1958; Holt, 1958; Wachstein et al., 1960; Tessenow, 1965) has been successfully employed for the examination of cellular elements in the vascular wall (Hüttner et al., 1967a). Since the lysosomal activity of the cells increases temporarily during the prenecrotic phase (DeDuve, 1963), both non-specific esterase (Plate LXIII/67) and acid phosphatase activity increase markedly prior to the development of the fibrinoid (Hüttner et al., 1967a). The reaction permits differentiation between the various phases of the necrobiotic state. The damaged vessel wall and the perivascular granulation present a characteristic picture (Plate LXIV/ 68–70).

In rats, the initial hypertensive strain of the vessel wall (Hüttner et al., 1965; Sótonyi et al., 1965; Gardner et al., 1967; El-Maghrabi et al., 1968) is indicated by the activity increase of the alkaline phosphatase-positive network at the borderline between media and adventitia (Hüttner et al., 1967b) (Plate LXIII/ 59–62). The activity decreases first segmentally, then around the entire circumference of the vessel wall after plasma protein deposition (dyshoria) has taken place and the media fibrinoid begins to develop (Plate LXIII/63, 64). Later, a distinct alkaline phosphatase activity appears in the perivascular granulation tissue, but in a granular rather than mesh-like distribution (Plate LXIII/65). The alkaline phosphatase-positive mesh can be observed in the adventitia of all arteries of the rat. A positive correlation between the intrinsic vascular wall pressure and the activity of the alkaline phosphatase-positive mesh was confirmed on infrarenally constricted rat artery: activity increased above the constriction and disappeared below it (Plate LXIII/66), while a broad, highly active meshwork appeared in the walls of the collateral vessels. Electron-microscopic examinations have shown that the reaction is produced by adventitial fibroblasts (Ishii et al., 1968) and to a much lesser degree by the pinocytotic vesicles of the smooth muscle cells. The rise of the intrinsic pressure probably enhances the intramural transport and thus the reaction may also serve as an indirect indicator of this phenomenon. In hypoxic rats where hypertension involved only the lesser circulation, the alkaline phosphatase-positive meshwork hypertrophied exclusively in that vascular area (Kerényi et al., 1971b). It is known that in the normotensive state the vascular calibre depends on the elastic elements, while in the hypertensive state it depends on the collagenous fibres (Fischer, 1965; Fischer et al., 1967). Thus it may well be imagined that the sensitive reaction signifies a rapid increase of fibroblast activity, aimed at the synthesis of newer collagen precursors, to compensate for the rising pressure (Plate XXXVIII/169, 170). Fibroblast activity may be enhanced not only by functional requirements, but also by drug action. For example, the segmental disappearance of the adventitial alkaline phosphatase-positive meshwork in acid-painted aortic segments became restored sooner and approximated the original localization more closely in animals treated with Solcoseryl than in those not so treated (Kerényi et al., 1970).

In summary, experimental acute hypertensive lesions serve as a model for various diseases. Apart from hypertension, additional factors play a role in their evolution such as hypoxia, electrolyte disturbance, permeability increasing substances, etc. The authors of this monograph believe that spasms, or rather the frequent alternation of vasospasm and vasodilation, play a decisive role in focal plasma protein deposition (dyshoria) and necrotic changes. Initial endothelial changes signify hypertrophy, hypoxia and disturbance of protein metabolism. Intramural plasma diffusion (dyshoria) takes place simultaneously or in succession. The localization of the vascular fibrinoid in the media or subendothelium determines the composition of the lesion and the proportions of its components. In small arteries with a strong, resistant IEL, the fibrinoid will develop subendothelially. The subendothelial fibrinoid consists chiefly of fibrin, the media fibrinoid chiefly of necrotic smooth muscle cells, and the bulk of the adventitial fibrinoid again consists of fibrin. Both the subendothelial and media fibrinoid contain characteristic crystal-like fibrin formations. The smooth muscle cell components of the media fibrinoid undergo an oedematous or an osmiophilic necrosis. The histochemical changes of the protein, lipid and carbohydrate components of the vessel wall cannot be recognized until the lesion has fully developed, whereas certain enzyme-histochemical reactions can indicate the damage prior to the appearance of any morphological alteration. In rat arteries, an increase in glucose-6-phosphatase and alkaline phosphatase activity precedes the development of the vascular wall lesion.

ACID MUCOPOLYSACCHARIDE (AMP) SYNTHESIS IN EXPERIMENTAL HYPERTENSION OF MUSCULAR-TYPE SMALL ARTERIES

The wall of the small arteries contains little AMP, predominantly chondroitin sulphate. In muscular-type arteries of rats, a delicate layer of AMP can be visualized around the smooth muscle cells and elastic membranes by Hale-PAS reaction or PAS-alcian blue staining (Crane, 1962a; Crane et al., 1964).

The observation that on parenteral administration maximum incorporation of [35]S (sulphate) took place in the sulphated AMPs (Dziewiatowski et al., 1949, Dziewiatowski, 1951; Layton, 1951), has enabled the follow-up of AMP metabolism in certain tissues and in vessels, by means of autoradiography and radiochemical methods. The amount of incorporated [35]SO$_4$ decreased proportionally with the calibre of the vessel. The aortic wall showed marked activity and muscular-type arteries showed moderate activity (Bescol-Liversac, 1963). The activity originated from the AMP-anabolism of vascular smooth muscle cells and adventitial connective tissue elements. Opinions have diverged on AMP-formation in the vascular endothelium. Experimental observations have recently favoured the ^{35}S-incorporating capacity of endothelial cells (Curran, 1957; Lindner, 1965; Kunz, 1968), although Stehbens (1962) has stated the opposite.

Examinations by means of labelled sulphur of human and experimental material have disclosed considerable new data, especially on ASC (Kowalewski, 1954; Buck, 1955, Dyrbye, 1959; Gerő et al., 1961a, b; Bescol-Liversac, 1963; Jakab et al., 1970), but also on experimental hypertension (Kocsár et al., 1961; Junge-Hülsing et al., 1963; Forman et al., 1968).

By virtue of the ability of their negative groups to enter into reversible bonds, the AMPs can play an important role in the control of water-electrolyte metabolism and diffusion. Moreover, mural electrolyte change may be a contributory factor in hypertensive lesions (Tobian et al., 1961; Koletsky, 1955, 1957; Koletsky et al., 1959; Gardner et al., 1963). Therefore, investigations into the biosynthesis of arterial AMPs may throw a light on the evolution of hypertensive vascular changes.

Investigations along this line have chiefly been conducted on the steroid hypertension model. *In vivo* (Crane, 1962a) and *in vitro* (Crane, 1962b) histochemical examinations have shown an increase of AMPs in the small arteries and arterioles of rats in connection with smooth muscle cell and fibroblast proliferation in DOC hypertension, and in lesions of large arteries in connection with arteritis or subendothelial fibrinoid deposition as well as in the fibrovascular tissue of the media.

In the same areas, the same author demonstrated radiographically an increased $^{35}SO_4$ incorporation compared to controls, and attributed it to smooth muscle cell and fibroblast activity. No labelled sulphate became incorporated into the subendothelial fibrinoid. A correlation was observed between blood pressure, degree of cardiac hypertrophy and degree of sulphate incorporation. Alterations were attributed to blood pressure rise, because according to Crane, DOC had no influence on arterial electrolyte composition.

Similar observations were made in adrenal-regenerative hypertension (Crane et al., 1964). Endothelial cells, smooth muscle cells and adventitial fibroblasts all bound the sulphate.

Gardner (1962a) demonstrated autoradiographically the incorporation of labelled sulphate into the media and adventitia of large muscular vessels affected by DOC-hypertension.

In this laboratory, incorporation of radioactive sulphur into muscular arteries was studied in albino rats with experimental renal hypertension (Konyár et al. 1971). Increase of AMP around the PAS-positive subintimal fibrinoid in the media and adventitia of mesenteric and coronary vessels could be demonstrated by Hale-PAS or alcian blue staining techniques after two weeks of hypertension (Plate LXIV/71). On autoradiographic examination, these vessels showed a distinct binding of $^{35}SO_4$ at the sites corresponding to the localization of the AMPs, so that binding can be attributed to smooth muscle cells and fibroblasts (Plate LXIV/72). No $^{35}SO_4$ became incorporated into the subintimal fibrinoid, and its activity was minimal above the endothelial cells. In some coronary arteries with undamaged tissue structure or only minimal smooth muscle cell enlargement, an increased medial muscle cell activity was observed without any histochemical indication of AMP increase (Plate LXII/43, 44). The same phenomenon was observed by Crane (1962a, b, 1964) in mesenteric arteries of hypertensive animals; it probably resulted from the enhancement of muscle cell activity by hypertension.

Thus autoradiographic examinations have shown an increased AMP synthesis by muscle cells of muscular arteries in both steroid and renal hypertension and by proliferating fibroblasts in lesions associated with arteritis. The relationship between the alteration of the barrier function of endothelial cells and the change of AMP metabolism in hypertensive vascular lesions requires further investigation.

MORPHOLOGICAL CHANGES OF SMALL VESSELS AFTER PAINTING WITH ACID

These examinations were conducted on small vessels damaged in the course of painting the aorta or femoral artery, and on those of rat uterus painted with different dilutions of hydrochloric acid.

The morphological changes of the vessel wall are described below in the temporal sequence of their appearance.

Depending on the degree of the damage, single smooth muscle cell necroses (Plate LXIV/86) appeared from one hour to two days after painting, and later fused to form a segmental necrosis of the vascular wall (Plate LXIV/87). The necrotic muscle cells showed an increased birefringence (Plate XXXVIII/171f) on polarization-microscopic examination, and showed a vivid greenish-yellow fluorescence on staining with choriphosphin or combined euchrisin-thiazinred stain, permitting their differentiation from plasma substances which in the meantime began to diffuse into the vessel wall (Plate LXIV/93). About 2–5 days after the damage, the margins of segmental and single muscle cell necroses lost definition in the surrounding plasma deposition (Plate LXIV/88), and the vessel wall assumed the homogeneous appearance of the characteristic fibrinoid necrosis (Plate LXIV/80). At this stage, the necrotic muscle cells could no longer be recognized on staining with azan, but they became apparent on the homogeneous red background, if M-stain was additionally used (Plate LXIV/90). With the progression of the process the entire vessel wall appeared homogeneous even on staining with the M-stain; the cellular elements practically disappeared (Plate LXIV/91) and the typical picture of fibrinoid necrosis became established.

Extensive vascular wall damage was followed by an increased intramural plasma diffusion, resulting in the involvement of the adventitia and perivascular area (Plate LXIV/92, 93). Thread-like or net-like fibrin structures appeared, showing a positive birefringence at a face difference of 35–48 mμ (Fig. 2); these were digestible by trypsin. A perivascular granulation, consisting of lymphocytes, histiocytes, many fibroblasts, fibrocytes and collagenous fibres, developed regularly around the several damaged vessels and, together with the mural lesions, it had a periarteritis nodosa-like appearance (Plate LXIV/94, 95).

In muscular-type small vessels which possess a thicker IEL and are consequently more resistant, the homogeneous eosinophilic substance, corresponding both histologically and histochemically with the fibrinoid, appeared also in the subendothelial space between the IEM and endothelium. While the necrotic area and the fibrinoid both stained homogeneously red with azan (Plate LXIV/96), the M-stain clearly differentiated the subendothelial fibrinoid from the necrotic smooth muscle cells of the media (Plate LXIV/97). The subendothelial fibrinoid showed the characteristic birefringence (Plate XXXVIII/171e) and the characteristic topochemical reactions of fibrin. When mounted in Canada balsam, the fibrinoid showed a positive birefringence of 35–48 mμ, which did not change after phenol or anilin reaction (Plate XXXVIII/171a, b, c). The positive birefringence of the necrotic medial muscle cells attained only 12 mμ. A 0.3 per cent trypsin solution digested the fibrinoid from a specimen fixed in Carnoy's solution within 60 minutes, after which the positive birefringence disappeared (Plate XXXVIII/ 171).

Thus painting muscular-type small vessels with acid elicited the same type of change—fibrinoid necrosis—as hypertension. The morphological resemblance of the lesions elicited by the two factors was so close as to permit no conclusion as regards their aetiology (Jellinek, 1970b). Certain micrographs are indeed practically identical (Plates LXIII/46–57; LXIV/86–96). In the small muscular-type vessels, smooth muscle cell necrosis is followed by intramural plasma diffusion of various degrees, depending on the extent of the damage and on the structure of the vascular wall. The plasma admixes with the necrotic smooth muscle cells to form

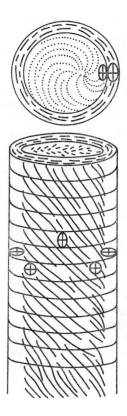

Fig. 2. Orientation of elementary elastic fibrils within the elastic fibre (a schematic presentation). Fibrils are arranged circularly in the external sheath, but in a spiral fashion within the central axis (after Romhányi, 1965)

the characteristic fibrinoid necrosis, but the two main components can be distinguished for a long period, to judge from the polarization optical analysis of hypertensive lesions and the disappearance of positive birefringence after trypsin digestion of the fibrinoid induced by painting with acid (Fig. 1).

Examination of lesions developing in experimental hypertension or after painting with acid suggests that various injuries elicit identical changes in given vascular wall structures. Hypertension and painting with acid uniformly elicit the formation of the characteristic vascular fibrinoid. Two further experiments, performed to substantiate this theory, are described in the next two sections.

NORADRENALIN-INDUCED LESIONS OF MUSCULAR-TYPE SMALL VESSELS

Noradrenalin plays an important role in the maintenance of vasomotor tone and blood distribution, but if large amounts are abruptly released into the blood stream, severe general vasospasm and hypoxia develop, with the possible result of acute vascular damage. The cardiac and small vessel changes associated with phaeochromocytoma are due chiefly to noradrenalin action (Szakács et al., 1958; Talbot et al., 1960). Similar changes may appear as a iatrogenic damage during the noradrenalin therapy of isovolaemic shock (Szakács and Cannon, 1958; Mond et al., 1959). In man, high doses of noradrenalin may elicit a shock accompanied by thrombotic changes of small vessels, if administration (infusion) is abruptly stopped (Whitaker et al., 1969). Vascular damage with noradrenalin infusion is enhanced by degenerative changes of the vessels which took place already during the state of shock (Ashford et al., 1966). The application of alpha-adrenergic blocking agents during infusion prevents the formation of thrombi; thus these clearly result from disseminated endothelial and mural impairment by vasospasm. The degree of vasospasm was measured quantitatively by Rossmann et al. (1967) and Birmingham et al. (1969). Elevation of the blood lipid level by noradrenalin, and ECG-changes during infusion, can be effectively prevented by beta-adrenergic blocking agents (Marchetti et al., 1968; Hoak et al., 1969). The noradrenalin sensitivity of the vessels depends on the age of the human or animal subject (Gey et al., 1965; Tuttle, 1966; Hruza et al., 1967), on ionic balance (Hiraoka, 1968), on presence of an advanced renal hypertension (Gardner et al., 1964), on sex and reproductive cycle (Carettero et al., 1967) and hormonal state of the animal (Honore et al., 1962). The action of noradrenalin may be modified by a toxic paralysis of the protein synthesis which may affect the patient under shock already at an early stage (Freed et al., 1968). A chemotherapeutic or surgical denervation of the vessel wall has no noticeable influence on noradrenalin action (Zimmermann, 1962), but it prevents the angiotensin-induced spasm.

Sámson (1932), Pugh et al. (1952) and Szakács and Cannon (1958) reproduced the noradrenalin-induced cardiac and vascular changes experimentally. The lesions bore a close resemblance to those elicited by painting with acid or experimental malignant renal hypertension (Hüttner et al., 1965, 1966a; Kerényi et al., 1965, 1966a) and their main characteristic was the development of a fibrinoid necrosis.

In this laboratory, 60 dogs of both sexes, weighing 6–12 kg, were given 300–450 or 700 gamma per kg body weight noradrenalin in 200 ml saline, in the form of a drop infusion administered in 45 minutes under chloralose anaesthesia. Pulse rate was checked before, during and after infusion, and blood pressure was recorded directly in the exposed femoral artery. During infusion, the blood pressure rose from an initial average 160–180 mm Hg to 260–280 mm Hg, heart contraction per minute fluctuated markedly (60–280) and the ECG record usually showed repolarization disturbances and extrasystole. The symptoms connected with noradrenalin treatment were observed by Pogátsa et al. (1963). Vascular changes were most distinct in the heart, hence these lesions were studied in more detail. Of the other organs, the kidneys, intestines and the pancreas showed slight vascular wall damage.

Treatment produced simultaneous changes in the heart muscle and in cardiac small vessels. Miliary necroses or small groups of necrotic fibres appeared in the muscle of both ventricles, depending on the amount of noradrenalin administered (Plate LXIV/74, 75).

Dogs killed 8–17 hours after the infusion showed no change of cardiac vessels, but after 48 hours the intramural small arteries, chiefly of the right ventricle, appeared damaged to varying degrees, depending on the dose of noradrenalin. The first light-microscopic change was the swelling and vacuolization of medial smooth muscle cells (Plate LXIV/79, 87). The necrotic muscle cells stained flamered with azan (Plate LXIV/78), reacted positively with PAS (Plate LXIV/79, 84) and bound PTA-haematoxylin more firmly than normal smooth muscle cells (Plate LXIV/81). They could be easily visualized by appropriate fluorochrome stains, but their birefringence was less and of a shorter duration than that shown by similarly changed muscle cells in hypertensive small vessels. Low doses of noradrenalin caused the necrosis of only a few muscle cells in relatively few vessels, but with the elevation of the dose the change became more extensive and involved greater segments, finally the entire circumference, of the vessel wall (Plate LXIV/83). Simultaneously with this process, the vessel wall began to show reactions characteristic of fibrinoid necrosis (Plate LXIV/80), but necrotic smooth muscle cells could still be visualized with M-stain amidst the abruptly appearing extensive plasma deposition (Plate LXIV/81). The extensive intramural plasma diffusion (dyshoria) was chiefly due to a severe endothelial damage (Altschul, 1957; Constantinides et al., 1969a–c). The endothelial cells became oedematous and showed structural disorganization. Although we failed to observe a disseminated thrombus formation in the vascular lumen (Whitaker et al., 1969), this might well result from an abrupt release from the endothelium of the granules promoting clotting (Burri et al., 1968).

The vessels of dogs treated with 700 gamma per kg noradrenalin showed, in addition to fibrinoid change of the media, a perivascular plasma diffusion, in which fibrin filaments were occasionally demonstrable by polarization microscopy or classical staining reactions (Weigert's fibrin stain, Endes' trichrome stain). Dogs killed no more than two weeks after treatment had much less muscle cell necrosis in the heart vessels than those killed after 48 hours; instead, there was an initial fibrosis around the damaged vessels and an increased fibre formation and cellular infiltration was seen.

The noradrenalin-induced lesions of cardiac muscular vessels developed in similar localizations to those found with hypertensive changes (Zollinger, 1959; Gorácz, 1963); this underlines the role of hypertension in vascular smooth muscle cell necrosis (Gardner and Brooks, 1963). Unlike hypertensive changes, however, the media showed only a slight birefringence and for a transitory period; this was probably due to the extreme degree of plasma diffusion, or perhaps the plasma proteins masked the myofilaments released from the disrupting muscle cells. A subendothelial fibrinoid (Plate LXIV/85) rarely developed after noradrenalin infusion; the coronary vessels, which became most severely damaged, possessed indeed a relatively weak IEL, with large pores (Plate LXI/2) (Reale and Ruska, 1965; Lang and Nordwig, 1966). Plasma diffusion often carried many red blood cells into the vessel wall, without leukocytes.

It is known that adrenergic neurohormones enhance the intracellular diffusion of sodium and this sensitizes the cells toward the renin-vasopressin system (Schmidt, 1962). The circumstance that angiotensin also possesses an indirect adrenergic action and the degradation products of intramurally deposited fibrin enhance the noradrenalin sensitivity of smooth muscle cell elements (Buluk and Malifiejew, 1969) complicates the understanding of these phenomena. Any vaso-active substance present in the plasma acts more directly in an intramural localization (Wurzel and Zweifach, 1966) than normally. Noradrenalin soon alters the electric activity of vascular smooth muscle cells (Nakajima and Horn, 1967; Somlyo and Somlyo, 1968) and, through the above interrelated mechanism, finally produces a typical fibrinoid vasculitis, a picture resembling periarteritis nodosa. Thus experiments with noradrenalin have again shown that the fibrinoid necrosis is the typical acute change of muscular-type small vessels in response to various kinds of damage and that the composition, localization and exten-siveness of the fibrinoid depend on the degree of damage and on the structural condition of the vessel wall.

SMALL VESSEL CHANGES ON HYPERSENSITIZATION

In a case report Kussmaul and Maier (1866) described, under the name periarteri-tis nodosa, a generalized vascular change characterized by inflammatory and degenerative lesions of medium and large arteries; nodules and aneurysms formed along the passage of the vessels and a diffuse nephritis and necrotizing enteritis were associated with the picture. This uniform-appearing syndrome was later subdivided into several entities on the basis of symptomatic and morphological differences: including various forms of allergic angiitis or granulomatosis, temporal arteritis and arteritis associated with collagenous diseases (Alarcon-Segovia and Brown 1964).

According to Arkin (1930), the periarteritis nodosa lesion has several stages which may be simultaneously present in one and the same subject. Oedema and exudation develop in the intima, causing a swelling and separation of medial smooth muscle cells and a constriction of the vascular lumen. This is followed by an inflammatory cell infiltration and a progression of the exudation to the adventitia, probably resulting in thrombus or aneurysm formation. In the third stage the inflammatory cellular reaction becomes chronic and a granulation tissue develops, followed by cicatrization and occasionally obliteration of the lumen. The lesions initially involve segments of the vessel wall, but later its entire circumference. Arterioles and veins do not become involved and no extravascular granulation develops around them.

The earliest change is an oedema and swelling of the media, followed by the deposition of an eosinophilic substance—very likely plasma proteins—in the subendothelial space. These phenomena precede the necrosis of the medial muscle cell layer which develops either segmentally or over the entire circumference. Cell infiltration appears in the wall and involves the adventitia in parallel with the impairment of the elastic membranes. Initially, the infiltrating cells are neutrophilic leukocytes and macrophages; later, chiefly monocytes, histiocytes, plasma cells and eosinophiles appear (Gardner 1965).

The probable direct role of viral, infectious, toxic and other injuries in vascular changes has received little attention as compared to hypersensitivity (Baló, 1924; Randerath, 1954). Gruber (1925) was the first to suggest an allergic mechanism on the basis of the frequent association of post-infectious periarteritis nodosa cases with asthma. Association of periarteritis nodosa with rheumatoid arthritis has also been observed (Ball, 1954; Sokoloff, 1957); according to Cruickshank (1954), this kind of arteritis can be distinguished from the true periarteritis nodosa; according to Schmid et al. (1961) and Finkbiner and Decker (1963), it is often indistinguishable, whether developing spontaneously or in consequence of the corticosteroid therapy of rheumatoid arthritis (Kemper et al., 1957; Slocumb et al., 1957), or if there is a difference, it is only quantitative (Radnai, 1969).

Occurrence of periarteritis nodosa in connection with drug therapy (sulphonamide, arsenic, etc.), or serum disease (Klinge, 1930; Rich, 1942; Rich and Gregory, 1943; Symmers, 1962) also seems to confirm that it is an immune or auto-immune condition, although the rise of the gamma-globulin level is not always demonstrable; the condition is interpreted as an analogue of rheumatic fever and it has been classified as an immunological connective tissue change (Gardner, 1965).

Examinations by immunofluorescence methods have served to support this theory; apart from human glomerulonephritis, lipid nephrosis and amyloidosis, the presence of gamma globulins in the intima and media could also be demonstrated in periarteritis nodosa lesions (Mellors and Ortega, 1956).

Albumin and fibrinogen have also been demonstrated by similar techniques (Paronetto and Strauss, 1962). According to Gitlin et al. (1957), at least part of the fibrinoid change consists of fibrin in rheumatoid arthritis, systemic lupus erythematosus, subacute or chronic glomerulonephritis, rheumatic fever, dermatomyositis and periarteritis nodosa. Thus not only an antigen–antibody reaction takes place, but also all serum proteins become precipitated in the lesion.

In accordance with the auto-immune theory, a search was made for vascular antibodies. Stefanini and Mednicoff (1954) demonstrated antivascular antibodies in patients with periarteritis nodosa; on the other hand, Fabius (1959) failed to detect precipitines to vascular antigens in 47 patients with vasculitis. Gardner et al. (1970) failed to prevent the development of hypertensive arteriolar lesions by immunosuppressive treatment.

Elevated blood pressure, cortisone and ACTH-effect have also been considered factors in the establishment of periarteritis nodosa (Haining and Kimball, 1934; Fahr, 1941; Selye and Pentz, 1943; Zeek et al., 1948; Masson et al., 1950; Baggenstoss et al., 1951; Ehrenreich and Olmstead, 1951; Zeek, 1952; Janssen and Michot, 1960; Moskowitz et al., 1963; Gardner, 1970).

Attempts at the experimental reproduction of human periarteritis nodosa lesions have been successful; almost identical changes were elicited in rabbits, rats, and other animals with 4-fluoro-10-methyl-1,2 benzanthracene (Hartmann et al., 1959), by sensitization with streptococci (Albertini, 1943) or staphylococci (Rajka et al., 1959), histamine (Heinlein et al., 1961), thiouracil (Marine and Baumann, 1945), thyrotropic hormone (Ranz, 1959), estrogenic implants (Cutts, 1966) or renal impairment (Loomis, 1946; Koletsky, 1955).

Experimental induction of periarteritis nodosa in rabbits with horse serum (Rich and Gregory, 1943; Kobernick and More, 1959; Germuth et al., 1957; More and McLean, 1949; More and Movat, 1959), horse serum + sulphathiazol (Saphir et al., 1962), bovine serum albumin (Vazquez and Dixon, 1958), or globulin (Hawn and Jeneway, 1947), etc. has indicated an allergic pathomechnism.

Studies with heterologous sera suggest that the lesion develops in response to heterologous proteins and is of the same nature as the cutaneous Arthus phenomenon (Kellaway et al., 1962; Rich and Gregory, 1943; Saphir et al., 1962).

In walls of changed arteries, gamma globulin (supposed to be an antibody) and vascular antigens and antibodies have been demonstrated by the immunofluorescence method (Vazquez and Dixon, 1958; Ohta et al., 1959; Cochrane et al., 1959; Beregi et al., 1963).

In view of the above findings, there would appear to be five possible ways in which periarteritis nodosa lesions and allergic vasculitis lesions might develop:

1. The lesion could arise from a local antigen–antibody reaction which, according to Taylor et al. (1961), can take place either on the reticular fibres or inside endothelial cells. Letterer (1956) has also mentioned the surface of smooth muscle cells and the collagenous fibres as possible additional localizations of hypersensitivity reactions.

2. A simultaneous precipitation of antigen and antibody could give rise to a permeability disturbance (Gardner, 1965).

3. Antigen–antibody complexes may form in the blood stream, as in anaphylactic shock or during the early phase of immune response in rabbits (Fennel and Santamaria, 1962; Sabesin, 1964; Beregi et al., 1964; Beregi, 1967; Beregi and Simon, 1967; Szilágyi et al., 1967 and others). Dixon et al. (1958) have observed that in experimental serum disease, the lesions evolve in the period when the complexes are circulating in the blood, and Cochrane and Weigle (1958) demonstrated a phlogistic action of the soluble complexes.

4. In addition to its phlogistic action, the complex may give rise to changes through the alteration of permeability (Ishizaka and Campbell, 1958; Benaceraff et al., 1960; Mellors and Brzosko, 1962).

5. Szinay (1968) has supposed that the damage of the complexes originates from their macromolecular nature.

In view of these dissimilar concepts, we initiated studies of the lesions making a comparison with the experimental models previously used (Kádár et al., 1965b). The following experiments were performed:

The evolution of vascular lesions was followed in rabbits immunized by the method of Rich and Gregory (1943). A group of the animals was exposed to cold for 5 minutes daily, as suggested by Beregi (1959). The temporal course of vascular changes was followed in the pulmonary, cardiac, renal, and intestinal submucosal vessels, among others, and different stages of the morphological alteration were observed simultaneously in the same animal.

The initial stage of the change was characterized by an intramural plasma diffusion (Plate XXII/98) and by vacuolization of endothelial cells, with subsequent appearance of vacuoles also in medial smooth muscle cells (Plate XXII/99). Although at this stage plasma deposition appeared also in the media, there was as yet no indication of a fibrinoid necrosis. Necrosis of single smooth muscle cells followed (Plate XXIII/100); the necrotic cells showed an increased affinity to PTA (Plate XXIII/101) and their nuclei became hyperchromatic (Plate XXIII/101). Later, the focal areas of smooth muscle cell necrosis fused with one another and, admixing with the intramural plasma deposition, they gave rise to a fibrinoid necrosis (Plate XXIII/102). At this stage the arterial wall stained homogeneously red with azan and became PAS-positive throughout its entire thickness, but the M-stain revealed confluent black patches which corresponded to the necrotic smooth muscle cells. The final stage of muscle cell necrosis was signified by the absence of nuclear staining; the wall stained yellow with M-stain, and a perivascular granulation developed, i.e. the regular microscopic picture of periarteritis nodosa appeared (Plate XXIII/103). Periarterial granulation often evolves simultaneously with the single muscle cell necroses. The structural relations of the periarteritis nodosa-like change depend on the calibre of the vessel wall. Plate XXIII/103 shows the complete homogenization of the wall of a small muscular artery not possessing an IEL. Plate XXIV/104 shows the alteration in a larger vessel with IEL. The subendothelial space has widened and does not contain fibrin, but a considerable amount of fibrin is present in the peri-adventitial granulation tissue (Plate XXIV/105) and the broadened intima contains many cellular elements (Plate XXIV/104).

Opinions differ concerning the priority of intramural plasma diffusion or medial muscle cell necrosis in experimental periarteritis nodosa lesions. Albertini (1943) suggests that the muscle cell deterioration is the initial change, whereas Rich and Gregory (1943) believe that medial cell necrosis is preceded by an oedema of the media and according to Kellaway et al. (1962), medial oedema follows upon the swelling of the endothelium.

In lesions induced by sensitization with horse serum in this laboratory, intramural plasma diffusion was the first demonstrable change, degeneration of vascular smooth muscle cells was the second step, and finally the admixture of necrotic muscle elements with plasma deposition resulted in the development of the characteristic fibrinoid necrosis.

At this stage the vascular wall change was in every respect similar to the fibrinoid necrosis induced by other methods and later, when perivascular granulation was established, to the microscopic appearance of periarteritis nodosa lesions resulting from other causes. The change was probably initiated by an antigen–antibody reaction: protein precipitation was followed by muscle cell degeneration and admixture with plasma substances resulted in the development of a fibrinoid necrosis. This model experiment has again provided evidence for the identity of arterial response to different damages (Albertini, 1943; Alarcon-Segovia and Brown, 1964; Jellinek, 1964) and has confirmed the view that the morphology of the vascular lesion is not conclusive with respect to the causative factor.

Thus the nature of allergic vascular lesions was essentially the same as that of lesions observed in experimental rat hypertension (Lőrincz and Gorácz, 1954), noradrenalin-induced hypertension of dogs (Jellinek et al., 1965a), and in direct vascular wall damage produced by painting with a caustic substance (Hüttner et al., 1965, Jellinek, 1965; Jellinek et al., 1965c).

Obviously, the development of the fibrinoid necrosis requires the interaction of plasma diffusion and muscle cell degeneration, because no such change evolved from plasma deposition in itself if muscle cell necrosis did not take place. Thus neither the components, nor the mechanism of evolution of the allergic vascular change differed from those of lesions induced by hypertension and other factors.

CHAPTER 7

CHRONIC LESIONS OF SMALL VESSELS (VASCULAR WALL TRANSFORMATION FOLLOWING ACUTE LESIONS OF SMALL VESSELS)

Analysis of vascular changes induced by different factors has clearly shown the fundamental identity of the acute vascular response to various kinds of damage. This chapter deals with the further development of acute lesions. Studies have shown that the nature of the causative factor plays no role in the chronic stage of the change, but that the severity of the damage is decisive, because this determines both the morphology and the course of the chronic lesion. The following description of chronic changes in the experimental models studied observes the same sequence as the previous discussion of acute changes.

CHRONIC SMALL VESSEL CHANGES AFTER HYPERTENSION

These may take place by two different pathomechanisms, although the final issue is identical:

1. Reparation of vascular wall after damage by malignant hypertension or temporary acute hypertensive states;
2. Benign hypertensive changes not resulting in acute damage.

Morphologically, the chronic vascular lesions may be of two types: (*i*) proliferative, or (*ii*) hyaline, and the establishment of one or the other type depends on the kind and size of the vessel, on the nature and duration of damage and on the organ in which the vessel is located (Jellinek et al., 1970*b*) (see Chapter 11).

Reparative reactions of the vascular wall are characterized by proliferation of endothelial and smooth muscle cells (Adams, 1964; Texon, 1967). Earlier investigators have agreed that the atheroma develops at the site of previous proliferative changes, through a partial degeneration of the latter (Esterly and Glagov, 1963; Imai and Thomas, 1968). Probably any local trauma or infection, which elicits an intramural plasma diffusion or a fibrin deposition on the endothelial surface, impairs the nutritional condition of the vascular wall and may thus become the source of later degenerative changes.

Hypertensive changes can be regarded as the primary cause of vascular damage. If the drug therapy for malignant hypertension is successful and the experimental animal survives, cellular elements seem to play a decisive role in the healing of the vascular fibrinoid lesion (Kojimahara, 1967) (see Chapter 8).

Of the three known phases of early arteriosclerotic change, two, the pre-proliferative and the proliferative phases (Thomas et al., 1968), resemble closely the proliferative type of chronic hypertensive lesions.

CHRONIC PROLIFERATIVE REACTIONS OF VESSELS DAMAGED BY A SINGLE TRAUMA OR BY AN ACUTE HYPERTENSIVE CRISIS

Hypertensive crisis gives rise to a diffuse vacuolization and degeneration of endothelial cells, it causes the opening of the endothelial junctions (Wiener et al., 1965) and promotes transcellular plasma diffusion (Bálint et al., 1970). As a result of acute damage, signs of an increased cellular activity (hyperplasia of endoplasmic reticulum and Golgi apparatus, increase in number of mitochondria) become constant, the subendothelial space widens, both endothelial and muscle cells extend cytoplasmic processes, and manifest focal degeneration of the cytoplasma (myelin figures, lipofuscin-like residual bodies) and microclasmatosis (fragmentation) can be seen (Plates XXXIX/172; XL/176, 177, 179). The basement membrane material increases, and cell detritus and newly formed, undifferentiated cells appear in it (Plates XXXIX/174; XL/176, 177; XLI/180). These structures are clearly visible in the subendothelial space if no extreme plasma diffusion takes place. Leukocytes also appear in the same location (Packham et al., 1967) (Plate XXXIX/175).

The endothelial cells undergo a focal proliferation during reparation, as also earlier in the chronic stage of hypertension (Plate LXV/109, 110). Proliferating muscle cells and fibroblasts (Plate LXV/107, 108) appear in the subendothelial space and media (Parker and Odland, 1966a, b; Kanisawa and Schroeder, 1969). These cells do not necessarily originate from the vessel wall in experimental animals. In rats, they appear first at the luminal side of the subendothelial fibrinoid, so that they may originate from the blood (Plates XLI/180–182; LXV/106, 107). Haust et al. (1960) believe that the smooth muscle elements of the intimal thickening arise from the endothelium. These smooth muscle cells with their cytoplasmic processes resemble fibroblasts and the basement membrane along them may be multiple, discontinuous, fragmented or absent (Geer et al., 1961; Imai et al., 1966) (Plate XXXVII/168). The presence of cells capable of differentiation to fibroblasts, smooth muscle cells or endothelial cells in the circulating blood of swine, has been confirmed experimentally (Stump et al., 1963). The modified, activated muscle cell components of the intimal thickening (Balis et al., 1964; Veress et al., 1969d) differ from the normal mural cell forms not only ultrastructurally, but also in physiological properties. Fibroblasts and muscle cells from proliferating lesions show a markedly different growth rate in tissue culture compared to normal vascular muscle cells and subcutaneous fibroblasts (Kasai and Pollak, 1964).

Ionizing irradiation causes marked endothelial cell damage, resulting in the increase of vascular permeability (Andres, 1963; Stearner and Sanderson, 1969). Simultaneously, muscle cell necrosis appears in the media.

In a recently described model of rabbit ASC, involvement of the coronary arteries was preceded by subendothelial oedema and increase of endothelial permeability. Finally, a complete obliteration may develop (Tjawokin, 1969). The animals, confined to special cages to limit movement, did not develop hypertension, and their serum cholesterol level rose only initially.

In this laboratory, dogs given a noradrenalin infusion simultaneously with isodihydroperparine showed a subendothelial plasma deposition in the intramural segments of the coronary arteries (Hüttner et al., 1966). The plasma deposition initially contained no fibrin, but later it became PAS-positive and PTA-positive, signifying that the plasma diffusion had reached such a degree of severity that fibrin also could gain access to the vessel wall. This damage occurred only in those cases in which isodihydroperparine could not depress the hypertensive action of noradrenalin. In addition to the haemodynamic factors, a relative insufficiency of the lymph circulation, signified by the distended lymph vessels, probably enhanced the development and maintenance of intramural plasma depositions (see Chapter 10).

If plasma diffusion is extensive, the lymph vessels are the only routes of drainage of extravasated albumin and lipoproteins, so that the preservation of intramural lymph vessels is essential for the disposal of plasma substances (Hollander, 1967; Veress et al., 1966b; Jellinek et al., 1970).

If extreme intramural plasma diffusion takes place during the acute stage, the subendothelial cell elements seem to play little role in the evolution of the lesion. Later, however, they aid the formation and disposal of the cell detritus which forms a part of the subendothelial fibrinoid (Plates XL/177; XLI/180).

Silver et al. (1969) observed human vascular lesions resulting from a single iatrogenic hypertensive injury. Application of high-pressure coronary perfusion during large vessel surgery resulted in the manifestation of angina pectoris after three months and in a fatal outcome within a year. At post-mortem examination, severe stenotic intimal thickenings were seen in the initial segment of the coronary arteries; microscopically, the IPs were identified as a fibrous tissue rich in AMP, but without elastic elements. The lesions were attributed to the uncommonly high pressure employed during perfusion: i.e. they resulted from a single hypertensive trauma. However, the role of mechanical damage by the cannula could not be excluded (Fishman, 1968).

Most IPs seen in human material have been post-thrombotic. Recently, however, thrombosis-associated endothelial damage, chiefly of the pulmonary arteries, has been observed after contraceptive medication. In these cases, too, the late change appeared in the form of an IP.

In man, subendothelial plasma depositions give rise to a subsequent fibrosis of the intima (Tallgren and Knorring, 1969), but this develops only after very severe damage.

Experimental mechanical damage of the veins is followed by the appearance of lipids in medial muscle cells located below the discontinuities of the endothelium (Hoff and Gottlob, 1967), and the lipid change always appears over a larger area than that originally damaged (Gutstein et al., 1963). The muscle cell components of the IP developing in response to mechanical damage originate from the media (Still and Dennison, 1967).

In addition to hypertensive changes, we examined IPs induced by acid or alkali painting of rabbit and rat aorta and of muscular-type small vessels in rat uterus (Hüttler et al., 1966a; Kádár et al., 1969b; Veress et al., 1969d; see later). Proliferation was frequent, but thrombotic processes were rare. Primary proliferative lesions were infrequent in small vessels, because the proliferative cells had first to absorb the relatively bulky intramural plasma deposition and its degenerative products (Plate XLI/180, 181). Therefore, the muscle cell components of small vessel proliferations were initially undifferentiated or showed a histiocytic rather than fibroblastic transformation. The initial absorptive proliferations of small vessels usually contained more extracellular substance than similar changes in large vessels. The vascular endothelial and smooth muscle cell elements were capable of an AMP-synthesis, in normal vessel wall and IP alike (Buck, 1958; Pease and Molinari, 1960; Ham, 1962; Kunz et al., 1968; Wissler, 1967, 1968). Rat arteriopathy connected with calciphylaxis could also be regarded as the reparative process of a simple vascular lesion; initially there was only an endothelial cushion, but shortly afterwards an IP developed, accompanied by an increase of AMPs, destruction of endothelium and chalk deposition (Seifert and Dreesbach, 1966). The AMPs and elastic fibres play a decisive role in both arteriosclerotic and calciphylactic vascular changes and often also appear in the reparative IP (Plate LXV/112, 114).

The physiological obliteration of the muscular-type segment of the rooster's ductus arteriosus is followed by a vigorous elastic fibre synthesis (Harms, 1967).

Experimental hyperkinetic pulmonary hypertension of dogs (Downing et al., 1963) results in the formation of fibrous mural plaques, which might arise by organization of earlier thrombi. Disseminated IPs are formed from organized microthrombi in bovine coronary arteries (Likar et al., 1969). The role of vascular injuries and thrombus formation in ASC have also been examined simultaneously (Mustard, 1967).

In summary, whether a single acute vascular injury induces a subendothelial or a media fibrinoid, the process always involves the mobilization and activation of endothelial and smooth muscle cells, which eliminate the destroyed elements and cope with the increased mechanical strain, while the final consequence of the change is always the development of an IP.

The reparation of the media is completed by the cicatrization of the proliferative tissue (Plate LXV/111, 112).

SMALL VESSEL HYALINIZATION AFTER AN ACUTE HYPERTENSIVE CRISIS OR OTHER SINGULAR DAMAGE

Late transformation of acute subendothelial fibrinoid often takes place by hyalinization rather than intimal proliferation (Plate LXV/113). The type of the advanced lesion depends greatly on the calibre of the vessel; in human cases a hyaline transformation is usually observed in vessels less than 100 μ in diameter. Some authors believe that hyalinization is related to intramural fat deposition (Wilens and Elster, 1950), while others think that it originates from the blood plasma (Duguid and Anderson, 1952; McKinney, 1962) or regard it as a product of muscle cells (Montgomery and Muirhead, 1954). The latter view has been supported by certain histochemical findings. Arterial hyaline has been regarded as a basement membrane-like substance, the most important component of which is fibrin (Stolpmann, 1967; Hüttner et al., 1970a, b), and increased endothelial cell activity is always associated with its formation (Plate XLII/185, 186, 187) (Hüttner et al., 1968). As a rule, fibrin is still demonstrable by fluorescence technique during depolymerization in the process of hyaline transformation (Skjørten, 1968). Subendothelial hyaline depositions are seen particularly often in human essential hypertension (Biava and Brynjolfsson, 1967). Hyalinized vessels have also been observed in hypertension associated with gouty nephropathy.

Oxygen supply to the subendothelial area is poor even normally (Moss et al., 1968); it is diminished when plasma diffusion takes place, and the cellular elements are unable to multiply and to differentiate into still more oxygen-requiring smooth muscle cells. This accounts for the observation that only cell debris is seen below the 2–3 rows of newly differentiated smooth muscle cells along the luminal side of the fibrinoid (Plate XLI/181, 182). Prior to the appearance of this superficial proliferation, the subendothelial fibrinoid becomes gradually disorganized, its fibrin undergoes depolymerization and loose structural definition, whereas the overlying endothelial layer becomes populated chiefly by young cells with a clear cytoplasm and an intense pinocytotic activity. Leukocytes migrating into the subendothelial space may signify a phagocytosis of fibrin, but intracellular fibrin decomposition does not seem to play a role in the elimination of fibrin (Hüttner et al., 1968) (Plate XLII/185, 186, 187). Aggregation of many cytofilaments in endothelial cells adjoining the hyaline change has often been observed, together with contents of hyaline density in pinocytotic vesicles and in the rough endoplasmic reticulum (Plate XLII/186, 187). Many lipid inclusions and lamellar myelin figures are present in the homogeneous subendothelial fibrinoid (McGee and Ashworth, 1963; Constantinides, 1968; Hüttner et al., 1968; Jellinek et al., 1969) (Plate XLII/188). Myelin figures have also been observed in hepatic hyaline (Biava, 1964). Occasionally medial damage is healed by hyaline cicatrization (Plate LXV/111).

Healing of radiation-induced extensive medial necrosis takes place by hyalinization in experimental animals (Kunz et al., 1965). Certain experimental conditions, e. g. administration of allylamine (Lalich, 1969), elicit a predominantly hyaline change, also involving a selective impairment of muscle cells.

In summary, in the chronic stage of change after a single vascular damage, hyalinosis takes place chiefly in small vessels, less than 100 μ in diameter, and it originates primarily from intramural plasma deposition. In addition to the hyaline transformation of intramural fibrin, there is cellular hyperactivity, and masses of cytofilaments appear in endothelial cells. The hyaline tissue contains lipid inclusions.

PROLIFERATIVE VASCULAR LESIONS IN CHRONIC BENIGN HYPERTENSION

Basic vascular changes in chronic benign hypertension correspond to those occurring in malignant hypertension, but intramural plasma diffusion is less intensive and more gradual. The muscle cell necrosis is disseminated and appears slowly. This accounts for the slow progression of regeneration and for the parallel appearance of early differentiated cell elements and later plasma deposition and cell degeneration within the same lesion.

As in proliferative arteriosclerotic lesions, endothelial cells show variable cytoplasmic density in the damaged areas (Plates XXXIX/172, 174; XL/177). The intercellular junctions stretch and the endothelial cells overlap one another considerably (Plates XXXIX/172, 173; XL/177); some of them become osmiophilic, or become detached entering the lumen (Plate XXXIX/174).

The main cellular component of proliferative, non-necrotic lesions in human ASC is the muscle cell (Geer et al., 1961; Haust et al., 1962; Scott et al., 1966).

The change contains preserved and damaged muscle cells and round, lipid-containing cells are probably macrophages (Plate LXII/30). Pre-senile vaso-motoric disturbances may play an important role in the pathogenesis of chronic hypertensive arterial lesions (Baráth, 1953).

The structurally preserved, non-dystrophic endothelium and the smooth muscle cell elements show signs of hyperactivity already in a very early phase of the change (Plates XL/178, 179; XLIII/190; XLIV/194, 198).

The rat is not a suitable model of benign hypertensive changes, because it is as a rule irresponsive to this condition, in contrast to its extreme sensitivity to malignant hypertension. Rats showed no vascular change after a prolonged, 2-year benign hypertension (Zollinger, 1959). Thus the well-known infiltrative, degenerative arterial lesions can rarely be induced in rats. Vascular sensitivity to malignant hypertension is a specific property of rats: periarterial granulation appears after 2–3 days of the condition, while in man it develops only after a very severe change (Okamoto, 1969).

However, benign hypertensive changes can readily be reproduced in rats if experimental renal hypertension is ameliorated by drug treatment (see Chapter 8). The early change is the subendothelial accumulation of a fibrillar substance of plasma density; this persists during the advanced stage, here and there forming basement membrane-like structures (Plates XXXIX/173; XL/176). Cells may also appear in the subendothelial space during the chronic stage (Hess and Stäubli, 1963a). Fawcett and Wittenberg (1962) report that the interendothelial junctions remain intact, whereas we observed that they became stretched (Plates XXXIX/ 172, 173; XL/177).

Arterial IP develops also in animals maintained on an atherogenic diet (Hoff and Gottlob, 1969). Intracellular lipids appearing in the lesion are more electron dense but less saturated than the lipid components of the diet, indicating a partial lipid modifying activity of the endothelium during the chronic stage of the change.

In essential hypertension of man and in experimental renal hypertension of rats, lipofuscin accumulates in the medial muscle cells of the renal arteries as well as in the intercellular spaces of the media and intima, and the muscle cells show membranaceous vesicular structures (Sinapius and Gunkel, 1964; Biava and Brynjolfsson, 1967; Weller et al., 1968). The latter phenomenon may be explained by microclasmatosis resulting from an increased membrane activity of smooth muscle cells and an *in toto* cell disruption (Plate XLIII/191).

Similar chronic vascular changes, involving smooth muscle celldisruption, deterioration of IEL, evolution of IP and elastic fibre formation have often been observed in the post-partum state of uterine arteries (Maner, 1959; Szinay and Jellinek, 1951) or in pulmonary arteries during mitral stenosis. Human essential pulmonary hypertension is accompanied by IP, obliteration of the muscular arteries, and slight, secondary inflammatory phenomena (Nagy and Gál, 1960).

Interstitial oedema, increase of ground substance, and proliferation of incompletely differentiated muscle cells were observed in infantile aortic coarctation. Like the activated smooth muscle cells of the hypertensive vascular wall, the muscle cells possessed a well-developed endoplasmic reticulum and many ribosomes (Balis et al., 1967). Increased synthesis of AMP and intimal thickening may appear in man as a senile change as early as at 30 years of age. Along with an extracellular fat deposition the latter probably participates in hypoxic vascular damage (Gerő et al., 1962; Papacharalampous, 1964).

The fibrinolytic activity of the vascular wall tends to decrease with age and this plays a decisive role in the reparation of vascular changes involving fibrin deposition.

Dystrophic processes involving lipid deposition may appear in the IP (Whereat, 1961) after the vessel wall has attained a critical thickness sufficient to impair oxygenation by diffusion (Kirck and Laursen, 1955a). The main characteristic of such lesions is the occurrence of unsaturated lipids in endothelial cells, intima and smooth muscle cells (Laperrouza, 1962; Martinez, 1964; Sinapius, 1964; Sinapius and Gunkel, 1964; Fuchs and Scharnweber, 1968), accompanied by the appearance of rare smooth muscle cell forms, nuclear pycnosis, and cytolysis in the media and a focal accumulation of cell debris rich in lipids.

In addition to cell debris, containing lamellar phospholipids (structural lipids), an AMP-containing delicate reticular substance (Plate XLIII/190) (Haust and More, 1967) also accumulates in the extracellular space. We regard this stage of the change as equivalent to the necrotic proliferative phase of the arteriosclerotic lesion, because each cell change observed in the former is present in the latter (Scott et al., 1967b; Florentin and Nam, 1968; Daoud et al., 1968; Imai and Thomas, 1968) and even the cell debris appears to be of the same nature as the cell necrosis products which form the bulk of the atheromatous plaque (Florentin and Nam, 1968). The damage is rendered more severe by the biphasic vascular reaction that follows hypoxia (Griesemer and Coret, 1960; Coret and Hughes, 1964). Rats with renal hypertension develop very severe changes when rendered anaemic by bleeding.

Certain authors think that medial damage is the primary change and the evolution of an IP is secondary (DeFaria, 1965b). In fact, in drug-suppressed rat renal hypertension viable muscle cells often showed herniation without simultaneous damage of the endothelium (Plates XXXIX/175; XL/178; XLII/189).

Dogs with an experimental pulmonary hypertension developed focal hyperplastic obliterative lesions in small arteries 50–200 μ in diameter (Esterly et al., 1968), and studies of the morphogenesis revealed a widening of the subendothelial space and a hyperactivity of intramural cellular elements. Prior to the proliferative phase, the pinocytotic vesicles of the endothelium increased and the cells extended villous processes towards the surface. The evolving IP arose from migrating smooth muscle cells of the media. Some endothelial cells covering the focal thickenings of the intima appeared degenerated, resembling the cell forms seen in arteriosclerotic proliferative changes of the miniature pig (Daoud et al., 1968). The basement membrane of the smooth muscle cells was fragmented; we observed a similar phenomenon around prenecrotic smooth muscle cells in hypoxic experiments.

The focal nature of the changes is probably explicable by circumscribed vasospasm resulting from focal innervation.

The form and extent of the fibrocellular obliterative reaction of pulmonary vessels in experimental hypertension of the lesser circulation cannot be modified by suppression of fibrous tissue proliferation (by combined treatment with heparin and corticosteroid), nor by fibrinolytic treatment. Increased blood flow in itself does not initiate IP, unless the blood pressure rises (Könn and Berg, 1965); the degree of vascular damage is parallel to the extent and duration of hypertension. Thus the hypertensive vascular lesion is a multifactorial change and, apart from the direct mechanical action of hypertension, the alteration of serum electrolytes (Szabó, 1962) and of innervation may play a substantial part in its establishment.

Hormone-induced experimental hypertension is as a rule benign (O'Steen et al., 1967). Administration of ACTH to rats for three months resulted in changes which served as a model of sclerotic lesions in human muscular-type arteries; they were characterized by an interlamellar oedema, elastolysis, muscle cell deterioration and chalk deposition (Buck, 1963). The oestrogens influence transudation through the vessel wall. Increase of the ground substance protects the vessel from spontaneous sclerosis (Dalldorf, 1963; Gostimirovich, 1968). Hypophysectomy effects a thickening of the IEL in the coronary arteries, and concomitant hypothyroidism predisposes to chronic vascular damage through elevation of the serum cholesterol level (Patek et al., 1963a; Hess and Stäubli, 1963a). Rats develop hypertensive vascular changes on administration of methyl-testosterone (Molteni et al., 1967).

Chronic congenital benign hypertension also alters the sodium, potassium and water content of the vessel wall (Phelan and Wong, 1968). The pituitary gland and the adrenal cortex influence mesenchymal functions through their hormonal activity (Bretán et al., 1954). Fluctuations of the blood glucose level may also result in the evolution of proliferative lesions (Magyar et al., 1954). Anti-insulin hormones (adrenalin, cortical hormones, diabetic pituitary hormones) probably bear a certain responsibility for vascular changes (Olsen, 1969b).

Vascular changes developing in chronic renal hypertension correlate well with the impairment of the juxtaglomerular cells in the essential hypertension of humans (Endes, 1963; Fischer et al., 1966).

Overdosage of vitamins A and D induces in the arterial media a calcifying chronic lesion, resembling the Mönckeberg sclerosis in man (Stearner and Sanderson, 1969; Selye, 1970). The chronic, proliferative, sclerotic vascular lesions show an increase in activity of both acid and alkaline phosphatase and of ATPase as well.

HYALINE VASCULAR CHANGES IN CHRONIC BENIGN HYPERTENSION

Since intramural plasma diffusion is less in benign than in malignant hypertension, no hyaline changes develop in large vessels in the former condition. The focal hyalinization occasionally present does not notably differ from similar changes taking place in the reparative phase of chronic lesions (Plate XLIII/193). This indicates that although the ground substance synthesized by endothelial and muscle cell elements indeed contributes to the lesion, the major part of the hyaline change arises from the intramurally deposited plasma, above all, from its fibrin content. Fresh recurrent diffusion of fibrinous material through the damaged endothelial cell row in each subsequent hypertensive crisis has been demonstrated in 75 per cent of human vascular wall lesions (Haust and More, 1963).

HYPOXIC VASCULAR CHANGES

Hypoxia has been shown to play a decisive role in certain cases of chronic vascular change and ASC (DeFaria, 1961; Kjeldsen et al., 1968; Kjeldsen, 1969; Terry et al., 1970). In such lesions, intramural lipid deposition originates partly from a disturbance of lipid metabolism and cell disruption (Müller and Neumann, 1959; Dixon, 1961), partly from an increased endothelial permeability (Kjeldsen et al., 1968). Since, regardless of its direct cause, chronic hypoxia is always associated with pulmonary hypertension, chronic lesions can be easily studied in the branches of the pulmonary artery (Hasleton et al., 1968). As hypoxia only infrequently causes a blood pressure rise in the greater circulation (Daugherty et al., 1967), this is the ideal site for the study of 'pure' hypoxic changes (Kerényi and Jellinek 1970).

Hypobaric hypoxia was induced in rats by keeping them under continuous negative pressure. After an initial adaptation period, atmospheric pressure was constantly maintained at a level of 300–260 mm Hg. The blood oxygen saturation of the animals was 40–60 per cent after 5 days. Red blood cell counts rose above 10 million. The vascular changes evolving in the course of hypoxia corresponded essentially to those taking place during a lasting benign hypertension. In addition to hypertrophy and parallel arrangement of the rough endoplasmic reticulum, residual bodies containing a considerable amount of unsaturated lipids appeared already early in the endothelial cells (Plate XLIV/195, 197, 198). The subendothelial space contained either a disorganized floccular material of plasma density, or a loose, parallel-arranged substance of basement membrane density (Plate XLIV/196). The muscle cells of the media showed initially a hyperplasia of the smooth and rough endoplasmic reticulum and an increase of the mitochondria (Plate XLV/199, 200). The activity increase of the muscle cells resulted in an increased basement membrane synthesis. Later the cells extended more and more cytoplasmic processes and osmiophilic prenecrotic forms and single cell necroses appeared (Plate LXII/25, 27). Lipofuscin-like granules were seen in the preserved hypertrophic smooth muscle cells (Laperrousa, 1962).

The high serum sodium level arising in consequence of a reduced sodium elimination probably acted as a sensitizing factor in the development of hypoxic vascular wall changes (Földi et al., 1954).

In summary, in chronic benign hypertension the endothelial cells show a variable electron density and considerable overlap. A floccular substance accumulates below the endothelium, and leukocytes may migrate into the subendothelial space. Nevertheless, smooth muscle cells arriving from the media play the decisive role in the evolution of the later IP. Lipofuscin-like inclusions appear in the smooth muscle cells, necrosis and oedema develop in the interstitial space, and cell debris and basement membrane increase. The endothelial and smooth muscle cells which have not been affected by dystrophy, show signs of hyperfunction and proliferation. The lesion most closely resembles the pre-proliferation and proliferative phases of ASC and degenerative absorptive and compensatory phenomena can be simultaneously observed in it. Animals affected by hypoxia develop similar vascular changes, it is, therefore, supposed that hypoxic-vascular damage may act as an important factor in the development of chronic hypertensive vascular lesions. The latter again are identical with the changes elicited by

7*

several other chronic vascular injuries. In chronic benign hypertension, vascular wall hyalinization develops less frequently than fibrinoid transformation of the intramural fibrin deposition.

CHRONIC TRANSFORMATION OF VASCULAR LESIONS INDUCED BY PAINTING WITH ACID, NORADRENALIN ADMINISTRATION OR SENSITIZATION WITH HORSE SERUM

The preceding chapters have dealt with the details of the acute and chronic stages of hypertensive vascular changes; this section is devoted to the further development of the chronic transformation of lesions induced in the other three experimental models. This seems important, because induction of vascular changes by painting with acid has not yet been reported in the literature, neither have the changes induced by noradrenalin or sensitization been followed morphologically beyond the granulation stage. Since in all the three models, transition to the chronic stage and the final morphological structure of the lesion were in every respect similar to those observed in chronic hypertension, only a brief description is presented to illustrate the analogies.

In chronic hypertensive lesions, the two types of fibrinoid change (subendothelial and media fibrinoid) had a decisive influence on the further development of vascular wall structure. Chronic changes resulted either in myo-elastofibrosis, or hyalinization of the vessel wall. The question was justly posed, whether the essential identity of acute vascular changes in hypertension and in the three other experimental models (painting with acid, noradrenalin administration, sensitization with horse serum) would persist during the chronic stage and what role the lipids might play in small vessel lesions.

No sharp distinction has as yet been made between 'fibrin' and 'hyaline' in the literature and a confusion in nomenclature still exists in this respect. A reasonable basis for differentiation is offered by the difference in staining affinity: the fibrinoid stains red with azan and black with M-stain, while the hyaline change assumes a blue and a yellow colour, respectively, with the same staining techniques. But staining affinity depends largely on the age of the lesion: the more recent the change, the more closely it resembles a fibrinoid, and the older, the more it assumes a hyaline character. Bell (1946) suggests that the onset of hypertension and the appearance of the acute and the hyaline change are interrelated. Fahr (1925, 1934) interpreted the hyaline transformation as the result of a benign lesion, and perivascular granulation as that of a malignant, more severe change. Dustin (1962) offers a similar explanation for hyalinosis and for acute vascular change.

The above considerations apply to the same extent to the chronic stages of the lesions induced in the three experimental models as they apply to the chronic hypertensive change. If, for example, painting with acid produced a milder damage owing to high dilution of the acid or a relatively distant location of the vessel from the painting site, the chronic lesion was proliferative; and if the damage was severe, a hyaline transformation occurred. Similar observations have been made after noradrenalin administration. Since the degree and effect of sensitization are undefinable, comparison was based on differences in the extent of tissue change.

Chronic transformation of lesions induced in small arteries by painting with acid depends on the severity of the damage. Vessels distant from the site of damage or treated with highly diluted acid show a uniform multilayered cell proliferation and a marked constriction of the lumen. The changed wall of the small artery consists of 4, 5 or 6 rows of cells (Plate LXV/115). Again, with milder damage, the deteriorated vascular wall portion undergoes a collagenous transformation (hyalinosis) and stains homogeneously blue with azan (Plate LXV/116). As in the hypertensive change, segmental necrosis of the media results in the development of a segmental IP, and complete vascular wall deterioration results in the formation of a complete one (Plate LXV/117, 118). The cellular components of the IP behave in every respect like smooth muscle cells, both in various staining reactions and on polarization optical examination after anilin reaction. Staining with resorcine-fuchsin often reveals the presence of a delicate meshwork of elastic fibres between the cells (Plate LXV/119), and sometimes even a newly formed IEL is seen. These phenomena closely resemble the picture of lamellar elastosis, described previously in connection with hypertension. A similar kind of proliferation takes place in uterine vessels, but there are thicker PAS-positive elastic fibres and clumps (Plate LXV/120), like those seen in human lesions (see Chapter 11). Proliferations of this kind show an increase of the AMPs, above all in the initial stage, when examined with Ritter–Oleson's staining technique. Later, the smooth muscle cell components of the proliferation diminish and collagenous fibres tend to increase.

In certain cases the fibrinoid necrosis persists in the new proliferation, while the adventitia already shows a thick, scar-tissue-like hyalinization (Plate LXV/121). This is analogous to the process of recurrent hypertension.

Reparation phenomena subsequent to the acute noradrenalin-induced change follow roughly the same course. In certain cases the homogeneous vascular wall undergoes a hyaline transformation (Plate LXV/121) and a marked fibrosis takes place in its surroundings. Segmental necroses, probably also slight injuries and plasma diffusion are followed by the evolution of an IP which proceeds toward the lumen and causes its constriction (Plate LXVI/123). The cellular and elastic fibre components of the IP are exactly the same as those observed in lesions resulting from other causes.

The reparative processes following the acute stage of vascular damage by sensitization are in every respect similar to the regeneration phenomena observed in the other lesions. However, the periadventitial granulation is accompanied by an extensive peri-adventitial cicatrization (Plate LXVI/124) and the reparation tendency is slighter. An IP develops, but the cellular components soon diminish and the dominant vascular wall change is cicatrization. It appears that sensitization causes more extensive damage than noradrenalin or painting with acid, and the inflammatory reaction involves a larger area, so that the nutritional condition and regenerative capacity of the vascular wall become seriously impaired.

*

It follows from the above observations that the reparative phenomena which succeed acute vascular lesions depend on the degree of damage and on vascular wall structure. Small vessels not possessing an IEL, or vessels in which an extreme intramural plasma diffusion takes place, are liable to hyalinization. If, on the other hand, the damage is slight, or the subendothelial fibrinoid becomes phago-cytosed, there develops an IP, composed of proliferating muscle cells, of elastic fibres synthesized by these cells, and later, when the cellular components diminish, of an increasing number of collagenous fibres.

Since vascular damage inflicted under four different conditions of experiment resulted in similar chronic changes, it may well be imagined that arteriosclerotic lesions represent the final stage of multifactorial changes not only in the large vessels, but also in the small ones.

CHAPTER 8

INFLUENCE OF DRUG THERAPY ON SMALL VESSEL CHANGES IN EXPERIMENTAL HYPERTENSION. PROBLEMS OF HEALING AND REVERSIBILITY

The decisive factor in hypertensive vascular changes is high blood pressure. This statement has been confirmed by investigations into the reversibility and healing of such lesions and into the action of hypotensive drugs. The correlation between the level of blood pressure and the degree of tissue reaction is a further aspect of the problem.

Various observations suggest that acute necrotic lesions are induced by an abrupt rise (Herbertson and Kellaway, 1960; Kellaway et al., 1962) or irregular fluctuation of blood pressure (Wilson and Byrom, 1941; Friedman et al., 1941; Byrom, 1964; Kóczé et al., 1970) rather than by its high level or persistence at that level (Wilson and Byrom 1939; Goldblatt, 1957; Zollinger, 1959). Additional factors to be considered are specific and individual variations in the response of experimental animals and technical variations such as the frequency of blood pressure measurements. Accordingly, the so-called threshold value of blood pressure required to initiate the evolution of fibrinoid necrosis is a fairly relative figure. Assessment of the quantitative relations of changes is hampered by various difficulties. Also, distinction between changes related to the so-called benign and malignant forms of hypertension is still a matter of controversy (see p. 91).

Hypertensive vascular change develops through exudative (fibrinoid deposition, inflammatory reaction), necrotic and proliferative processes. The latter take place in the intima, media and adventitia and become predominant under the influence of drugs.

Intima. The hypertensive IP of the muscular arteries is either a primary change, and as such can be regarded as a regenerative phenomenon developing in response to various endothelial damages, or it is secondary, developing in the course of absorption processes aimed at the *phagocytic* elimination of the intramural deposition of various extravascular substances, such as fibrinoid, basement membrane fragments, etc. (Allison et al., 1967; Kojimahara, 1967; Hatt et al., 1968) (see p. 91). Increase of AMPs in the proliferation is followed by the synthesis of reticulum-, collagenous and elastic fibres (Kojimahara, 1967).

Media. In addition to muscle cell hypertrophy, which plays a decisive role in the thickening of the wall, the hypertensive change involves also a hyperplasia of the medial smooth muscle cells. Crane and Dutta (1963, 1964), and Crane and Ingle (1964) observed in DOCA-hypertension an increased incorporation of ^{3}H thymidine below the intima fibrinoid; this indicates an enhanced DNA-synthesis by the medial smooth muscle cells and endothelial cells of the area. These hypertrophic and hyperplastic changes are due either to hyperactivity or vasoconstriction, or to absorptive processes directed toward the elimination of intramural plasma substances and cell degeneration products (Hatt et al., 1968).

Adventitia. The increase of adventitial fibroblasts is probably an early secondary reactive phenomenon (Hüttner, personal communication). Fibrosis of the media and adventitia has been described in hypertensive vascular changes of rats (Huber, 1960), rabbits (Campbell and Santos-Buch, 1959) and dogs (Muirhead et al., 1951a) as a reparative phenomenon.

Vascular response to benign and malignant hypertension differs only in the degree of permeability disturbance; this is slight in the benign lesions which are predominantly hyperplastic, and more distinct in malignant lesions in which intramural plasma diffusion and degenerative phenomena are prevalent, but also proliferative processes occur (Hatt et al., 1968). The latter require a certain time to develop: in experimental rabbit hypertension proliferative phenomena appear after about 6 days (Allison et al., 1967).

Healing. On elimination of the constriction of the renal artery in rabbit renal hypertension, Daniel et al. (1954) observed only a slight thickening of the vessel. In a similar model, Allison et al. (1967) observed after release of the ligature a fall of blood pressure followed by the disappearance of acute lesions: the necrotic fibrinoid changes demonstrated previously by biopsy, were gradually replaced by vascular wall fibrosis and elastic elements inreased.

Reversibility. According to Pickering (1945), removal of the ischaemic kidney of rats after unilateral constriction of the renal artery for 7 weeks did not result in the normalization of blood pressure and a necrotizing arteriolitis and myoelastofibrosis developed in the contralateral preserved kidney. On removing after 5 days the rubber capsule placed on the kidneys of rats to induce experimental perinephritic hypertension, Gorácz (1963) observed a fall of blood pressure and the evolution of vascular wall fibrosis without any early change; appearance of the early changes after 7 days, nevertheless, suggested that reversibility is time-limited, and a simultaneous rise in blood pressure indicated the role of extrarenal factors (vascular lesions) in the hypertension. Fekete (1970a, b) was able to induce hypertension by unilateral ligation of the renal artery and the blood pressure did not normalize on removal of the ischaemic kidney after 20–40 days.

Hypotensive drugs. The fibrinoid necrosis developing in various forms of experimental hypertension is a suitable model for the study of hypotensive drug action. The sites of action and the pharmacological effects of the available hypotensive preparations are varied. Among others hydralazine (Apresoline) reduces the diastolic pressure and enhances renal blood flow through its central, direct renal and peripheral actions. Reserpine acts through depression of the vasomotor centre, etc. Similar effects of various substances on hypertensive vascular changes suggest that they act through a lowering of the blood pressure.

Continuous treatment of experimental animals with hydralazine during hypertension induced by partial renal infarction resulted in a considerable amelioration of the lesions as compared to controls (Masson et al., 1958, 1959). A single daily administration of the drug prevented the development of necrotic phenomena, i.e. fibrinoid necrosis, in steroid hypertension (Gardner, 1960; Takatama, 1960). Hydralazine treatment had similar results in hypertension developing after regeneration of the adrenals (Gardner and Brooks, 1962), and it prevented local permeability change in acute hypertension induced with angiotensin, methoxamine or noradrenalin (Giese, 1966).

Reserpine produced a hypotensive action also in animal experiments: it reduced the degree of renal hypertension in rats (Dutz and Voigt, 1957) and prevented the evolution of the fibrinoid necrosis (McQueen and Hodge, 1961). Administration of the sympathicolytic Bretyliumtosylate reduced the frequency of arteriosclerotic lesions (Gardner, 1962b), and the combined use of reserpine and hydralazine suppressed their evolution (Gaunt et al., 1955; Kojimahara, 1967).

Apart from the prevention of fibrinoid necrosis, hypotensive preparations may modify the tissue changes. Drug treatment after the establishment of hypertension has an effect similar to that of eliminating constriction of the renal artery, because it induces sclerotic and fibrotic changes (Masson et al., 1959). Medication with the anti-fibrinolytic compound E-aminocaproic acid during hypertension, induced by a bilateral compression of the renal arteries, effected following a fall of blood pressure the evolution of periarteritis nodosa-like changes (Ooneda et al., 1962). Animals with an established fibrinoid necrosis showed an adventitial fibrosis after treatment, owing probably to permeability-reducing action of the drugs. The author observed the development of an IP exclusively in the medicated animals. Kojimahara (1967) treated rats with a combination of Apresoline (hydralazine hydrochloride) and Serpasil (reserpine) after 4 weeks of experimental hypertension induced by constriction of the renal artery; he observed absorption of the fibrinoid, which was replaced by a fibrocellular proliferation; the elastic elements increased and fibrosis developed in the media and adventitia; in fact, Kojimahara saw the transition of the fibrinoid necrosis to an arteriosclerotic change. Non-medicated animals also showed the above phenomena, but new necrotic lesions appeared continuously in the affected vessels. Intermittent medication resulted in an aggravation of the tissue changes.

Experiments in this laboratory. Anti-hypertensive drugs with various sites of action were tested in the perinephritic hypertension model of Lőrincz and Gorácz (Lőrincz and Gorácz, 1965; Konyár and Jellinek, 1973). Sanegyt (EGYT) has an adrenergic action, Sanotensin (guanethidine sulphate) (EGYT) is a ganglion-blocking agent and the benzyl-isochinolin derivative designated BTF (Ch) is a spasmolytic. The alkaloid Vincamin (Chemical Works of Gedeon Richter Ltd.) resembles in effect the *Rauwolfia* derivatives.

A common property of the above preparations is their hypotensive action. In the experimental model used, all preparations reduced, or occasionally almost normalized, the high blood pressure of the rats and simultaneously reduced the frequency, or delayed the evolution, or slightly modified the appearance, of periarteritis nodosa-like lesions in large muscular arteries and of fibrinoid necrosis in the arterioles.

For example, treatment with 15 mg per kg Sanegyt (EGYT) for 1 or 2 weeks resulted in a less distinct development of fibrinoid necrosis or subintimal fibrinoid deposition, as compared to controls on a statistical basis (Plate LXVI/ 125).

Apart from the numerical decrease of exudative or necrotic vascular changes, the depression of hypertension was suggested by the predominance of medial muscle cell hyperplasia or hypertrophy in those arteries in which no fibrinoid necrosis developed. This phenomenon was observed with a 7.5 mg daily dose of BTF and 15 per kg daily dose of Sanotensin (guanethidine sulphate) (Plate LXVI/126, 127).

Untreated hypertensive rats showed an absorptive IP with remnants of the fibrinoid deposition (Plate LXVI/128); a few animals showed this change after 7–10 days, and almost all showed it by the 21st day. In rats treated with 20 mg per kg Vincamin, the change appeared after 10–14 days in more animals than in the control group, and fibrosis or sclerosis of the media and adventitia appeared about 7 days earlier (Plate LXVI/129).

Drug influence in experimental hypertension is essentially similar to the action of hypotensive preparations on vascular lesions in man. On chemotherapeutic depression of human malignant hypertension, Harington et al. (1959) observed a fibrosis of the arterioles and a newly formed IEL. McCormack et al. (1958) observed a subintimal fibrosis and obliteration of renal arteries, but only sporadic arteriolar and glomerular changes, 4–48 months after the hypotensive treatment of human malignant hypertension.

In summary, hypotensive drugs may reduce or even normalize the elevated blood pressure and may modify the vascular lesions depending on the degree of the fall in blood pressure, on the species and the reaction of the experimental animal and on the mode of medication.

1. If hypotensive treatment is introduced simultaneously with the induction of hypertension, the drug may prevent, depending on its potency, the development of periarteritis nodosa-like lesions and of fibrinoid necrosis, ameliorate the exudative or necrotic lesions and/or defer their evolution. Reduction of hypertension may also result in the establishment of a so-called benign hypertensive change, characterized by thickening of the vascular wall and proliferation of smooth muscle cells and fibroblasts.

2. If hypotensive treatment is applied after the malignant hypertensive lesions have become established, its effect resembles that of the release of a ligature of the renal artery or of the removal of the compressing capsule from the kidney: the lesion heals via fibrocellular-sclerotic transformation, involving all three layers of the vascular wall. Lasting hypotensive treatment may prevent the exacerbation of the fibrinoid necrosis. These experimental data have been confirmed by observations on human material.

3. The results of an intermittent hypotensive medication have been differently interpreted by the various authors; this may be explained by the non-uniformity of the experimental animals and drugs used.

CHAPTER 9

CONCLUSIONS FROM AVAILABLE EXPERIMENTAL DATA ON THE ROLE OF VASCULAR STRUCTURE IN THE MORPHOLOGY OF VASCULAR LESIONS

Examinations of the two main types of vessels have shown that elastic vessels respond to damage by muscle cell necrosis and IP, while small muscular vessels respond by the development of a fibrinoid necrosis, followed in each case by a hyaline transformation of the IP or fibrinoid. As noted above, the elastic lamellae of the vascular wall have in certain cases a decisive influence on the progress of the acute vascular wall change. Let us refer to Plates LXII/28–30; LXIII/54–57; LXIV/85, 89, 90, 96, 97 which illustrate the evolution of fibrinoid necrosis in small vessels; these clearly show the barrier behaviour of the IEL on plasma diffusion into the vessel wall. A well-developed IEL prevents plasma diffusion (Jellinek, 1970b), consequently the plasma substances become deposited in the subendothelial space. The accumulating plasma lifts the endothelial cell row, hence the name subendothelial fibrinoid. This change can be temporarily distinguished from the other form of fibrinoid change, which arises from necrotic smooth muscle cells of the media, hence the name media fibrinoid. Admixture of the two kinds of fibrinoid results in the characteristic lesion known generally as fibrinoid vascular wall necrosis. As a matter of fact, the two kinds of fibrinoid arise from entirely different components. The necrotic products of smooth muscle cells form the media fibrinoid, which later admixes with plasma to form the fibrinoid necrosis. The plasma substances which form the subendothelial fibrinoid differ in every respect from the components of the media fibrinoid.

The subendothelial fibrinoid initially consists of fluid plasma and can be regarded as a subendothelial oedema. Later, albumin, globulins and finally fibrinogen enter the vessel wall, depending on the degree of damage. The intramural diffusion of these plasma constituents has been demonstrated experimentally (More and McLean, 1949, Movat and More, 1957; Vazquez and Dixon, 1957, 1958; Movat and Fernando, 1963a). In the subendothelial fibrinoid, fibrin arises from the fibrinogen, as demonstrated by various staining techniques, polarization microscopy (Fig. 1), phase-contrast microscopy (Plate XLV/201, 202) and electron microscopy (Plates XXXV/160; XXXVI/161–164).

The two types of fibrinoid are responsible for the often dissimilar structural relations in the chronic stage of the vascular wall change. The subendothelial fibrinoid initially contains precipitated proteins in a delicate granular distribution and organized fibrin molecules; these later aggregate to form the characteristic periodic bodies appearing in the phase contrast micrograph as clumps (Plate XLV/201, 202); the clumps fuse with one another, incorporating the globular proteins and tend to lose the periodic structure (Plates XXVIII/121; XXXVI/163) until they transform to hyaline. At this stage, the periodic structure of fibrin disappears entirely and lipid-like substances are demonstrable ultrastructurally in the homogeneous hyaline tissue (Plate XLIII/188). The hyaline transformation of the subendothelial fibrinoid has been observed in both small and large, muscular- and elastic-type vessels (Plates LXII/30, 31; LXV/113, 116, 120–122).

The media fibrinoid, i.e. the necrosis of the muscle cells, initiates the regeneration of the muscle-cell layer. The dividing muscle cells migrate toward the intima of the deteriorated vascular wall portion to form the IP (Plates LXV/109, 110, 112, 114, 117, 119; LXVI/123). The IP represents a reparative process of the vascular wall, in which smooth muscle plays the main role. This reparative process takes place in both types of vessels, but it is more distinct in small vessels where the IP results in the characteristic myoelastofibrosis than in large vessels where subendothelial fibrinoid formation and hyalinization are predominant. The subendothelial fibrinoid as a foreign body may itself initiate an IP by eliciting of its phagocytosis; in fact, phagocytosis of subendothelial fibrin by the cells of the proliferation has been demonstrated ultrastructurally (Plates XLI/180; LXV/106, 107). In the advanced lesion, the phagocytic cell proliferation can no longer be differentiated from proliferating cells produced to compensate for muscle cell necrosis in the media fibrinoid.

The proliferating cells are muscle cells and they synthesize elastic fibres, in the manner described and illustrated in the preceding chapters.

The decisive role of the elastic elements is particularly conspicuous when an acute injury simultaneously affects both elastic and muscular-type vessels. Plate LXVI/130 illustrates such an instance; on painting with acid, cell deterioration has begun in the aorta, but no plasma diffusion has taken place, owing to the barrier effect of the dense fibres; in contrast, the small muscular-type vessel branching of the aorta shows on the one hand a distinct muscle cell necrosis, clearly visualized by PTA (Plate XLVI/131), and on the other, a characteristic fibrinoid necrosis (Plate LXVI/132) resulting from an intramural plasma diffusion. Obviously, the thin elastic membrane of the small muscular-type arterial branch failed to prevent the deposition of plasma in the deteriorated media. This observation stresses again the decisive importance of the elastic membrane in the development of vascular change and its influence on vascular fibrinoid formation.

Further evidence of this is that in elastic-type vessels, the necrosis of muscle cells located between the elastic fibres can be demonstrated for several days after painting with acid, by PTA staining technique (Plate LXVI/133) and polarization optical examination, but since intramural plasma diffusion is prevented by the strong IEL the typical staining reactions of the fibrinoid necrosis fail to appear.

In addition to these changes, substances carried by the diffusing plasm apparently become adsorbed onto the surface of the IEL, because this first stretches, then becomes rigid and fragmented and the discontinuities promote further plasma diffusion at a later stage (see below). The surface adsorption of plasma substance seems to be supported by the finding that in the presence of subendothelial fibrinoid the digestibility of the IEL by elastase increases as compared to the normal, i.e. the IEL becomes more resistant (Nagy et al., 1970). This may explain its greater liability to fragmentation as it has lost its elasticity (Plate LXVIII/ 152–155).

In the case of small vessels, perivascular granulation and cicatrization, which appear after a rapid vascular wall deterioration, play the same barrier role as the

IEL in large vessels. If hypertension persists, plasma will deposit above the perivascular scar tissue and give rise to a subendothelial fibrinoid-like structure (Plate LXIII/53).

Differences between the conditions of flow across the walls of small and large vessels are further explicable by dissimilarities of the endothelial lining and external coat. Examinations with ruthenium red in this laboratory have shown that the aortic coat is more resistant to hypertensive damages than the internal coat of small vessels. This can account for the observation that under identical conditions of hypertension, aortic changes appear considerably later than the small vessel changes (Plate LXII/31).

It follows that the conditions of transmural flow play a primary role in the evolution of the various vascular wall changes, and the following chapter is therefore devoted to the discussion of all factors which affect vascular wall changes, with special regard to those controlling transmural flow and permeability.

CHAPTER 10

PROBLEMS OF TRANSPORT ACROSS THE VESSEL WALL

INTRODUCTION

Increase of the permeability of vascular endothelium is a phenomenon accompanying all fundamental vascular changes. By making possible intramural plasma diffusion and deposition of plasma substances in the vessel wall, increased vascular permeability promotes the establishment of functional and lasting morphological changes. The importance of permeability conditions in vascular pathology was already pointed out by Schürmann and McMahon in 1933.

Permeability disturbance resulting from inflammation was first observed by Cohnheim (1867, 1873) more than 100 years ago and has been extensively restudied ever since, most recently by electron microscopy using tracer methodology (Majno and Palade, 1961; Movat and Fernando, 1963d).

The intramural deposition of lipid-like substances, above all of large-molecular lipoproteins, is the decisive event in the evolution of arteriosclerotic vascular lesions; after the pioneer investigations of Anitschkow (1913) and Aschoff (1924), several workers (Page, 1954; Gerő, 1962, 1969; Gofmann and Young, 1965; French, 1966; Adams, 1967; Adams et al., 1967; Virágh et al., 1968 and others) have brought forth evidence in support of the filtration hypothesis.

The role of permeability changes in hypertensive vascular lesions has been pointed out by Giese (1964), Still (1967), Still and Dennison (1969), Jellinek et al., (1967a, 1969) and Wiener et al. (1969).

Gardner (1965) described the role of increased intramural plasma diffusion in vasculitis associated with auto-immune diseases. The vascular changes contained gamma globulin (Gitlin et al., 1957) and albumin (Paronetto and Strauss, 1962).

In sum, it appears that the various vascular damages elicit changes varying with the type of vessel, type and duration of damage, but similar in their final morphology (Jellinek, 1965). A common factor in the evolution of lesions is the intramural diffusion of plasma, plasmatic vasculosis (Lendrum, 1963, 1967). Since, however, different teams of workers have dealt with a different aspect of transport across the vessel wall, the designation of these phenomena as vascular permeability easily gives rise to misunderstanding.

Intramural plasma diffusion, the transport across the vessel wall proceeds in three steps, which follow from the structure of the vessel wall:

1. Intimal structure determining the intramural diffusion of plasma substances (endothelial permeability).

2. Medial structures determining the further disposition (transmural flow) of plasma constituents which gained access to the vessel wall.

3. Adventitial structures responsible for the drainage of substances which diffuse across the vessel wall.

In this manner transport across the vessel wall is understood as a complex of the phenomena of permeation through the endothelium, transmural flow across the media and drainage through the adventitia.

1. Permeability of the vascular endothelium is understood as the transcellular and intercellular passage of substances controlled by endothelial cells, intercellular junctions and the so-called extracellular amorphous substances (external coat, basement membrane).

2. The components controlling the intramural passage of materials are constituents of the media (smooth muscle cells, collagenous and elastic elements, and the AMP matrix coating the fibres).

3. The adventitial components responsible for the drainage of materials passing across the vessel wall are the adventitial connective tissue and lymph gaps.

In addition to the morphological structure of the vessel wall, changes in the proportion and absolute amount of circulating plasma components influence the transmural transport.

Finally, pressure, flow and microcirculation factors influence the transmural passage of material (Table 1).

TABLE 1

Factors determining transport across the vessel wall

1. Structure of vessel wall
   (a) permeability of intima
       (transcellular permeability, junctions, external coat, basement membrane)
   (b) flow across the media (smooth muscle cells, collagen, elastic elements, AMP-matrix coating the fibres)
   (c) drainage through adventitia
       (adventitial connective tissue, lymph channels)
2. Alteration of proportions, or absolute amounts of plasma components
3. Pressure, flow and microcirculation factors

METHODS OF TRACING THE TRANSMURAL PASSAGE OF MATERIAL. COLLOIDAL TRACERS

Morphological and other techniques for the examination of vascular permeability and transmural flow are continually improving. Bloch (1963) has established criteria for the ideal method as follows: 'The ideal method is expected to visualize the passage of the molecule across the vessel wall, to inform simultaneously on the extent of hydrostatic and osmotic pressures and to detect the energy requirement of the transmural passage.'

Stains. As early as 1971 McGill et al. observed the subendothelial appearance of Evans blue after injury of the aortic intima. Systematic study of the passage of colloidal stains into the vessel wall was initiated by Petroff in 1922, using trypan blue or lithium-carmin solutions as tracer substances. Ten years later Duff (1932), also using trypan blue, inferred aortic endothelial or capillary permeability from the degree of staining affinity. Cohnheim (1867, 1873) had already

111

used aniline blue to examine inflammatory permeability disturbance in the previous century. Arnold was able to locate India ink in the intercellular junctions as early as in 1873. India ink—colloidal carbon—has been widely employed as a tracer substance ever since. On examining the factors responsible for the blackening of the vessel wall, Cotran and Karnovsky (1967) have pointed to the role of certain vascular and plasmatic components. India ink was used along with other dyes (Ewans, 1915; Brickner, 1927; Jancsó, 1947) to examine the RES and its relationship with the endothelium.

The application of electron-microscopic tracer substances has resulted in considerable methodological improvement. In addition to India ink, ferritin, saccharated iron oxide, colloidal gold, silver, mercury sulphide, thorotrast, polystyrene-latex, lipids, dextran, horseradish peroxidase, human myeloperoxidase or bacterial suspension have been used to detect permeability (Table 2).

TABLE 2

Common colloidal tracer substances

Tracer	Particle size (Å)	Mol. wt
India ink (colloidal carbon)	200–300	
colloidal gold	100–150	
colloidal silver	100–500	
thorium dioxide	100–250	
mercury sulphide	70–350	
saccharated iron oxide	30–100	
ferritin	100	
peroxidase	50–50	40,000
human myeloperoxidase		
		160,000–180,000
bacterial suspension		
lipid chylomicron	5,000	
lipoprotein	500	
serum protein		
albumin	50–150	69,000
haemoglobin	70	68,000
globulin	40–210	156,000
lipoprotein	50–250	200,000
lipoprotein	200–200	300,000
globulin	50–150	90,000
fibrinogen	50–600	400,000

Movat and Fernando (1963a) observed the passage of carbon particles across the vessel wall in acute inflammation. Majno and Palade (1961), by means of colloidal carbon, detected permeability disturbances induced by histamine or serotonin. Chambers and Zweifach (1947) and Stehbens and Florey (1960) studied the intravascular precipitation of intravenously administered India ink. On the basis of earlier observations and their own experience, Brånemark et al. (1968) have outlined the errors of this method. These result from the fact that carbon does not form a stable emulsion in a protein suspension. The colloidal carbon aggregates and the emboli thus formed give rise to microcirculation disorders which may result in an abnormal increase of permeability in circumscribed areas. Despite this disadvantage, the tracer substance is often helpful in detecting permeability disorders resulting from various causes in capillaries and large vessels (Giese, 1964; Cotran et al., 1967).

Ferritin and saccharated iron oxide are easily visualized by Prussian blue reaction for both light- and electron-microscopic purposes. Saccharated iron oxide (Ferrlecit) is demonstrable by this reaction also in a 1 mμ thick section after the araldite has been removed. This permits the cutting of properly oriented ultra-thin sections (Nagy, 1971). The tracer substances pass across the basement membrane more easily than the carbon particles (Cotran et al., 1967). In addition to vesicles and multivesicular dense bodies, free ferritin may appear also in the cytoplasm of endothelial cells (Florey, 1966, 1967). Saccharated iron oxide precipitates on the endothelial surface, and from there pinocytotic vesicles carry it across the endothelium (Florey, 1966). On analysing the passage of saccharated iron oxide and colloidal gold into mesothelial or endothelial cells, Staubesand (1963) found that the gold particles appeared in the form of independent dense particles, while the iron from the same gold-iron suspension precipitated to form spots of a lower density. Electron-microscopic identification of saccharated iron oxide particles may be hampered by the fact that the ribosomes are of the same size. Jellinek et al. (1969) have shown that the electrophoretic mobility of Ferrlecit corresponds to that of alpha$_1$- and alpha$_2$-globulin and prealbumin. Bálint et al. (1970) failed to demonstrate by immuno-electrophoresis the linking of the tracer substance with protein (Plate XLV/203, 204). The iron preparation proved to be more sensitive than India ink for the detection of hypertensive vascular lesions (Plate LXVII/156, 157) (Nagy et al., 1968; Jellinek et al., 1969). Peroxidase has been used for the examination of capillary permeability (Karnovsky, 1967), mesothelial permeability (Cotran et al., 1967) and alveolar capillary permeability (Schneeberger-Keeley and Karnovsky, 1968). Protein of a molecular weight of 40,000 can be easily detected by both light- and electron microscopy after an appropriate histochemical reaction. In addition to horseradish peroxidase, Graham and Karnovsky (1966) employed also human myeloperoxidase, 4–5 times higher in molecular weight than the former, for the study of glomerular permeability. According to Kluge (1969), peroxidase has no influence on permeability, while Cotran et al. (1967) demonstrated by means of colloidal carbon that intradermally, intraperitoneally or intravenously injected peroxidase causes a local permeability increase in venules and this effect can be prevented by antihistamines. Kluge and Hovig (1968) have proved the passage of peroxidase across the tight junctions.

Alksue (1959) has used mercury sulphide to detect histamine-induced permeability increase in cutaneous capillaries. He believes that this tracer substance can also pass across the normal capillary wall, but histamine enhances the transmural flow. Hampton (1958) observed that the mercury sulphide particles become coated by fibrin, thus intramural passage of the tracer substance means passage of fibrin as well. Casley-Smith (1964) combined various tracer substances (chylomicron, India ink, lipoprotein, thorium dioxide, ferritin) to examine the permeability of the lymphatic endothelium and found that larger corpuscles can also pass across it if the injury has been severe. Besides the common thorotrast and carbon techniques, Casley-Smith and Reade (1965) used a bacterial suspension——*E. coli* on account of its high lipopolysaccharide content—for membrane permeability studies on liver cells from foetal and adult rats. Suter and Majno (1965) used lipid chylomicron for vascular permeability studies in newborn rats. Grotte (1956) and Arturson and Kjellmer (1964) analysed the blood–lymph barrier and capillary permeability, respectively, by means of dextran preparations of different molecular weights; the quantity of dextran drained by the lymph was measured in both experiments. Finally, mention should be made of Ascheim's (1964) work in investigating the permeability conditions of the capillary endothelium by radioactive albumin and [86]Rb.

In summary, in addition to India ink, various stains, metal salts, and protein-, lipid- or carbohydrate-like substances have been used during the past 10 years as tracer substances to detect vascular permeability. Examinations have chiefly been performed on capillaries, and the results are often contradictory, owing partly to methodological differences, partly to an eventual modification of permeability conditions by one or another tracer substance. Thus, generalizations to other types of vessels should be drawn with proper caution and critical sense. The known tracer substances, although they have furnished valuable information, are by no means perfect indicators of vascular permeability changes.

FACTORS RESPONSIBLE FOR INTRAMURAL TRANSPORT

FACTORS CONTROLLING PERMEABILITY

TRANSCELLULAR PERMEABILITY

Transport of material across the endothelium can take place by intercellular or transcellular routes. Casley-Smith and Reade (1965) have differentiated between three forms of transcellular transport, taking place through pores (*i*), organelles (*ii*) or by direct penetration (*iii*) through the cell membrane. Gárdos (1968) defines the forms of transport across the cell membrane as follows: simple or thermic diffusion, activated diffusion, penetration by means of carriers, and endocytosis. Arterial or venous endothelial cells possess no pores (Reale and Ruska, 1965), thus transport through them takes place either by direct transcellular penetration or by means of cell organelles. Direct penetration plays a role in ion or water transport, and only a severe impairment of this mechanism by osmotic changes, pH changes or other injury can be demonstrated morphologically as cellular or intracellular oedema, reduction of cellular enzymatic activity, or cell death (Constantinides and Robinson, 1969*a*, *b*, *c*).

Casley-Smith and Reade (1965) detected in the free cytoplasm a large amount of ferritin and smaller amount of thorium dioxide, which according to these authors were not artefacts. The amount of these substances increased considerably the disruption of the cytoplasmic membrane. Such swollen pale cells were permeable to particles of India ink which could not normally enter the cytoplasm. The most easily definable form of transcellular transport is that furnished by the endothelial pinocytotic vesicles. Such vesicles, 50–75 μ in diameter, frequently fuse with the cell membrane and later with the membranes of the cytoplasmic vesicles. Pinocytotic vesicles were first observed by Palade (1953) and their numbers and location indicate the pre-fixation state. Their functions are nutrient uptake micropinocytosis, material transport, cytopempsis (Moore and Ruska, 1957), uptake of macromolecules, phagocytosis, release of material from the cell (reverse micropinocytosis). Bennett (1969) has proposed the terms 'encystosis' and 'excystosis' to indicate the trend of material transport. Florey (1966) regarded the pinocytotic vesicles as surface-increasing factors and attributed an important role to caveoles and intracellular vesicles in transport to and from the lumen. Casley-Smith and Reade (1965) distinguished between large and small vesicles and thought that only small vesicles play a role in transport. Alksue (1959) characterized the vesicles and caveoles as manifestations of active material transport. Jennings et al. (1962) introduced salt solution and tracer substances (thorium oxide, saccharated iron oxide, ferritin) into isolated heart preparations to study their transport across the vessel wall. The first two tracers appeared chiefly within endothelial vesicles, while ferritin occurred also freely in the cytoplasm. Passage across junctions played a rather secondary part under these conditions of experiment. Two forms of vesicular transport were observed, one effected by a single vesicle and another taking place by the coalescence of vesicles (membrane flow) (Bennett, 1956). Shea et al. (1969) analysed the transport function of pinocytotic vesicles by mathematical-statistical methods.

Occasionally cytoplasmic processes extending from the endothelial surface towards the lumen have been observed. They probably play the same role as the undulating membranes in plasma intake. Cytoplasmic invaginations occur less often, the larger the vessel (Reale and Ruska, 1965); according to Florey (1966), they appear when large molecules have to be taken up, but their exact function is essentially unknown.

ENZYMATIC PHENOMENA ACCOMPANYING ENDOTHELIAL PERMEABILITY

Transport of sodium from the cytoplasm to the extracellular space takes place against an electrochemical gradient. It is an energy-requiring process and energy is derived from ATP. The circumstance that active ion transport across the cell membrane requires ATP, while the membrane itself contains ATPase has suggested a relationship between the two processes. Schatzmann (1962) has postulated that the lipoprotein structure is responsible, on the one hand, for the stabilization of the protein chain, on the other for a reinforcement of the fixation of ATP to the active centre of the enzyme. The importance of K^+–Na^+ activated ATPase in active material transport is supported primarily by biochemical evidence. The morphological evidence is equivocal, primarily for methodological reasons. Presence of ATPase activity in the surroundings of pinocytotic vesicles has, however, been unequivocally shown (Wallace and Campbell, 1968). Shakhlamov (1969) observed a greater ATPase activity in micropinocytotic vesicles 350–500 Å in diameter, as compared to those 700–1500 Å in diameter, and concluded that the small vesicles are actively involved in material transport. In addition to other oxidative enzymes, ATPase also decreases under conditions of hypoxia (Adams, 1967). The pinocytotic activity of vessels and smooth muscle fibres is accompanied by an ATPase activity (Hoff and Graf, 1966.) Hoff (1968) located ATPase in the vesicles during the energy-dependent transport process in endothelial and smooth muscle cells. Günn et al. (1968) investigated the role of ATPase in the maintenance of cellular homeostasis.

INTERCELLULAR (GAP-JUNCTION) TRANSPORT

Capillary interendothelial juctions open easily depending on functional requirement, thus permitting the extravasation of serum and corpuscular blood elements (Suter and Majno 1965; Karnovsky, 1967). Coupling structures of various types have been observed in the interendothelial junctions (Virágh, 1968). Patent junctions are normally rare. Saccharated iron cannot penetrate beyond the tight junctions (Florey, 1966). Patent junctions increase in number after an endothelial injury (Casley-Smith and Reade, 1965). In analysing vascular changes associated with experimental pancreatitis, Nagy et al. (1970) demonstrated in muscular-type small arteries (Plate LXVI/134) the formation of gaps, filled by the applied colloidal tracer substance (Plates XLVI/205; XLVII/206). Suter and Majno (1965) showed electron microscopically that the intercellular gaps of the vascular endothelium are wider in young than in adult rats, permitting the penetration of chylomicrons. Others (Palade, 1961; Bruns, 1963) also failed to detect tracer substance in intact junctions, but horseradish peroxidase, the relatively low-molecular weight protein introduced by Karnovsky, is able to pass across intact junctions.

Intercellular transport of material takes place through patent junctions or intercellular gaps. A considerable amount of protein diffuses through the inter-endothelial gaps, to judge from detections by tracer substances (French, 1966). In capillaries of the corpus luteum, the rapid transmural passage of ferritin and carbon indicates a considerable protein transudation (Morris and Sass, 1966). Passage of carbon particles across intercellular gaps has also been demonstrated in vessel buds formed during wound healing (Schoefl, 1963), which are known to be highly permeable to proteins. Under pathologically altered conditions, intercellular gap formation takes place in the normally continuous endothelium, accompanied by a local increase of intramural protein flow. These changes appear most characteristically in inflammatory flow disturbances. Majno and Palade (1961) observed that histamine and 5-hydroxytryptamine cause separation of the venous endothelium thereby permitting the intramural passage of certain large-molecular tracer substances (mercury sulphide, carbon or chylomicron). Marchesi (1962), Ham and Hurley (1965) and Cotran (1965) made similar observations in inflammatory disturbance of permeability induced by various substances. Hurley and Ryan (1967) used colloidal iron to detect the permeability-increasing effect of histamine, turpentine and rabbit serum on diaphragmatic vessels of the rat. Movat and Fernando (1963) consider that gap formation is still poorly understood, while Majno and Palade (1961) attribute it to the distension of the junctions. Florey (1964) observed intercellular gaps in renal glomeruli and demonstrated the passage of ferritin through them.

EXTRACELLULAR AMORPHOUS SUBSTANCES.
EXTERNAL COAT, BASEMENT MEMBRANE

The basement membrane, external coat and matrix of the supporting tissues form the three groups of extracellular amorphous substances (Oláh, 1968). These are of a mucopolysaccharide nature and play an important role in the regulation of transport across the vessel wall.

Voltera (1925) was the first to attract attention to the non-cellular, argentophilic, amorphous pericapillary structures responsible for the control of vascular permeability. Later, Chambers and Zweifach (1940) pointed to a similar role of the intercellular cement synthesized by endothelial cells. Florey et al. (1959) studied the intercellular cement electron microscopically and observed deposition of silver in the junctions and to cell surfaces after fixation in osmium tetroxide and treatment with silver nitrate.

EXTERNAL COAT

The external polysaccharide coat of the cells, or glycocalix as Bennett (1963) called it, has the function of filtration.

Brandt and Pappas (1960) observed in experiments on amoebas that the filamentous substrate of the external coat bound thorotrast particles or ferritin molecules and pinocytosis followed. The best known and most important property of the external coat is the binding or large molecular-weight substances, followed by the invagination and pinching-off of the membrane (Marshall and Tachmias, 1965).

Investigations by Pease (1966) have suggested that the external coat not only participates in the transport of large molecular-weight substances, but also stores water by virtue of its water-binding capacity. The latter property permits the acceleration of the diffusion of ions and small molecules. A morphologically easily definable glycocalix has been observed on the luminal surface in several invertebrates, among others in *Lumbricus terrestris* (Hama, 1960).

BASEMENT MEMBRANE

The larger arteries of invertebrates possess only traces of a subendothelial basement membrane, if any (see Chapter 1). Smaller arteries, however, always possess one, the smaller their calibre, the more so. At a given vascular size, the absence of subendothelial basement membrane facilitates the nutrition of the internal third of the vessel wall (Reale and Ruska, 1965). The basement membrane appears homogeneous in non-counterstained preparations, but counterstaining reveals that it contains randomly oriented filaments, $3-4 \mu$ in diameter. The filter property of the basement membrane in capillaries and venules has been confirmed experimentally in several instances, and Farquhar and Palade (1960) showed the same for the glomerular basement membrane, using ferritin as tracer substance.

The fundamental investigations of Pappenheimer (1953) have shown that ions, molecules and macromolecules can pass across the capillary wall. He observed

117

that the capillaries possess perforated cylindriform pores, 60–90 Å in diameter and pore distribution is 1/5–10 × 10 Å of capillary surface. Nothwithstanding this pore size, several workers, among them Grotte (1956) and Shirley et al. (1957), demonstrated the passage of substances of more than 400,000 molecular weight through the pores. Bennett (1963) correlated these data with the structural properties of the basement membrane and concluded that the capillary acts as an osmotically active filter, regulating transmural passage according to molecular size; it prevents the rapid penetration of large molecules, but permits slow passage. Owing to its uniform structure, the basement membrane is overall permeable to such particles or molecules. The expandable pores observed by Shirley et al. (1957) correspond essentially to the filtration canals of the basement membrane; according to Bennett (1963), the latter is permeable to small molecules, but it retards intramural protein diffusion. No transversal chains connect the filaments, thus these distend easily. The permeability of the basement membrane depends on the pore diameter of the meshwork and on the amorphous substances inside the pores. Mathematically, the pore size is about 29 ± 10 Å, thus substances of 80,000–90,000 molecular weight would represent the upper limit of the filtrable molecular size range. Gekle et al. (1966) demonstrated by means of ^{14}C inulin, polyvinylpyrrolidone and ^{131}I that the distribution coefficient of molecules in the basement membrane is inversely related to the molecular weight, i.e. the lower the molecular weight, the greater will be the molecule's capacity to penetrate the basement membrane. Apart from molecular size and pore diameter, the penetration capacity of the molecules depends on their solubility in lipids. The distribution coefficient of molecules in the basement membrane is much higher for lipid-soluble substances than for those not soluble in lipid.

GROUND SUBSTANCE

The third extracellular amorphous substance is the connective tissue ground substance. This will be discussed in the following section on factors controlling transmural flow.

COMPONENTS CONTROLLING TRANSMURAL FLOW

GROUND SUBSTANCE

Changes of vascular AMPs have mostly been dealt with in reports and monographs on ASC (Gerő, 1962, 1969; Gerő et al. 1961a, b, 1962; Gerő and Székely 1968). This section is a summary of some data on the transmural flow-controlling function of AMPs. While in capillaries, small arteries and venules either the basement membrane or the external coat plays the leading role in the control of transmural flow, in larger vessels the connective tissue AMPs also participate in this function. The presence of chondroitin sulphates A, B, C, hyaluronic acid, heparin, heparitin sulphate and of less well-defined neutral AMPs has been demonstrated in the aortic wall (Zugibe, 1963). The composition of AMPs changes with the type of the vessel and with aging as well (Table 3).

118

TABLE 3

AMP contents in the various types of vessels
(after Zugibe, 1963)

Hyaluronic acid	various amounts in aorta and coronary arteries
Chondroitin sulphates A, C	free or bound to collagen, diminishes with age
Chondroitin sulphate B	part bound to elastic elements, part gradually links with collagen; increases with age
Heparin, heparitin sulphate	spot-like distribution in intimal area

The interrelationships between water, AMPs and collagenous and elastic elements are important from a functional point of view; they determine permeability among other things. The relationship between water and AMP is indicated by a sedimentation coefficient. The viscosity of the filtering solution depends on that of the material responsible for this property (Fessler, 1960). Hyaluronic acid is highly polymerized and its molecular weight is usually of the order of a million. It is postulated that at a physiologic concentration of hyaluronic acid (1 per cent), the polysaccharide molecules form a three-dimensional structure with water. The sulphated polysaccharides of the ground substance have a lower molecular weight, but the protein bonds they form are similar in molecular weight to hyaluronic acid. It follows that these also form a three-dimensional structure. Such structures become stabilized by fibrin and inhibit the penetration of water to a considerable extent and influence or control the diffusion of various colloidal macromolecules (Laurent, 1966). Laurent and Persson (1964) verified the filter effect of the ground substance by examining the sedimentation rate of alpha-crystalloid and human serum albumin in the presence of various polymers (dextran, ficol, dextran sulphate, methylcellulose, etc.). The sedimentation rate of the larger molecules tended to decrease steadily. The inhibitory effect of the polymer is greater, the higher its degree of polymerization and the fewer side chains it possesses. Polymers with an electric charge have a greater retarding capacity than neutral ones. Day (1952) also recognized the decisive role of hyaluronic acid in permeability. Ogston and Sherman (1961) examined the diffusion of various substances through a filter in the presence or absence of hyaluronic acid and found that it reduced markedly the diffusion of glucose, polyglucose and serum albumin (fibres 8 Å in diameter). The reduction was proportional to the amount of hyaluronic acid present and to the size of the diffusing molecules. Collagenous gel had scarcely any effect on diffusion (fibre 500,000 Å in diameter). Probably a permeability change of ground substance AMPs was responsible for the intramural diffusion. This phenomenon became more pronounced during aging or under pathologically altered conditions (Schallock, 1962). Addition of hyaluronidase, which acted on hyaluronic acid as well as on chondroitin sulphates A and C, increases arterial permeability, as judged from observations on rabbits fed cholesterols (Seifert et al., 1953). Böttcher (1964) believed that a de-polymerization of the AMP results in an increase of vascular wall permeability. Sobel (1968) concluded from studies of vessel-wall diffusibility that this alters with aging, resulting in a change of small ion molecule and oxygen transport. According to Friedman and Byers (1962), the newly formed capillary endothelium contains a greater amount of lipids or lipoproteins than the old one. Evans blue or trypan blue more readily permeate the aorta of young than of old rabbits.

Dees (1923) concluded from experimental observations that the IEL itself is impermeable and only the fenestrae allow passage of material. According to Lendrum (1963, 1967), the plasma proteins may obstruct the fenestrae of the arterial elastic fibres, thus retarding lipid or lipoprotein in the vessel wall. The intramural diffusion of cholesterol is also filtered, or retarded, by the aortic elastic fibres, thus labelled cholesterol aggregates at the inner side of the latter (Adams and Moym, 1966). Williams (1956) observed that in human lesions, the diffusion of lipoprotein and cholesterol is markedly inhibited by the fibre components, but very little by medial smooth muscle cells. Jellinek et al. (1964, 1969) and Jellinek (1970c) found that the IEL acts as a barrier to intramural diffusion during the development of the vascular fibrinoid in hypertensive changes, and that the intramural transport of plasma or tracer substances can take place exclusively through the fenestrae (Plate LXVII/150, 151). Fuchs and Claus (1967) observed that the fenestrae of the IEL undergo a constriction or diminution during aging and inferred that this change may play a role in senile vascular lesions. On investigating hypertensive lesions by means of colloidal carbon or labelled gamma-globulin techniques, Olsen (1969a, b) found that the IEL inhibits penetration; in vessels with a stretched IEL intramural diffusion of plasma or tracer substance was detected exclusively at those sites at which the IEL was discontinuous. Gaps in the elastic membrane permit the diffusion of plasma proteins from intima to media (Ooneda et al., 1965; Kojimahara, 1967). Jellinek (1967) explains the impairment of the IEL by transport disturbances as follows: 'Disorders of plasma transport, resulting in a local deposition of plasma constituents, may promote the ASC-enhancing action of elastase described by Baló and Banga (1949a).' Olsen (1969a, b, c) has expressed a similar view, suggesting that plasma enzyme (elastase) activity may be regarded as an additional factor responsible for the damage of the IEL. Nagy et al. (unpublished observations) have, however, found that the stretched IEL is more resistant to elastase than the unstretched IEL (Plate LXVII/152–155).

In this laboratory, rats were rendered hypertensive by the method of Lőrincz and Gorácz, and after 7 days paraffin-embedded sections were secured from their small mesenteric and subserosa arteries and resistance of normal and stretched IEL by exposure to elastase was examined for various periods. The stretched IEL, covered by a subintimal fibrinoid deposition resisted the digestive action of the enzyme; apparently, the plasma proteins depositing on the surface of the IEL modify not only its shape, but also its structure in such a manner that it becomes inacces sible to enzymatic effect.

SMOOTH MUSCLE CELLS

The function of these cells has been analysed in detail in other parts of this monograph; the subject of this section is their role in mural transport. According to Rhodin (1962) plasma constituents have a fairly direct access to smooth muscle cells through the myoendothelial junctions. Local metabolites, hydrogen ions, osmotically active substances, biogenic amines and peptides may also act on muscle cells through these junctions. The many vesicles lying immediately subjacent to the cytoplasmic membrane increase the cell surface by about 25 per cent through their contact with the latter and/or with membranes of other vesicles (Rhodin, 1962). The vesicles play an important role not only in cytopempsis, but also in intercellular transport (Reale and Ruska, 1965), and are involved in transport phenomena related to contraction-associated enzymatic activity (reverse pinocytosis). High ATPase activity in these areas signifies an intensive material transport (Hinke et al., 1964; Santos-Buch, 1966). A discernible, although not significant, increase of muscle cell ATPase activity precedes the development of fibrinoid necrosis in experimental hypertension. Rise of ATPase takes place not only in arteries and arterioles, but also in the aorta (Oka and Angrist, 1962, 1967).

FACTORS RESPONSIBLE FOR DRAINAGE OF PLASMA SUBSTANCES

Materials entering the vessel wall pass into the intercellular space and lymphatic system. The relation between blood vessels and intramural lymph vessels has been relatively little studied. Lymph capillaries have been demonstrated in the aortic adventitia (Hoggan and Hoggan 1883; Lee, 1922; Rényi-Vámos, 1960; Setti, 1965) and in the wall of the pulmonary artery of newborns (Papamiltiades, 1952). Papp and Jellinek (1961) studied the relationship between large veins and lymph vessels. Veress et al. (1969c) have observed distended lymph vessels in the aortic adventitia of rats maintained on an atherogenic diet. Wernze et al. (1965) observed an increased lymph drainage in angiotensin-induced hypertension. According to unpublished data from this institute, in addition to the vascular changes, a marked distension of lymph vessels takes place in drug-treated chronic experimental hypertension.

Arterial lymph drainage has not been dealt with in fundamental monographs on the lymphatic system (Yoffey and Coirtice, 1956; Rusznyák et al., 1960). The following experimental observations were described in order to throw light on the functional and morphological relations of lymph drainage inside the arterial wall.

INCREASE OF PERMEABILITY IN ASSOCIATION WITH LYMPH STASIS

It has been observed that experimentally induced insufficiency of the lymph circulation results in myocardial damage (Földi et al., 1954b; Rusznyák et al., 1960) and cardiac lymph circulation plays a substantial role in the evolution of fibrosis and other alternative changes (Kline, 1960).

Veress et al. (1966b) and Jellinek et al. (1966) observed that lymph stasis damages the coronary arteries. In dogs injected with Evans blue to visualize the lymphatic system, pericardial lymph nodes and lymphatic channels were constricted by a suture and the thoracic duct was ligated. Cardiac lymph stasis developed in 3 days (Plate LXVI/135) and the following coronary changes took place: in some small branches the endothelial cells became vacuolized and plasma depositions, staining blue with azan, appeared subintimally, causing the protru-

121

sion of the endothelium into the lumen (Plate LXVI/136). Occasionally, plasma was deposited also in the media (Plate LXVI/137, 138). If the lymph stasis was extensive, muscle cell necrosis occurred and a characteristic mural fibrinoid (Plate LXVI/139) necrosis developed in due course. The process affected chiefly the medium and small arteries of the ventricles, hence the lesions appeared primarily in those branches which might play a role in collateral circulation. The severity of the lesions was closely related to the extent of disseminated, focal muscle cell necrosis, so that coronary constriction seems to be an important factor in the evolution or progression of these changes. In the above experimental model, vascular lesions were induced by the obstruction of lymph drainage.

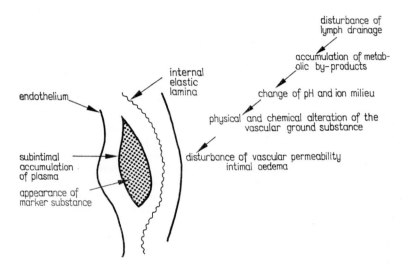

Fig. 3. Hypothetical course of vascular permeability change consequent upon mechanical lymph stasis

In another series of experiments, Hüttner et al. (1966) treated dogs with 300, 450 or 700 g per kg noradrenalin, administered by drop infusion for 40 minutes, and added 10 mg per kg dihydroperparine (No-Spa, Chinoin) to the infusion solution to potentiate the vasodilator effect. Vacuolization of endothelial cells (Plate LXVI/145) and subintimal deposition of plasma (Plate LXVII/146, 148) also appeared under these conditions, but since the duration of the damage was relatively short, the plasma disappeared from most vessels and only the loosened mural structure indicated the sites where it had been present (Plate LXVII/149). In certain vessels, however, a pronounced mural oedema and prolonged lymph stasis were followed by smooth muscle cell and fibrinoid necrosis. Lymph stasis was always signified by marked dilation of cardiac lymph vessels and interstitial oedema. In this experiment, lasting vascular changes were due to a functional insufficiency of lymph drainage, resulting from an increased intramural flow.

In analysing the above experiments, it was questioned why, on a mechanical blocking of the lymph circulation, the plasma depositions should appear subendothelially rather than in the adventitia although changes of the latter ought to precede involvement of the media and subendothelium. Nagy et al. (1969) attempted to clarify this problem by the colloidal iron tracer method. Lymph stasis was produced mechanically as in the foregoing and subsequently Ferrlecit was administered intravenously. The tracer substance accumulated in the damaged vessels at sites corresponding to the PAS-positive plasma deposition (Plate LXVI/ 140, 142), after which it formed large spots in the subendothelium (Plate LXVI/ 143) and smaller ones in the media (Plate LXVI/141). These changes were attributed to an increase in permeability of the coronary arteries and the following pathomechanism was inferred: lymph stasis interferes with the normal drainage of plasma diffusing into the vessel wall and this transport disturbance results in the retardation of cell metabolic products, the accumulation of which gradually alters the pH and the ion milieu. These changes affect the filter function of the mural AMPs and basement membrane, resulting in an increase of permeability (Fig. 3).

Nagy et al. (1970) further examined arterial wall permeability in dogs under conditions of lymph stasis in the extremities, to substantiate the above hypothesis. Ligation of inguinal lymph nodes or vessels in one hindleg produced a well-defined lymph stasis in 3–5 days. On subsequent administration of Ferrlecit, the positive Prussian blue reaction of the examined small muscular arterioles (Plate LXVI/144) indicated a permeability disturbance similar to that observed in the coronaries.

In summary, a close functional relationship of vascular permeability changes to disturbances of mural lymph drainage or transmural flow seems quite probable.

INTRAMURAL DIFFUSION OF VARIOUS PLASMA SUBSTANCES

SERUM PROTEINS, LIPIDS, LIPOPROTEIN AND IONS

Previously, Meyer (1949) observed the infiltration of fibrin and other proteins into the intima and later More and Haust (1961) reported similar findings. Duncan et al. (1962) observed that a greater amount of lipoprotein penetrated the proximal than the distal portion of the dog aorta. On studying the penetration of proteins labelled with ferritin or fluorescein into post-mortem human aortic segments under a luminal pressure of 15 mm Hg, Hirst and Gore (1962) found that the intima was permeable to albumin or colloid of 69,000 mol. wt and less permeable to globulin (186,000 mol. wt) and ferritin (500,000 mol. wt).

Examinations by tracer substances, autoradiography, and fluorescence and immunofluorescence tests have shown that the vessel wall is normally permeable to various plasma constituents. Adams and Moym (1966), who followed the intramural passage of ^{3}H-labelled cholesterol, ^{125}I-labelled albumin or globulin and ^{32}P-labelled lipid with special attention to cholesterol transport and evolution of the atheromatous plaque, concluded that intramural plasma diffusion also takes place in normal vessels. Christensen (1961, 1967) and Duncan et al. (1959) confirmed this opinion by examinations with ^{32}P-labelled lipoprotein. Intramural diffusion of albumin and beta- or gamma-globulin can take place from the adventitial side through the vasa vasorum (Adam, 1967), but in vascular lesions, including arteriosclerotic changes, direct diffusion from the luminal side is predominant. Biggs and Kritchevsky (1951) and later Dayton (1961) observed in certain diseases that the bulk of intramural cholesterol originates from the blood stream. On examining the intramural passage of labelled beta-lipoproteins, Virágh et al. (1968) observed species differences and correlated them with the actual amounts of mural AMPs. Cholesterol transport has been extensively studied owing to the key role of lipids in arteriosclerotic changes (see p. 60). Of the many investigators dealing with this problem, Adams (1964) pointed to the decisive importance of transport from the luminal side, on the basis of studies of the *in vivo* intramural passage of cholesterol. Jorgen (1967) studied the intramural diffusion of ^{14}C-labelled cholesterol, in connection with vascular metabolic activity.

On the basis of the observations of Mancini et al. (1962), Duncan et al. (1963), and their own experience, Walton and Williamson (1968) regard the diffusion of plasma proteins into aortic and arterial walls as verified. Serum lipids, in contrast, cannot pass through the intact intima in the form of chylomicrons, only in a soluble form such as high-density or low-density lipoproteins or albumin-bound fatty acids. Low-density lipoprotein is the most important barrier protein of all plasma components (Walton and Williamson, 1968), and intramurally deposited beta-lipoproteins and fibrinogen play the leading part in the evolution of vascular lesions (Steward, 1962).

In their studies of sodium and chloride flow from intima to adventitia in the wall of aorta and hollow veins, Sawyer and Valmond (1961) observed that vessel wall damages affect the ion transport. Kirck and Laursen (1955b) examined the diffusion coefficient of nitrogen, oxygen, carbon dioxide, lactate, iodide and glucose in human aortic endothelial membrane preparations and found that the diffusion coefficient, or permeability, tended to increase with age.

The intramural diffusion of lipids has been much disputed and it is still not clear in all details. Experimental animals show no discontinuity of endothelium after an atherogenic diet or intravenous administration of lipid. As no lipid appeared in the intercellular gaps or pinocytotic vesicles, Shoefl and French (1968) have supposed that the passage of lipid across the endothelium is preconditioned by a hydrolysis (lipase activity). In experiments with ^{32}P-labelled lipoprotein, Christensen (1961) concluded that lipids enter the vessel wall in a lipoprotein form. Gaps enabling a direct passage are found exclusively in the endothelium of the hepatic vessels (Ashworth et al., 1960). Williamson (1964) suggests that free fatty acids become absorbed via the pinocytotic vesicles; non-esterified fatty acids pass from vesicle to vesicle until they reach the inside of the cell. ATPase appears on the endothelial cell organelles (Hoff and Graf, 1966; Hoff, 1968).

Moore and Ruska (1957) and Bierring and Kabayashi (1963) have observed an increased endothelial pinocytotic activity during intramural lipid diffusion and recently Bálint et al. (1970) observed intramural lipid transport by macrophages (see p. 62).

Electron-microscopic studies of Kaye et al. (1965) suggest that small molecules, such as sodium, can pass directly through the endothelial cell membrane. Davson and Oldendorf (1967) have demonstrated that the diffusion of small molecular substances from the blood corresponds with their diffusion coefficient in water. Among proteins the haemoglobin molecule represents the upper limit of permeability (70 Å); larger molecules pass slowly, via pinocytosis. According to Kent (1969), ions and molecules can enter the cell by diffusion, pinocytosis, phagocytosis or active transport. He examined permeability disturbance with fluorescein-labelled, anti-rat IgG after damaging the cell membrane with lecithinase C and found that non-demonstrable quantity of plasma protein is present intracellularly under normal conditions. The intracellular diffusion of plasma proteins always signifies a disturbance of cell membrane permeability. On analysing the transport function of pinocytotic vesicles, Stehbens (1965a) found that vesicles of higher density are involved in protein transport and the two vesicle types are responsible for selectivity.

Adams et al. (1967) have distinguished two types of changes by analysis of intramural depositions in human lesions. The first category includes the changes showing typically the nature and staining properties of plasma proteins, while the second one includes the endogenous degenerations of the vascular wall. Substances released from endogenous lesions modify the staining properties of intramural plasma substances. The following protein depositions belong to the first category: ASC (hyaline change of spleen, diabetic or hypertensive changes of the kidney), malignant hypertensive changes of vessels, auto-immune arteritides, vascular amyloidosis, and glomerular exudation in diabetes and auto-immune diseases. The second category covers arteriosclerotic vascular changes, diffuse hyaline change of glomeruli in diabetes, Kimmelstiel–Wilson's glomerular and nodular change and nonfibrinoid wire-loop glomerular changes in SLE.

Tryptophane, tyrosine, cysteine and cystine are important components of plasma proteins, particularly of globulins and fibrinogen, but they occur in relatively small amounts in the connective tissue of the normal vessel wall. In changes of the first category, the intramural presence of these amino acids results from plasma filtration. It should be noted that the conventional M- and azan staining techniques are unsuitable for the differentiation of plasma components. The fact that the intramural plasma depositions or the fibrinoid necrosis stain sometimes blue, sometimes red with azan signifies not so much the predominance of one or another component (albumin, fibrinogen), as the actual physicochemical (colloidal) state of the proteins.

As to lipid depositions, most exudative lesions of the first category contain cholesterol, triglyceride, phospoglyceride and phospholipid (lecithin, cephalin). The lipid composition resembles that of the plasma lipoprotein. Sphingomyelin is not a typical plasma component, but it occurs in the vascular arteriosclerotic plaque; this suggests its endogenous local synthesis. Sudanophilic neutral lipids often associate with protein depositions, while part of the phospholipids originate from muscle cells or macrophages. Neutral lipids enter the vessel wall, or the arteriosclerotic plaque lipoprotein-bound, from which they then dissociate. Lesions of the second category contain no such lipids, probably because their cell components do not synthesize neutral lipid. As to AMPs, both types of lesions show a PAS positivity, suggesting the presence of mucoprotein, lipoprotein or

125

neutral polysaccharide. Exudative lesions of the first category contain little if any AMP, whereas lipoprotein originating from the plasma is always present. AMP being a substantial component of the collagenous matrix, all degenerative processes of collagen result in AMP release as found in lesions of the second category.

EFFECTS OF ABNORMAL ACCUMULATION OF VASOACTIVE AMINES
AND HORMONES, AND OF HYPOXIA AND pH-CHANGE ON PERMEABILITY

The integrity of the vascular endothelium involves the presence of a coating fibrin film over its surface (McFortane, 1964). Activation of plasminogen by streptokinase or urokinase increases vascular permeability probably through the removal of the endothelial fibrin barrier by plasmin (fibrinolysin) action. As already noted in the foregoing sections on tracer substances, vasoactive amines have been extensively used in permeability model experiments, hence under this heading only a brief reference is made to the investigations of Alksue (1959), Majno and Palade (1961) Movat and Fernando (1963a, c, d) and others, which have shown that administration of exogenous histamine or serotonin elicits a widening of the junctions, or a gap formation (see p. 128).

Constantinides (1969) has summarized the effects of vasoactive substances as follows: (i) tyramine, chlorisondamine and allylamine disrupt and destroy the cytoplasmic membrane; (ii) angiotensin causes endothelial cell contraction and consequent opening of the intercellular junctions; (iii) epinephrine and dopamine cause an intra- and extracellular oedema and (iv) serotonin and bradykinin cause distension of the junctions and concomitant oedema.

Buckley and Ryan (1969) examined the *in vivo* effects of histamine and serotonin on mesenteric vessels of rats. After the administration of histamine, the presence of colloidal carbon indicated an increase of capillary and venous permeability with the vascular calibre intact. Serotonin caused vasospasm, less distinctly in veins than in arteries. Buckley and his co-workers are of the opinion that histamine-type mediator substances directly affect the endothelial cells. Nikulin and Lapp (1965) and Nikulin and Schiemer (1965) have observed that histamine liberator substances effect an increase of transcellular permeability, as judged by the enhanced cytopempsis. Nikulin and Walther (1964) have differentiated two types of histamine effect: induced histamine, synthesized very likely by the vascular intima, rises and falls slowly in the blood; whereas bound histamine is abruptly released on stimulation and decomposes rapidly. Ischaemia and histamine liberators promote the release of bound histamine. Serum histamine level rises markedly in a state of general hypoxia, showing an initial maximum of 480 gamma per ml. Tissue ischaemia promotes the release of bound histamine, but it suppresses the action of induced histamine. According to Goodman (1968), the biochemical mechanism of histamine effect is the activation of either intracellular phosphodiesterase, or of cyclic adenosine 3', 5'-monophosphate production. Smooth muscle cells and capillary and venous endothelium are extremely sensitive to diesterase. Nikulin and Lapp (1965) and Nikulin and Schiemer (1965) describe three phases of histamine action under the influence of histamine liberators. The first phase is the protective response to histamine release: platelet agglutination in the capillaries and endothelial plasma insudation. This results in a permeability disturbance, i.e. in an impairment of controlled active transport, so that plasma diffuses into the endothelium, while proteins and electrolytes leak from it. This is followed by the restoration of the semipermeability of endothelial cell membranes and restoration of active transport. Nikulin and his co-workers attribute these phenomena to a direct histamine effect. The next phase are regeneration and *restitutio ad integrum*. Hurley and Spector (1965) induced inflammatory disturbance of permeability by intrapleural administration of turpentine. Permeability increase occurred chiefly in the veins and took place in two phases, the first of which could be inhibited with antihistamines, the second with sodium salicylate. Fuchs and Claus (1967) observe by tracer technique a histamine- or serotonin-type permeability disturbance in dextran oedema.

Antihistamines suppress the evolution of experimental atheromatosis through inhibition of histamine-induced permeability increase. Harman (1962) was able to ameliorate ASC of cholesterol-fed mice by chlorphenylamine treatment and Shimamoto et al. (1966) found a significant reduction in size of atheromatous lesions on administration of anti-bradykinin at an unchanged serum cholesterol level.

Proteolytic and glycolytic enzymes disrupt the endothelial cell membrane. Lipolytic enzymes have no noticeable effect, but surface-active substances cause a distinct endothelial destruction (Constantinides, 1969) (Plate XLVIII/207). The last cited author found that anoxia induced by cyanide or aortic constriction for 16 minutes caused no significant change in endothelial cell membranes, but did cause a striking widening of interendothelial junctions. Müller and Locwenich (1961) emphasize in their review the importance of hypoxia as a factor in arteriosclerotic change. Kjeldsen et al. (1968) report that hypoxia increased the severity of experimental atheromatosis. Saphir et al. (1962) observed an increased insudation of *in vivo* cholesterol-incubated aortic segments after blocking the oxidative enzymes with sodium cyanide or potassium chloride. Yoffey and Coirtice (1956) found an increase of endothelial permeability in an anoxic environment. On analysing osmolarity changes, Constantinides (1969) found that 3,000 mOsm caused no endothelial change, whereas 0 mOsm (distilled water) effected an opening of the junctions. Both acid and alkaline pH result in widening of the junctions. Cervos-Navarro (1964) induced increase of capillary permeability in the central nervous system of monkeys by X-ray irradiation. The vesicles multiplied in the endothelial cells and the basement membrane became wider.

Irradiation with 185 MeV caused distension of the endothelium, microvillus formation on the luminal side and nuclear damage (Andres, 1963). Forty-two hours later a granular substance appeared in the subendothelial portion of the artery. Intramural cell necrosis and fibrin and fat deposition were seen in places. Thus, the appearance of necrotizing vasculopathy corresponded with that of intramural plasma diffusion or hypoxic damage. Post-irradiation changes of arteries, including intramural depositions, were also analysed by Kirkpatrick (1967). Altmann et al. (1962) reported that irradiation of the elements of circulation induced an overall increase of permeability, resulting in plasma diffusion into the impaired segments of larger vessels. Zollinger (1960) has termed this change 'plasmatic radiation vasculopathy'.

127

PRESSURE AND FLOW FACTORS

A thorough analysis of vascular permeability changes includes the study of intra-vascular, hydrostatic, colloidal and osmotic pressure conditions and microcirculation factors. Yoffey and Coirtice (1956) have pointed to the role of filtration pressure in the intra-endothelial passage of proteins, lipoproteins, chylomicrons and other blood components. Duncan et al. (1962) inferred the importance of the pressure gradient from a follow-up of the intramural diffusion of labelled albumin. In his *in vitro* experiments on intramural lipid diffusion, Steward (1962) maintained pulsation by means of a Dale–Schuster pump, to reproduce the pressure conditions indispensable for mural insudation. Texon (1960), Wosolowsky et al. (1965) and Blumenthal (1967) have emphasized the role of haemodynamical factors in the local manifestations of various vascular changes. Turbulence, high frequency vibration and the coagulation-promoting dead spaces of flow also are important factors (Heberer, 1966). Texon (1960) regarded fluid dynamics so important that he explained the development of intimal oedema in the early phase of the arteriosclerotic plaque by Bernoulli's flow dynamics law and concluded that the negative pressure developing in the bifurcations has a decisive influence on the evolution of the changes. Langen (1953) postulated that an intramural pressure gradient, diminishing from the intima towards the adventitia, might play a role in transmural transport.

French (1966) thinks that pressure changes are decisive in the milking effect of pulsation waves acting from the lumen towards the endothelium. Byron and Dodson already in 1948 pointed to the mechanical effect of blood pressure rise on hypertensive lesions.

EFFECT OF HYPERTENSION ON TRANSPORT ACROSS THE VESSEL WALL

HYPERTENSIVE DISTURBANCES OF TRANSMURAL FLOW IN SMALL ARTERIES*

Hackel (1930) was one of the first to describe vascular permeability disturbances in hypertension. He produced hypertension by ligation, adrenalin treatment, and nerve stimulation and observed the intramural passage of trypan blue. Rise of blood pressure caused diffusion of plasma into the aortic intima, and not only the stain but also colloidal plasma components entered the vessel wall. Since then many efforts have been made to elucidate the mechanism of evolution of the vascular (subintimal and media) fibrinoid (see pp. 74, 76) (Byrom, 1954; Esterly and Glagov 1963; Giese, 1964, 1966; Ooneda et al., 1965; Jellinek, 1965, 1967; Still

* Dr. Hüttner, the author of this section, was a Research Fellow of the Canadian Arthritis and Rheumatism Society at the Department of Pathology, McGill University, Montreal, during the preparation of this manuscript.

The original report of this study was partly published in the *American Journal of Pathology* **61**, 357–370 (1970) in collaboration with Dr. Robert H. More, Chairman and Professor, and Dr. George Rona, Associate Professor, Pathological Institute, McGill University. The author wishes to express his appreciation for permission to incorporate this paper into the monograph.

1967; Still and Dennison, 1969; Hüttner et al., 1968; Wiener et al., 1968, 1969; Olsen, 1969).

Jellinek et al. (1969) studied hypertensive permeability changes by means of India ink or colloidal iron (Ferrlecit), of which the latter proved more sensitive (Plate LXVII/156, 162). Wistar albino rats were rendered hypertensive by the method of Lőrincz and Gorácz and 7 days after surgery they were given either 0.5 ml India ink or 0.8 ml Ferrlecit per 100 g body weight and killed. Mesenteric and subserous small arteries were examined. A positive Prussian blue reaction indicated permeability disturbance prior to its microscopic detection by India ink or PAS-reaction. Electron microscopically, iron clumps were seen located in intracellular vacuoles and in depositions within the widened subendothelial space (Plates XLIX/208; L/209).

In the early phase of the hypertensive change the endothelium becomes discontinuous, the junctions widen and intercellular gaps become established. These changes can in themselves account for the increased intramural diffusion of tracer substances. Additional endothelial damages are the swelling of the cells and increase of cytoplasmic electron density. Thus, endothelial degeneration is one component in the widening of the junctions. The cisternae of the rough endoplasmic reticulum distend and an electron-opaque substance fills them, which is probably related to the increased basement membrane synthesis. The rise of intraluminal pressure may enhance the passage of tracer substance, plasma substances, cells and cell fragments into the vessel wall. Swelling of endothelial cells, distension of junctions, and deposition of plasma and fibrin in the subendothelial space and media are the main characteristics of the early hypertensive lesion (Plates XLIX/208; L/209). Similar observations have been reported by Ooneda et al. (1965) and Hüttner et al. (1968). In angiotensin-induced hypertension, Giese (1966) observed an alternation of dilated and constricted vascular portions and detected permeability increase in the former by means of a combined tracer–in vivo microscopy technique. Wiener et al. (1969) explained permeability increase by the renin-angiotensin mediated transmural flow enhancing action of blood pressure rise. Other non-pressor substances originating from the kidney also gained access to the vessel wall (Asscher and Anson 1963; Yasamura, 1967). The increased transmural flow carried an increased amount of electrolytes (Tobian et al., 1961). Wernze (1965) measured an increased amount of lymph in the thoracic duct and Veress et al. (Personal communication) observed distension of lymph vessels around the mesenteric arteries of rats kept hypertensive for 3 weeks by the method of Lőrincz and Gorácz and treated with an experimental preparation (BTF). These observations indicate that both transmural flow and lymph drainage become enhanced under conditions of hypertension and their roles in the pathogenesis of permeability increase are inseparable (Nagy et al., 1969).

In early hypertension, Veress et al. (1969a, b) detected a sudanophilic substance exclusively in damaged medial smooth muscle cells and explained its appearance by phanerosis. The subendothelium showed no sudanophilia, but the perivascular granulation did and this reaction was attributed to plasma lipoproteins (Plate LXIV/73). Olsen (1969) followed the subsequent fate of proteins labelled with colloidal carbon or fluorescein after angiotensin-induced hypertension. They passed into mononuclear cells and into the surrounding connective tissue. The elastic membrane inhibited transmural flow. Still (1967) observed in experimental animals the passage of mononuclear cells into intra- and subendothelium under the influence of blood pressure rise. The cells entered the vessel wall through the many endothelial gaps, along with the diffusing plasma substances. Earlier, Esterly and Glagov (1963), Still (1963), Still and O'Neal (1962), Still and Mariott (1964) and Still and Prosser (1964) made similar observations in experimental ASC. In glomerular changes associated with steroid hypertension, Still and Dennison (1969) observed the aggregation of the same granular substance as occurs in the large elastic-type vessels of the subendothelium.

POST-HYPERTENSIVE PERMEABILITY DISTURBANCE OF AORTA

Insudation of plasma proteins into arterial walls (Giese, 1961; Trillo et al., 1970) and increased permeability to different tracers (Giese, 1964; Jellinek et al., 1969) have been repeatedly found in experimental hypertension. The few studies (Wiener et al., 1969) concerned with the structural basis for this increased endothelial permeability have described the occurrence of gap formation. It has been suggested that endothelial cell contraction or degeneration occurs, similarly to that found in other experimental models resulting in increased arterial permeability (Constantinides and Robinson 1969a–c). Although observations reported in some studies hinted to some correlation existing between the physiologic passage ways of the vascular endothelium and the mechanism of early plasma insudation (Still, 1968; Florey, 1970), we were unable to find in the literature any structural studies that gave evidence for this suggestion.

The previous fine structural studies in experimental hypertension were carried out in mesenteric and coronary arteries (Kerényi et al., 1966a; Jellinek et al. 1967a, b; Hüttner et al., 1968 1969c; Jellinek et al., 1969).

The aorta, however, appeared to be a preferable vessel for the investigation of this problem (Hüttner and More, 1970). Accumulation of plasma proteins in the relatively closed subendothelial compartment of the aorta represents a constant early change in diverse experimental hypertensive models (Still, 1967, 1968; Veress et al., 1969d). Furhermore, the aortic wall lends itself readily to technical procedures, such as time studies with tracers, used in our experiments. The experiments were carried out in adult male rats of the Sprague–Dawley strain, weighing 300–400 g. Arterial hypertension was produced by unilateral renal ischaemia with complete ligation of the aorta between the origin of the renal arteries (Rojo-Ortega and Genest, 1968). Blood pressure was measured directly in the carotid artery by manometric method. On the second post-operative day, rats found to be hypertensive were used for tracer experiments along with controls. Horseradish peroxidase (Type II, Sigma Chemical Co.), ferritin (double crystalline, horse spleen, cadmium free) and colloidal carbon (Pelican, Gunther Wagner) were used as tracer molecules.

Light microscopy (using 1 μ sections stained with toluidine blue) of the upper (subdiaphragmatic) part of the abdominal aorta showed widened subendothelial spaces as compared with controls. These spaces contained homogeneous material, darkly staining clumps and occasional mononuclear cells. This change was associated with smooth muscle cell hypertrophy in the media and fibroblastic swelling in the adventitia.

130

In hypertensive rats the subendothelial spaces were widened and contained granular material (Plates LI/210, 211, 212; LII/213), polymerized fibrin (Plate LII/214) and focally, macrophages and lymphocytes (Plate LIV/219). The granular material was consistent with plasma proteins. The interendothelial junctions morphologically appeared normal. The endothelial cells displayed striking structural changes: the cells were enlarged, the nucleus was crenated, its chromatin uniformly dispersed and the nucleoli were prominent. In the cytoplasm of the endothelial cells much rough endoplasmic reticulum as well as many free ribosomes appeared. The Golgi complexes were prominent and augmented in number and size. The cytoplasm contained many dense bodies (Plate LIII/215, 216, 217, 219). The number of plasmalemmal vesicles also appeared to be increased. Occasionally, lymphocytes were found passing through the endothelial cell layers, apparently through the cytoplasm of endothelial cells (Plate LIV/219).

In the smooth muscle cells of the media, rough endoplasmic reticulum and Golgi complex components were found in a strikingly increased quantity as compared with controls. In the Golgi regions, many dense granules appeared (Plate LV/220, 221).

TRACER STUDIES

PEROXIDASE EXPERIMENTS

In the aorta of control rats 1.5 minutes after horseradish peroxidase injection, peroxidase reaction product was seen on the luminal surface of the endothelial cells, in endothelial cell junctions and within some of the plasmalemmal vesicles, particularly those at intercellular junctions. A low density reaction product was discernible in the subendothelial space (Plate LVI/222). As observed at 6 minutes and at 30 minutes after injection, peroxidase reaction product increased in intensity in the subendothelial space, appeared in plasmalemmal vesicles at the subendothelial surface of the endothelial cells and was found on the medial side of the IEL. In some endothelial cells reaction product appeared in larger vesicles and in vacuoles probably representing coated vesicles and multivesicular structures. In some rats the subendothelial space appeared to be widened and occasional subendothelial macrophages were seen with peroxidase-containing vacuoles.

In the aorta of hypertensive rats 1.5 minutes after horseradish peroxidase injection, peroxidase reaction product was found as in the controls, on the luminal surface of the endothelial cells, in the interendothelial junctions, and within some of the plasmalemmal vesicles. There was a more intensive reaction for peroxidase in the widened subendothelial space intermingled with the accumulated plasma material and this was also seen on the other side of the IEL in the extracellular compartment of the media (Plate LVI/223, 224). The distribution of peroxidase reaction product was similar in aortas fixed at both 6 minutes and 30 minutes after peroxidase injection.

FERRITIN EXPERIMENTS

In the aorta of control rats, at both 6 minutes and 30 minutes after ferritin injection, ferritin molecules were seen in small numbers within plasmalemmal vesicles of the endothelial cells and in the subendothelial space (Plate LVII/225). Groups of ferritin molecules occurred within dense bodies or multivesicular structures of the endothelial cells. Ferritin molecules were not encountered within interendothelial junctions.

In the aorta of hypertensive rats the distribution of ferritin molecules at 6 minutes and at 30 minutes was similar to that of controls. However, the number of ferritin molecules strikingly increased within plasmalemmal vesicles and in the subendothelial space (Plates LVII/225–227; LVIII/228–231). Moreover, ferritin molecules appeared markedly increased within dense bodies and multivesicular structures of the endothelial cells (Plate VIII/228, 229). A few ferritin molecules were seen in the extracellular space of the media close to the fenestrae of the IEL. In the endothelial cells it was not always possible to establish whether ferritin molecules were located within plasmalemmal vesicles or overlying cytoplasmic matrix. Although ferritin molecules were not encountered within endothelial junctions, occasionally mononuclear cells, which penetrated the endothelial cell layer, led to a gap formation containing ferritin molecules.

COLLOIDAL CARBON EXPERIMENTS

Colloidal carbon was not encountered during the period under study (from 6 to 30 minutes) in the endothelial cells, nor in the subendothelial space of controls. In hypertensive rats carbon particles were found infrequently in a few areas of the subendothelial space.

Physiological studies of the permeability of capillaries have measured the rate at which molecules leave the intravascular compartment or are transferred from blood to lymph. This has led to the 'pore theory' of capillary permeability (Starling, 1896; Landis and Pappenheimer, 1963) which assumes the existence of two pore systems, one small (diameter 90 Å) and the other large (diameter 250–700 Å). The large pore system has been suggested as the sole passage way for molecules with a diameter larger than 80 Å, such as most plasma proteins.

Electron-microscopic tracer techniques have utilized horseradish peroxidase (mol. wt 30,000, diameter 50 Å) as a probe molecule for the small pore system (Straus, 1967) and ferritin (mol. wt 500,000, diameter 110 Å) comparable in size to most plasma proteins (Höglund and Levin, 1965), for tracing the large pore system. Colloidal carbon (diameter 250–500 Å), while too large for tracing the pore systems, has been found useful for detecting discontinuity of the endothelial cell layer. Studies utilizing these techniques have confirmed the structural equivalent of the two pore systems in certain types of capillary endothelium (Karnovsky, 1967; Bruns and Palade, 1968; Clementi and Palade 1969). The morphological equivalent for the small pore system in capillaries with continuous endothelium has been suggested to be the endothelial cell junction (Karnovsky, 1967) and, for the large pore system, the plasmalemmal vesicles (Bruns and Palade, 1968). It has further been suggested that the structural basis for increased capillary permeability is a transient opening of interendothelial junctions achieved by chemical mediators producing either endothelial cell contraction (Majno et al., 1969) or an effect on the protein–polysaccharide complexes at interendothelial junctions (Clementi and Palade, 1969).

In arteries, normal endothelial transport processes resemble those of capillaries with continuous endothelium (Florey, 1967, 1970). The structural equivalent of the two pore systems is, however, not yet established in arterial endothelium. In experimental hypertension models, insudation of plasma proteins into the arterial wall (Giese, 1961; Trillo et al., 1970) and increased permeability to different tracers (Giese, 1964; Jellinek et al., 1969) have been verified. However, only a few of these studies were designed to investigate the structural basis of the increased endothelial permeability (Wiener et al., 1969). It has been suggested that gap formation, i.e. endothelial cell separation, is responsible for plasma insudation.

A recent tracer study in experimental hypertension showed peroxidase passage through cerebral artery endothelial junctions, with no leakage of carbon particles (Giacomelli et al., 1969).

Our study revealed that in control rats peroxidase reaction product appeared in aortic endothelial cell junctions and within plasmalemmal vesicles, particularly those communicating with junctions or cell surface. On the other hand, ferritin molecules were not present in endothelial cell junctions, but were found mainly within plasmalemmal vesicles. These results indicate that in aortic endothelium of normal rats, as in capillaries with continuous endothelium, the structural equivalents of the small pore system are the endothelial cell junctions and those of the large pore system the plasmalemmal vesicles of endothelial cells.

In hypertensive animals the point of entry for peroxidase and ferritin did not change. Ferritin molecules, however, were strikingly increased within plasmalemmal vesicles and both tracers appeared to be increased in the subendothelial space. Moreover, markedly increased amounts of ferritin were found within dense bodies and multivesicular structures of the endothelial cells. These results indicate that in the early stages of experimental hypertension tracer molecules enter the aortic intima in increased amounts through physiologic pathways. Furthermore, these results and the presence of plasma proteins in the subendothelial space support the view that the increased permeability of endothelium to plasma proteins in the early stages of hypertension is related to an enhanced physiologic transport rather than to gap formation. Molecules of a similar size to peroxidase pass through cell junctions whereas molecules of a size similar to ferritin, such as most plasma proteins, are transported by plasmalemmal vesicles. The high metabolic activity in the endothelial cells, as reflected by an increased amount of rough endoplasmic reticulum, free ribosomes, Golgi complex and other organelles during hypertension, tends to support the specific role of endothelium in protein transport. These morphological signs of active protein synthesis in endothelial cells may be partly related to the membrane regeneration required for the enhanced vesicular transport. The increased number of dense bodies and multivesicular structures in endothelial cells could possibly reflect an intracellular barrier function.

The mechanism of changes indicating hyperplasia of smooth muscle cells and fibroblasts awaits elucidation. The high metabolic activity of these cells may be secondary to an overload elicited by the high intraluminal pressure or may be a reactive process to increased passage of plasma constituents through the aortic wall. This latter possibility is in agreement with the conclusion of other studies on hypertensive medial aortic lesions (Salgado, 1970). Whatever the mechanism may be, the high metabolic activity in these cells probably represents a prelude to production of new connective tissue.

It has been described (Karnovsky, 1967) that horseradish peroxidase causes histamine release in different species, including the rat and thus may produce endothelial leakage. However, observations concerning histamine effect have been made only on venular endothelium (Karnovsky, 1967; Majno et al., 1969; Florey 1970). In the present experiments, in a few control specimens, at both 6 minutes and 30 minutes after peroxidase injection, widened subendothelial spaces were found with occasional subendothelial macrophages. Although this finding may be related to histamine release, the consistent difference between the control and hypertensive groups at 1.5 minutes, when there was no widened subendothelial space in any of the controls, indicates that there is increased peroxidase passage in the hypertensive rats that is not secondary to any effect of the peroxidase.

This study gave information concerning the passage ways of protein molecules through aortic endothelium in experimental hypertension. The primary cause responsible for the increased protein transport remained, however, unknown. High blood pressure alone may produce increased protein passage, as molecules move, at least in part, by diffusion-dependent hydrodynamic forces along both physiologic avenues of the vascular endothelium.

Although the described results do not exclude the role of gap formation in plasma insudation, particularly in advanced hypertensive vascular injury, the tracer studies indicate that there is enhanced passage of protein molecules through physiologic pathways which represents a constant permanent mechanism in the early stages of hypertension. This mechanism may permit the passage of all plasma proteins including fibrinogen. The finding of occasional carbon particles, macrophages and lymphocytes in the subendothelial space suggests that gaps undoubtedly occur, but clearly they do not account for the continuous enhanced passage of proteins in this stage.

*

Thus the fundamental factor in hypertensive vascular changes is clearly plasma insudation, which occurs in all affected vessels independently of type.

Various descriptions of permeability disturbances support the view (Jellinek, 1965) that the vascular system responds stereotypically by similar morphological changes to various kinds of injury (vasculitis, hypertension, ASC, X-ray irradiation, etc.) and the one main functional event is always the disturbance of vascular permeability, transmural flow and drainage of plasma materials.

ARTERIOSCLEROSIS AND MURAL TRANSPORT

ROLE OF PERMEABILITY IN ATHEROGENESIS

According to the filtration theory of atherogenesis (Gofmann and Young, 1965), increase of endothelial permeability and the consequent greater than physiological insudation of plasma components into the vessel wall are the fundamental changes by which the arteriosclerotic vascular lesions develop (Constantinides, 1965). A similar explanation has been offered by Doerr in his work entitled *Per-*

Fusionstheorie der Arteriosklerose (1963). He differentiates two forms of ASC, the common form in which the changes arise from a disturbance of perfusion (mural transport, as we would call it) and the uncommon form in which local metabolic disturbances arising at sites of preference give rise to the arteriosclerotic plaque.

Many newer findings during the last decade have been in support of the filtration theory. There are two possible approaches to the problem:

1. verification of the increase of endothelial permeability;
2. demonstration of plasma components in the vessel wall.

Normally endothelial cells are impermeable to intravenously administered vital stains (Petroff, 1922; Okuneff, 1926) and to thorium oxide (Efskind, 1940, 1941) as well. Rabbits kept on an atherogenic diet, however, showed in contrast to controls a marked accumulation of intravenously administered colloidal thorium in endothelial cells (Duff et al., 1954). Colloidal [110]Ag was further detected in arteriosclerotic lesions of rabbits, while normally fed rabbits had no aortic silver deposits (Felt, 1960). Similar observations were made with Evans blue (Friedman and Byers, 1963); the stain did not appear in the aortic wall of control animals. Accumulation of ^{131}I-labelled albumin was observed in the inner third of the aortic wall (Adams et al., 1968). The severity of evolving lesions could be diminished by administration of permeability-reducing antihistamines (Harman, 1962; Shimamoto et al., 1966).

There is also electron-microscopic evidence of permeability increase. Colloidal thorium appeared in endothelial cells and in the deeper layers of the atheromatous plaque (Still, 1964; Still and Mariott 1964, Still and Prosser, 1964). Accumulation of a large amount of thorium particles was observed in the aortic subendothelial space and media of a hyperlipaemic parrot (Hess and Stäubli, 1969), while in the control aorta only a few thorium granules appeared in pinocytotic vesicles of endothelial cells, signifying physiologic transport. Still and Prosser (1964b), however, failed to observe any parallel between accumulation of lipid and thorotrast. Iwanaga et al. (1969) utilized peroxidase to demonstrate the increase of endothelial permeability in rats and rabbits maintained on an atherogenic diet.

In this institute, a colloidal iron tracer technique was developed which permitted the detection of permeability increase by both conventional and electron microscopy (Nagy et al., 1968; Jellinek et al., 1969) (see Chapter 10). Utilizing this method, permeability increase was unequivocally demonstrated in rats after 3 weeks of an atherogenic diet. Iron granules were located in aortic endothelial cells and subendothelial space by their positive Prussian-blue reaction (Plate LXII/32, 33). Electron micrographs verified the light-microscopic findings: aggregated iron granules within endothelial cells were surrounded by a membrane (Plate XXXII/142). No similar phenomena occurred in control animals.

Demonstration of those plasma components which do not normally deposit in the vessel wall further supports the filtration theory. Investigations along this line have repeatedly been carried out since the early 'sixties, utilizing radio-isotope techniques and immunomorphological methods. Labelled plasma proteins and lipoproteins were detected in the vessel wall (Gerő et al., 1961b; Watts, 1961; Christensen, 1962; Duncan et al., 1962, 1963; Newman and Zilversmit 1962, 1964; Davis et al., 1963; Adams et al., 1968).

Fibrin and low-density lipoproteins were demonstrated in human and experimental arteriosclerotic lesions by Woolf and Crawford (1960), Gerő et al. (1961a), Haust et al. (1964, 1965), Woolf and Pilkington (1965), Koo and Wissler (1965), Walton and Williamson (1968) and Wissler (1968).

In summary, increase of endothelial permeability during an atherogenic diet has been confirmed by light- and electron microscopy and by immunohistochemical and biochemical methods as well. Nevertheless, present knowledge is not sufficient to account for the true cause of permeability increase, nor for the mechanism of its evolution.

ROLE OF LYMPH CIRCULATION IN EXPERIMENTAL ARTERIOSCLEROSIS OF THE RAT

Constantinides (1965) writes on page 14 of his monograph: ' . . . the metabolic needs of most of the arterial wall . . . are served by a continuous diffusion of fluid through it from the lumen towards the lymphatic channels of the adventitia.' This view has been generally accepted, but relatively few authors have dealt with the role of the adventitia (Williams, 1961; Lusztig, 1970) and aortic lymph vessels in ASC. Hoggan and Hoggan (1883) utilized silver impregnation to demonstrate lymph channels in the aortic adventitia. Lee (1922) detected by Prussian-blue reaction one superficial and one deep lymphatic plexus in the adventitia of the ligated cat aorta. Papamiltiades (1952) found lymph capillaries in the wall of the pulmonary artery of newborns. Rényi-Vámos (1960) demonstrated lymph channels draining the dog aorta by means of India ink applied at the border between media and adventitia. Recently Setti (1965) have dealt with aortic lymph drainage.

Atherogenic diet elicits an abnormal increase of endothelial permeability (see p. 134), resulting in an abnormal increase of fluid passing across the vessel wall. Electron micrographs of the aorta of rats maintained on Loustalot's (1960) diet revealed a network of lymph channels in the adventitia (Jellinek et al., 1970) (Plate XXXIII/143). After 9 weeks of the experimental diet, the lymph channels distended considerably and contained in places a plasma-like substance of medium electron density (Plate XXXIII/147, 152, 153). Simultaneously, many pinocytotic vesicles appeared in the endothelial cells of the lymph vessels and some of the intercellular junctions opened (Plate XXXIII/144–147, 149). Neutral lipid droplets were also present (Plate XXXIII/148, 150, 153), like in aortic endothelial cells. These morphological changes were clearly unrelated to intestinal food absorption, because the animals had been starved for 18 hours prior to extermination.

Our observations on the relation between aortic changes and lymph drainage during the atherogenic diet might explain Williams' (1961) finding, who observed severer lesions in aortas deprived of adventitia than in those not deprived; he might well have removed the lymph channels along with the adventitia and the absence of lymph drainage might have been the cause of the extraordinarily enhanced fat deposition. The recent observation of Lusztig (1970) that adventitial mast cells of rabbits become degranulated after 9–10 weeks of an atherogenic diet suggests a new approach to the problem. Active substances released during degranulation were shown to enhance the permeability of the lymph vessel endothelium (Virágh et al., 1966).

Distension of adventitial lymph vessels and accumulation of lipids in lymph vessel endothelial cells of rats during an atherogenic diet suggest that general or local lymph drainage disorders resulting from any cause might deleteriously affect the severity of arteriosclerotic lesions through the insufficiency of drainage of pathologically increased depositions of extramural substances.

CHAPTER 11

STUDIES ON HUMAN VASCULAR DISEASES WITH REGARD TO OBSERVATIONS IN MODEL EXPERIMENTS

EVALUATION OF ACUTE SMALL VESSEL LESIONS

Fibrinoid necrosis of the vessel wall has long been known in human pathology, but opinions have differed concerning the mechanism of its evolution. It follows from the name of the change that is has been attributed to vascular wall necrosis subsequent to fibrin insudation. Initially, the swelling and alteration of collagenous fibres were held responsible for its evolution, but later studies have disclosed that vascular fibrinoid differs considerably from connective tissue fibrinoid and from Neumann's (1896) interpretation of a fibrinoid as well.

The vascular fibrinoid had been characterized by its staining properties, viz. that it stains homogeneously with haematoxylin and eosin, and with azan, and fibrin is demonstrable in it by specific stains (e.g. Weigert's fibrin stain). Later, it was questioned whether it contains fibrin at all and what its components might be. Several authors believed that the change arose from plasma insudation, while others attributed it to vascular muscle cell deterioration. Recent observations suggest that plasma insudation and vascular wall deterioration are jointly responsible for the establishment of the vascular fibrinoid. Fibrinoid changes of this type were first observed in periarteritis nodosa (Kussmaul and Maier, 1866), and so the fibrinoid necrosis and the surrounding periadventitial granulation were regarded as characteristic of that condition. Later, similar vascular lesions, with a nearly indentical morphology, were demonstrated in several other diseases [basilar meningitis, hypertension, Wegener's granulomatosis (1970), various collagenoses and allergic manifestations]. Recent immunohistological studies suggest that the variation of lesions with the type of disease is less pronounced than originally thought (Miescher and Müller-Eberhand, 1968–1969). The structural similarity of lesions developing in various forms of necrotizing angiitis hampers their aetiological and diagnostic differentiation; conditions generally classified in this category are periarteritis nodosa, hypersensitivity arteritis, granulomatous angiitis, malignant hypertension and giant-cell arteritis (Takayashu's disease). SLE has been segregated as a different disease group, but the vascular changes caused by it do not fundamentally differ from those associated with angiitis, and their chronic stage serves to affirm the identity of reparative processes following upon identical lesions. Similarity of lesions and difficulties of diagnostic differentiation have been discussed in connection with periarteritis and hypersensitivity angiitis by Wilbrandt et al. (1969) and Jellinek (1970).

Nevertheless, the classical periarteritis nodosa-type lesions have so much been associated with this particular condition that muscular biopsy is still being performed to confirm the diagnosis. We have long been sceptical about the value of diagnosis based on histological examination of biopsy specimens from alleged periarteritis nodosa cases. The tissue changes would uniformly suggest a periarteritis nodosa, while later post mortem would often reveal a different condition, e. g. Wegener's granulomatosis, as the basic disorder. We, therefore, decided to analyse those conditions which have been reported to cause a periarteritis nodosa-like fibrinoid necrosis and added a few others from our own experience, as follows:

Periarteritis nodosa	8 cases
Wegener's allergic granulomatosis	4 cases
Tuberculous basilar meningitis	5 cases
Malignant hypertension	6 cases
Collagenoses	5 cases
Allergic tuberculous granulomatous inflammation	1 case
Rheumatic vascular changes	3 cases
Purulent inflammation	3 cases
Pyelonephritis	9 cases

Only those cases were investigated in detail in which the changes met all criteria of the classical fibrinoid vascular wall necrosis. The analysis of these cases led to the conclusion that the vascular lesions were in every respect similar to one another in each condition studied and also that the mechanisms of evolution of the lesions could be correlated. The literature usually deals only with the characteristics of the established lesion, without describing the stages of its evolution. Since we had observed the entire course of the change in experimental models, it was easy to identify the same stages of progression in human lesions resulting from various causes but identical in morphological appearance.

In addition to the complete vascular fibrinoid change, single muscle cell necrosis occurred in some small muscular arteries in connection with Wegener's allergic granulomatosis, hypertension, lupus erythematosus, periarteritis nodosa (Plates LXVIII/163, 164; LIX/232, 233 234) and basilar meningitis (Plate LXVIII/165). Apart from the conditions associated with periarteritis nodosa-like lesions, single vascular muscle cell necroses have been observed in the wall of uterine arteries during involution (Plate LXVII/166, 167), in acute infectious diseases in the spleen of a dead child and in a small artery of a septic spleen (Plate LXVIII/168, 169).

The latter change was reminiscent of the initial single or diffuse muscle cell necroses observed in model experiments (Plates LXIII/46, 49; LXIV/78–81, 86, 87; LXV/100, 101).

Segmental muscle cell necroses known from the model experiments (Plates LXIII/47, 50; LXV/82, 83, 87, 88, 102) as a more advanced stage of the lesion occurred in allergic granulomatosis and hypertension (Plates LIX/235, 236; LXVIII/163, 164, 170).

These changes were the prelude to complete vascular wall degeneration, fibrinoid formation and subsequent periadventitial granulation. In human lesions, fibrin deposition (Plates LIX/237, 238, 239; LXVIII/170, 171, 173) and periadventitial granuloma were in every respect similar to those observed in model experiments after experimental hypertension, sensitization with horse serum or noradrenalin treatment (Plates LXIII/51, 53, 57; LXIV/94, 95; LXV/103, 105).

All stages of evolution of fibrinoid necrosis inferred from model experiments have thus been encountered in human lesions. The reasons for disregarding these changes in earlier studies might have been, on the one hand, the concentration on the periarteritis nodosa-like picture for diagnostic purposes; on the other, the eventual modifying effects of specific drug therapy which might prolong, or temporarily suppress, the process. A vascular fibrinoid necrosis was in fact observed in all conditions listed above, and illustrations for some have been omitted only for lack of space.

Variation of the change with the vascular structure was essentially the same in human cases as in model experiments. Both subendothelial fibrinoid (Plates LIX/240; LXVIII/172, 173) and media fibrinoid (Plate LXVIII/168, 169, 173) developed in muscular-type human arteries possessing a distinct IEL. The latter has obviously a barrier function also in human vessels and being better developed than in experimental animals, human lesions may often be more distinct. Muscle cell necroses of the media fibrinoid could be clearly distinguished from the subendothelial space (Plate LXVIII/168, 169,173), which usually widened to a greater degree than in the model experiments (Plates LXIII/52, 54, 56; LXIV/81, 97). The fibrinoid change stained homogeneously with azan, as in experimental animals, but necrotic smooth muscle cells were seen for a longer period in human lesions (Plate LXVIII/166–169).

Thus the hypertensive changes of small vessels are essentially the same in human and experimental hypertension. The characteristic fibrinoid necrosis always arises from medial muscle cell necrosis and intramural plasma deposition, and later transmural extravasation of plasma elicits a periarteritic inflammatory reaction. It follows that the evolution of the vascular fibrinoid takes the same course in humans as in experimental models, depending on the degree and duration of injury and on vascular structure.

CHRONIC LESIONS OF SMALL VESSELS

The specimens used for the study of acute vascular injury by various diseases also permitted conclusions on chronic lesions, because various stages of acute-to-chronic transition of vascular changes were encountered in all pictures investigated.

In certain cases the segmental necrosis of the vessel wall was followed by a segmental, regenerative cell proliferation (Plates LIX/241; LXVIII/174) resulting in a unilateral reduction of the lumen, as in the model experiments (Plate LXV/108, 117, 118). In other cases, cell proliferation took place along the entire circumference of the vessel, reducing the lumen uniformly to a high degree (Plate LXVIII/175, 176). The bulk of the lumen-reducing growth consisted of cellular elements, most of which were identified as smooth muscle cells (Plate LXVIII/177) by polarization microscopy and various staining techniques. Between the cells, newly formed elastic fibres of varying number and size were detected by staining with resorcin-fuchsin (Plates LIX/243; LXVIII/178–181), as in experimental lesions (Plate LXV/114, 118, 119). Thus the newly formed vessel wall, which developed above the deteriorated IEL, consisted initially of smooth muscle cells and elastic fibres. Later, part of the cellular components (degenerated and collagenous fibres appeared in their place (Plate LXVIII/182). Thus the regenerative proliferation of the vessel wall was first of a myoelastotic, later of a myoelasto-fibrotic nature. The periadventitial inflammatory change became gradually replaced by collagen-rich scar tissue (Plate LXVIII/175).

The above phenomena of acute-to-chronic transition of vascular change had not previously been observed. Recently, proliferative growths reducing the lumen nearly to obstruction have repeatedly been encountered, above all in cases surviving under a specific prednisolone therapy (Plate LXVIII/176). The progression of the regenerative lesion to this extreme degree is clearly related to the once unprecedented prolongation of the patient's life by drug therapy. It should be, nevertheless, noted that in certain cases prednisolone or other cortisone derivatives elicit through vascular permeability-increasing action a fibrinoid change and even haemorrhage. The question is, therefore, justly posed whether the IP might originate from thrombus organization. This can be excluded in the first place by the fact that thrombosis was never observed in the cases studied by us, secondly, by the frequent presence of an IP already in the acute stage of the change (Plate LXVIII/183).

The hyaline transformation of the human subendothelial fibrinoid took the same course as in the experimental lesions, to judge from the staining reactions, i.e. red-to-blue and black-to-yellow colour transitions with azan and M-stain, respectively. The most typical examples of hyaline transformation have been observed in splenic arteries, in which antigen–antibody reactions greatly enhance the intramural diffusion of plasma, and this often becomes hyalinized directly, without an intermediate fibrinoid change.

Apparently, the evolution of the vascular fibrinoid in humans can be divided into successive stages, of which the appearance of the fibrinoid itself is the last. Muscle cell necrosis plays a decisive role in vascular wall injury (Gardner 1960, 1963; Kojimahara, 1967), but the microscopic detection of such cells is often hampered by the presence of already established lesions. Initial single muscle cell necrosis can be detected only in those vessels in which the injury has been recurrent. In any case, muscle cell necrosis and subsequent plasma insudation were seen in all conditions studied, although less distinctly than in established lesions. Since all diseases studied were slowly progressive, early vascular changes were hardly discernible at the time of examination. The early lesions did not contain fibrin; this appeared only with the progression of vascular wall degeneration.

These findings accord well with the observation made in four different hypertensive experimental models that the vascular fibrinoid can be induced by various aetiological factors (Gardner, 1960; 1962a, b, c; Jellinek, 1967, 1970) and that its evolution takes place through different, morphologically definable stages.

Recent reports in the literature have referred to the identical nature of the vascular fibrinoid developing in response to different diseased conditions and have accordingly questioned its value in aetiological differentiation. Among others Goldberger (1959) has pointed out the difficulty of diagnostic differentiation between periarteritis nodosa and rheumatic arteritis as well as between hypertension and periarteritis, and Boyd (1957), Fischer (1957) and Bosch (1960) have reported similar problems in the relation of rheumatic fever and periarteritis nodosa. Koszewski (1958) and Koszewski and Hubbard (1957) held the view that periarteritis nodosa and Takayashu's disease represent one and the same picture according to Jäger (1932), periarteritis nodosa and Buerger's disease, and to Fischer and Hellstrom (1961), Cogan's and Buerger's disease are histologically indistinguishable. Most authors, however, agree that the vascular fibrinoid is a typical lesion in several of these conditions. As to the evolution of the fibrinoid, some authors have attributed the primary role to plasma insudation (More and McLean, 1949; Movat and More, 1957; Movat and Fernando, 1963a; Vazquez and Dixon, 1957, 1958; Zollinger, 1959; Cohen and Sapp, 1959; Veress et al., 1966b; Jellinek, 1969, 1970b; Jellinek et al., 1967a, b, c; Fuchs, 1970), while others have implicated medial muscle cell necrosis (Arkin, 1930; Muirhead et al., 1951a, Muirhead and Grollman, 1951a; Montgomery et al., 1953; Montgomery and Muirhead 1954; Gardner, 1962c, 1963; Churg, 1963; Veress et al., 1966a). Vazquez and Dixon (1957, 1958) and Winsor (1958) have published micrographs showing the presence of fibrin in the vessel wall, to affirm the association of this lesion with certain diseases. It is, however, clear from the analysis of human and experimental vascular lesions that the fibrinoid necrosis of muscular-type small arteries is a common change in several diseases and, therefore, not characteristic of any of them, and for the same reason, the dominant morphological features of the vascular lesions have no diagnostic value either. Various degrees of vascular wall injury have consistently been encountered in all diseases studied, and the morphological appearance of the lesions depended exclusively on the duration of the condition. If the disease is prolonged the microscopic picture is dominated by the fibrin-containing fibrinoid necrosis and early changes are detected with difficulty. If the disease takes a short, fatal course, many early lesions can be seen. In view of these observations we disagree with the concept that fibrin-containing vascular lesions are typical of certain diseases. A further objection to this view is that microscopic periarteritis nodosa lesions may not only be identical with those caused by Wegener's granulomatosis, but they are in fact histologically indistinguishable from those arising in noradrenalin-induced experimental hypertension Jellinek, 1966b). Similar, if not identical, vascular changes may also occur in human and experimental hypertension.

Chronic proliferation, lamellar elastosis and myoelastofibrosis occurred in the same form in human lesions as in the experimental models. Formerly, such chronic changes were rarely reported and their recent greater frequency may well be ascribed to the prolongation of the patient's survival time by modern therapeutic measures. The occasional presence of such changes in various organs was probably responsible for the earlier view that they were manifestations of an organic Buerger's disese.

CORRELATION OF HUMAN LARGE VESSEL LESIONS WITH SIMILAR CHANGES IN EXPERIMENTAL ANIMALS

Large vessel changes in humans originate primarily from Buerger's disease. The pathomorphology of lesions associated with this condition was analysed by Jäger (1932) who also reported the occurrence of periarteritis nodosa-like lesions in visceral organs in a typical case of Buerger's disease. He suggested that these two vascular diseases probably represent different vascular manifestations of the same damage. The truth of this assertion has since been verified by the experimental evidence that vascular response to various injuries is essentially uniform, independently of the type of the vessel. Some experimental observations made earlier in this institute should be discussed in this context. Rats kept hypertensive for 70 days under the usual experimental conditions of the Lőrincz–Gorácz model showed, in addition to a fibrinoid change of small vessels, mesenteric large vessel lesions reminiscent of Buerger's disease. The vascular lumen was reduced by fresh or organized thrombi, inflammatory cells infiltrated the media and adventitia and there was a distinct perivascular granulation (Plate LXVIII/184).

Necrosis of the intima, thrombus formation and organization as well as fibrosis of the IEL have been known as the characteristic pathomorphological changes of Buerger's disease. Experiments on muscular-type vessels have suggested that any kind of vascular injury is followed by an elastomuscular transformation—regeneration—of the vessel wall, whether or not thrombus formation has taken place. The periarterial changes observed by Jäger (1932) in Buerger's disease may also appear around muscular-type large arteries and initiate in them a regenerative process consisting of cell proliferation and of a reduplication of elastic fibres. Naturally, an allergic factor may also play a role in the process and according to certain authors, may initiate a fibrinoid transformation of the intima which will again result in proliferation and further reduction of the lumen.

Changes reminiscent of Buerger's disease may appear in the conditions studied if these take a prolonged course. Muscular type vessels become affected in the same manner as large muscular arteries under experimental conditions. Frequent investigations of biopsy specimens from cases with Buerger disease-like symptoms have convinced us that a histological diagnosis of this condition is often impossible, while diseases of a different symptomatology may often appear histologically as Buerger's disease as, e.g. in the following case:

Male patient, aged 23, a football team member. After training in melting snow, circulation stopped in both legs, this was accompanied by severe pain, and finally both legs had to be amputated for gangrene. Grossly, the amputated parts showed gangrene of the toes and tarsal area and a lamellar detachment of skin in other regions. Microscopically, the vessels contained a loose, partly recanalized and vascularized fibrous tissue originating from thrombus organization, the vessel walls showed secondary dystrophic changes and occasional fresh thrombi. The gangrene resulted from a cold-induced powerful vasospasm of constricted and recanalized vessels and a slight fresh thrombotic complication aggravated the picture.

Various inflammatory conditions may initiate an IP and a reduction of the lumen. In a case of Takayashu's disease (Jellinek et al., 1963), specific giant-cell proliferation (Plate LIX/242) resulted in the formation of an IP which practically obliterated the lumen; the IP was composed of smooth muscle cells (Plate XL/177) and newly formed elastic fibres (Plate LIX/243) like the similar experimental lesions (Plates LXI/7, 10–12; LXII/41).

The secondary role of vasoconstriction is supported by the observation of Seeliger and Schopper (1969) that in 33 cases of digital gangrene, obliteration of the vascular lumen was consequent to proliferation. The same authors consider that the term endangiitis is erroneous, because inflammation is rare in such conditions. Although the cell proliferation may be initiated by inflammation, it may as well result from any other cause that affects the nutrition of the vascular wall, such as, e. g. innervation disorders. Bednar (1970) has justly opposed the use of the term angiohypertrophic myleomalacia (Foix-Alajonanine), at least until more details become known about the aetiology and pathogenesis.

On analysing 137 cases of non-syphilitic aortitis from 14 countries, Restrepo et al. (1969) concluded that although the causative factors were various, the mechanism of vascular-wall transformation was essentially similar. Aortic injury and reparation often follow upon a primary injury of the vasa vasorum (Jellinek et al. 1969; Kemnitz and Willgeroth, 1969).

A non-specific response of the vessel may be elicited by high perfusion pressure during surgery (Silver et al., 1969). Certain authors have tried to distinguish such changes from sclerotic lesions, but this seems fairly difficult. For example, homocysteinaemia may elicit a mural reaction which may be modified in its course by the presence of the damaging substance, but its final issue is the same as in the above pictures (McCully, 1969).

The many correlations in the causation and pathogenesis of small and large vessel lesions are well illustrated by the following case report:

Female patient, aged 22, developed arthritic complaints 1 month after delivery. The small joints of the arms and legs exhibited a painful swelling and reddening. A temporary improvement resulted from treatment with Rheosolone (2 mg prednisolone and 100 mg phenylbutazone, Kőbányai Gyógyszergyár) but the pain was recurrent and a diagnosis of SLE was established after one and a half years. Two years after the onset of the disease, gangrene of the fingers and toes developed, followed by impaired renal function, acute abdominal pain, and circulatory and respiratory insufficiency.

Post-mortem diagnosis: Systemic lupus erythematosus with generalized organic changes and a dominant vascular injury resulting in infarctions, necrosis and gangrenes. Very remarkably, the large branches of the visceral and peripheral arteries showed an endarteritis obliterans-type vasculitis. The phases of the clinical course were more or less precisely reflected by the vascular changes (Plate LXVIII/187), which represented all stages from an acute fibrinoid necrosis to an arteriosclerotic plaque (Plate LXVIII/185–188).

Apart from an acute fibrinoid change (Plate LXVIII/185), some vessels showed a periarteritis-like proliferation (Plate LXVIII/185), larger ones showed a proliferation reminiscent of Buerger's disease (Plate LXVIII/186, 187). The changes produced several vascular layers (Plate LXVIII/187) in accordance with the clinical phases and symptoms. The aortic subendothelial fibrinoid deposition, showing the initial signs of an IP (Plate LXVIII/188) resembled in every respect the subendothelial lesions of hypertensive experimental models (Plate LXVII/28, 29) and chronic hypertensive changes (Plate LXII/25). Lipid-like substances were demonstrated in the aortic lesion by specific stains.

These proliferative vascular changes account for the association of gangrene with SLE, which is usually rare, and also confirm the variation of lesions with the vascular structure in response to a given injury: in small vessels a fibrinoid necrosis, in muscular vessels a Buerger-type change and in the aorta arteriosclerotic lesions were simultaneously present in the terminal stage of the disease.

It appears that according to Jäger's (1932) concept, apart from acute small vessel lesions, similar but minor changes arise in large arteries which progress to a proliferative process. The periarteritic changes described above were of this type, as were the proliferative phenomena observed in a streptomycin-treated case of chronic basilar meningitits. Proliferative changes of large muscular vessels also occur in malignant hypertension and after the drug therapy of collagenoses.

The comparison of experimental hypertensive changes with human lesions has served to confirm the conclusions inferred from experimental observation. It appears that the vascular changes developing in response to various injuries are morphologically similar. In small vessels a characteristic fibrinoid necrosis develops which undergoes a myoelastofibrotic-sclerotic transformation during the stage of repair. In large vessels, the progression of the lesion is greatly influenced by the mural structure, but the fundamental phenomena of the change are essentially the same as in small vessels. Elastic elements of the vessel wall retard, or even inhibit plasma insudation and the development of fibrinoid necrosis. In vessels with a distinct IEL, the latter divides the intramural fibrin deposition into two morphologically distinguishable forms, the subendothelial and media fibrinoid. In large vessels with a strong IEL, intramural plasma deposition and fibrinoid change are retarded in the subendothelial space and subsequent hyaline transformation of the subendothelial fibrinoid serves as a basis for the hyaline arteriosclerotic plaque. In small vessels with a weak IEL, plasma insudation intermingles with the necrotic smooth muscle cells of the media to give rise to the media fibrinoid, which initiates a regenerative proliferation of the intima, serving as a basis of the cellular arteriosclerotic plaque. Secondary fat deposition in both types of fibrinoid change results in the establishment of the typical atheroma which is no longer conclusive as to the causative factor originally responsible for the change.

APPENDIX

DESCRIPTION OF SURGICAL METHODS AND FIXING AND STAINING TECHNIQUES FREQUENTLY REFERRED TO IN THIS BOOK

RAT EXPERIMENTAL HYPERTENSION MODEL ELABORATED BY LŐRINCZ AND GORÁCZ

The experimental rat hypertension model proposed by Lőrincz and Gorácz (1954; Gorácz, 1963) is a perinephritic form of the so-called renal hypertension. The working principle of the method is that foreign bodies placed in the surroundings of the kidney cause tissue irritation, inflammation and scar formation, resulting in compression of the kidney and, in some cases, even in hypertension, if the surgical intervention is bilateral. Dunihue (1941) and Gross (1958) suggested the role of the renin-angiotensin mechanism in perinephritic hypertension, whereas Bohle et al. (1953), Omae et al. (1961) and Endes (1963) have doubted the importance of renin and of the juxtaglomerular system. Gorácz (1963) observed that no normalization of the blood pressure took place after the elimination of renal ischaemia.

SURGICAL PROCEDURE

A single operation is performed. An incision is made in the back of the rat along the dorsal median line, then the kidneys are exposed and the renal capsules are removed, taking care not to injure the adrenals. A perforated rubber sheet, prepared from a surgical glove, is placed on each kidney by gently drawing the kidney through the opening, avoiding compression of the hiluses. The kidney is then wrapped in the rubber sheet and the casing is fixed by tying the ends of the sheet below the renal pole (Plate LX/244, 245). Compression can be adjusted by making taut the sheet, as required. After the rubber casing is set 20,000 IU penicillin, dissolved in 0.5 ml saline, is sprayed into the operation field by a syringe, then the muscles are united by a silk suture, and the skin is closed by clamps after sprinkling Ultraseptyl (sulphamethylthiazole) powder on the subcutis. Solanid in an 0.1 ml per 100 g dose is administered i.m. at surgery and on two subsequent days. The operated animals are given a synthetic rat feed (LATI) and drinking water ad libitum. Hypertension becomes established 2–3 days after the operation or by 14 days at the latest. The rubber casing rapidly elicits blood pressure rise through direct compression of the kidney. One layer of connective tissue overgrows either side of the rubber capsule, one separating it from the kidney itself, the other from the visceral organs. Blood pressure measurements on the operated animals were carried out under aether anaesthesia by Bonsman and Balogh's photoelectric cell method, by an Oscillometre Enregisteur type FC 12 apparatus made in France and by a piezoelectric signal transformer constructed by Oravetz et al. (1971). Compression by the rubber casing elicited a blood pressure rise of 58–80 mm Hg from a normal level of 80–115 mm Hg.

RAT EXPERIMENTAL HYPERTENSION MODEL ELABORATED BY ROJO-ORTEGA AND GENEST (1968)

Rats of both sexes, weighing more than 300 g, are used. Abdominal incision is made to expose the abdominal cavity and the intestines are drawn aside to find the aorta in the retroperitoneal cavity. The aortic segment between the two renal arteries is then ligated, resulting in atrophy of the left kidney, which gives rise to hypertension in 90 per cent of the operated animals.

AZAN STAINING TECHNIQUE AS MODIFIED BY KRUTSAY

Rinsing of de-paraffinized section in distilled water and 0.5% Orange G solution	3 min
Rinsing in 2% acetic acid, 0.1% acid fuchsin	5 min
Rinsing in 2% acetic acid, immersion in 5% filtered PTA	2 min
Rinsing in 2% acetic acid, 0.5% aniline blue solution	10 min
Rinsing in 2% acetic acid, 96% ethanol	
Dehydration; mounting in Canada balsam	

MALLORY'S PHOSPHOTUNGSTIC ACID HAEMATOXYLIN STAINING TECHNIQUE (MODIFIED)

Treatment with sublimate is necessary for formalin-fixed specimens.

De-paraffinized section is rinsed in distilled water, placed in saturated sublimate (56 °C) for 3 hours;
Washing in distilled water, incubated in Lugol solution for 3–24 hours;
Placed in 5% Na-thiosulphate, until brown colour vanishes;
Soaking in 0.25% potassium permanganate for 5 minutes;
Washing twice in distilled water;
Placed in 5% oxalic acid for 5 minutes;
Rinsing in distilled water or soaking, if required, placed in phosphotungstic acid-haematoxylin for 24 hours at room temperature;
Rinsing in distilled water for 1–3 minutes, dehydration and mounting in Canada balsam.

MAYAHARA'S ALKALINE PHOSPHATASE REACTION FOR LIGHT-MICROSCOPIC INVESTIGATIONS (MODIFIED)

Incubation solution:

0.2 M TRIS-HCl buffer, pH 8.5 (final conc. 28 mM)	2.8 ml
0.1 M Na-beta-glycerolphosphate (final conc. 20 mM)	4.0 ml
15 mM magnesium phosphate (final conc. 3.9 mM)	5.2 ml
Saturated alkaline lead citrate solution, pH about 10.0	8.0 ml

Preparation:

0.464 g $^{20}Pb(OH)_2$ (0.1 M)

0.474 g Na_3 citrate   (0.133 M)

in 10 ml distilled water;

shake, and filter several times.

8% sucrose

pH is adjusted to 9.2–9.4 by addition of 0.1 N NaOH or 0.1 N HCl,

Incubation solution is filtered;

Incubation: unfixed sections for 2–5 min at 20 °C

            fixed sections for 10–40 min at 20 °C

Incubated sections are washed in 0.2 M Tris-HCl buffer, pH 8.5; developed in ammonium polysulphide for 2–3 min, washed twice in distilled water and mounted in glycerol gelatin.

PROCESSING OF SECTIONS FOR ELECTRON-MICROSCOPIC EXAMINATIONS

1. Fixation for 2 hours in 6% glutaraldehyde-containing Holt's fixing solution:

       19 ml Holt's fixing solution

       +6 ml glutaraldehyde

2. Washing in Holt's washing solution for 24 hours

3. Fixation in 1% osmium tetroxide   2 h

4. Washing in Millonig buffer   10 min

5. Dehydration in graded ethanol:

       30%   ethanol   10 min

       50%   ethanol   10 min

       70%   ethanol   15 min

       75%   ethanol, containing

       0.5% uranyl acetate   1 h

       90%   ethanol   10 min

       96%   ethanol   15 min

       absolute ethanol   45 min, twice exchanged

       propylene oxide   20 minutes, once exchanged

        1 : 1 mixture of propylene oxide and Araldite

6. Embedding:

    Araldite, twice for 1 hour at 37 °C (in incubator)

      embedding in capsule, or in a paper boat, then incubation for 24 hours at 37 °C (incubator)

7. Staining of sections:

    Immersion in 6% uranyl acetate dissolved in 50% methanol for 20 minutes (solution must be filtered prior to use)

    Rinsing three times in concentrated methanol

    Staining with lead citrate for 20 minutes

    Rinsing three times in double distilled water

Chemicals: Holt's fixing solution
        750 g glucose
         85 g Na_2HPO_4
         25 g KH_2PO_4
         1 litre formalin to 10 litres distilled water
Holt's rinsing solution (same as fixing solution except for formalin component)
        Millonig buffer, pH 7.4
         A + B + C + D solutions:
        solution A: 2.26% NaH_2PO_4
        solution B: 2.523% NaOH
        solution C: 5.4%   glucose solution
        solution D: 83 ml A + 17 ml B
Buffer: mixture of 90 ml D and 10 ml C solution
Osmium also is diluted in Millonig buffer
Araldite mixture (Fluka AMC, Switzerland)
        7.5 ml A
        7.5 ml B
        0.7 ml C
        0.4 ml D
Preparation of lead citrate:
        1.33 g $Pb(NO_3)_2$ and 1.76 g $Na_3(C_6H_5O_7) \cdot 2\,H_2O$ are dissolved each in 15 ml distilled water, mixed and shaken for 1 hour; then 8 ml NaOH is added and the mixture is made up to 50 ml with distilled water.

Preparation is difficult, because the material is very sensitive, but a well-mixed solution keeps for a long time in the refrigerator.

WATER-SOLUBLE DURCUPAN EMBEDDING (DURCUPAN, FLUKA, SWITZERLAND)

Durcupan is supplied in the form of 4 separate components of which only one is completely water soluble. This component is used to dehydrate tissue by diluting to graded percentages.

Embedding schedule:
      50% component A in H_2O 2 h
      70% component A in H_2O 2 h
      90% component A in H_2O 2 h
   100% component A in H_2O 3 h
                            (3 × 1 h changes)
Tissue is then placed in the following mixture overnight at 4 °C:

Complete resin:
      Component A   5   ml
      Component B   11.7 ml
      Component C   1.4 ml
      Component D   0.3 ml

Immersion in fresh mixture for 4–6 hours follows overnight incubation, then the mixture is exchanged for a third time and allowed to polymerize for 24–48 hours at 48 °C, with the tissue block embedded.

ELASTASE DIGESTION PROCEDURE

Porcine pancreatic purified elastase (Worthington) is used at a concentration of 6.4 IU per ml (1 mg elastase contains 80 IU) in a carate buffer solution (0.025 M, pH 8.8). Ultra-thin sections mounted on copper grids are immersed in the enzyme solution and incubated for 15 minutes at 37 °C, rinsed several times in distilled water and stained with uranylic acid or PTA.

HUGEN–BORGERS' ALKALINE PHOSPHATASE REACTION FOR ELECTRON-MICROSCOPIC INVESTIGATIONS (DIRECT LEAD METHOD)

The specimen is fixed in 6% glutaraldehyde-containing TRIS-maleate buffer (pH 8.2) for 2 hours
100 μ sections are cut
Sections are washed in 0.33 M glucose containing TRIS-maleate buffer, pH 8.2, and incubated for 30–60 minutes at 37 °C.

    Incubation solution:

TRIS-maleate buffer pH 9	2 ml
1.25% Na-beta-glycerolphosphate	2 ml
distilled water	4.7 ml
lead nitrate, 1%	1.3 ml

After incubation, the sections are dehydrated and embedded. The incubation solution is allowed to stand after mixing for 30 minutes each at 37 °C and at room temperature.

The TRIS-maleate buffer is prepared according to the method of Barka and Anderson.

Processing is essentially the same for light-microscopic investigations, only 10 μ sections are cut, distilled water is used for rinsing after incubation and developing is made in ammonium sulphide for 2–3 minutes, followed by repeated rinsing in distilled water.

The sections are mounted in glycerol-gelatin.

RUTHENIUM RED (FLUKA, SWITZERLAND; PURIFIED ACCORDING TO BROOKS) TREATMENT FOR ELECTRON-MICROSCOPIC EXAMINATION

1. Fixation: 1.2% glutaraldehyde dissolved in 0.067 M, pH 7.3, Na-cacodylate containing 1 mg per ml ruthenium red, for 1 hour at room temperature
2. Washing: in 0.15 M, pH 7.3 Na-cacodylate buffer, for 10 minutes at 4 °C

3. Immersion in 2% Na-cacodylate (0.067 M, pH 7.3), containing 1 mg per ml ruthenium red, for 3 hours at 20 °C
4. Washing in Na-cacodylate buffer (0.067 M, pH 7.3), and embedding for electron-microscopic examination

RUTHENIUM-RED STAINING TECHNIQUE (LUFT METHOD)

1. Specimen is immersed in 6% distilled glutaraldehyde made up in 0.1 M, pH 7.2 cacodylate buffer, containing 1 mg per ml ruthenium red (Lepkin and Williams Ltd., England) for 1 hour at 4 °C
2. Washing in 0.1 M cacodylate buffer for 15 minutes (3 changes)
3. Postfixing in Veronal-buffered (pH 7.2) 1% OSO_4, containing 1 mg per ml ruthenium red, for 3 hours
4. Embedding for electron microscopy

METHOD OF EXPERIMENTS WITH PEROXIDASE, FERRITIN AND COLLOIDAL CARBON

Experimental animals under ether anaesthesia received by injection into a femoral vein 8 mg peroxidase in 0.5 ml per 100 g saline, for 100 g body weight, or 100 mg ferritin in 0.1 ml per 100 g saline, for 100 g body weight, or 0.1 ml colloidal carbon for 100 g body weight.

The aorta was perfused directly (Forssmann, 1969) with fixative, through the left ventricle of the heart, 1.5, 6 and 30 minutes after peroxidase injection and at 6 and 30 minutes after administration of ferritin or colloidal carbon. Perfusion fixation was carried out under 120 mm Hg pressure for 5 minutes, using a mixture of 1% freshly prepared paraformaldehyde and 1.25% purified glutaraldehyde (Fahimi and Drochmans, 1965), in 0.1 N Na-cacodylate buffer (pH 7.4), containing 5% sucrose (final osmolality: 750 mOsm). Small aortic blocks secured from the subdiaphragmatic segment of the abdominal aorta were used for electron-microscopic examination and accordingly postfixed for 2 hours in a mixture of 2% paraformaldehyde and 2.5 per cent glutaraldehyde, in the same buffer (final osmolality: 900 mOsm) (Karnovsky, 1965, 1967), and washed for 2 hours at 4 °C in 0.1 N Na-cacodylate buffer (pH 7.4), containing 11.25% sucrose (final osmolality: 380 mOsm). Then tissue blocks were incubated in the Graham–Karnovsky medium (0.05 TRIS-HCl buffer, pH 7.6, 10 ml, containing 0.01 per cent H_2O_2 and 10 mg 3,3'-diaminobenzidine tetrahydrochloride) (Graham and Karnovsky, 1966) for 30–60 minutes at room temperature, washed three times in distilled water, postfixed for 90 minutes with 1% OsO_4 in Palade buffer, pH 7.4, containing 4.9% sucrose (final osmolality: 430 mOsm) and washed again in the buffer solvent of the fixative (final osmolality: 380 mOsm). Specimens secured from the aorta of ferritin-treated or colloidal carbon-treated rats were processed as above, except for incubation in the peroxidase-containing medium. After each procedure, tissue blocks were dehydrated in graded ethanol and embedded in Epon (Luft, 1961). Ultra-thin sections were cut with diamond knives. Unstained sections and sections stained with ethanolic uranyl acetate and lead citrate (Venable and Coggeshall, 1965) were examined for the tracers.

PUBLICATIONS BY THE EDITOR AND HIS TEAM

Bálint, A., Nagy, Z. (1971): Permeability traces and serum proteins. *Experientia (Basel)* **27,** 175.

Bálint, A., Veres, B., Kóczé, A., Nagy, Z., Jellinek, H. (1970): Az aorta permeabilitásának fokozódása atherogen diéta hatására (Increasing aortic permeability by atherogenic diet). *Morph. Ig. Orv. Szemle* **10,** 2.

Bálint, A., Veress, B., Nagy, Z., Jellinek, H. (1971): Role of lipophages in development of rat atheroma. *J. Atheroscler. Res.* **15,** 7.

Csillag, I., Gergely, R., Jellinek, H. (1955): Experimental data of the pathogenesis of gastric haemorrhage. *Acta morph. Acad. Sci. hung.* V/1 **2,** 183.

Csillag, I., Jellinek, H. (1959a): Regeneration des Wanddefektes grosser Venen nach homo-, hetero- und alloplastischem Ersatz. *Zbl. allg. Path. path. Anat.* **100,** 173.

Csillag, I., Jellinek, H. (1959b): Über die Verwendung von Pflanzenstoffen zur Versorgung der Wanddefekte grosser Venen. *Zbl. allg. Path. path. Anat.* **100,** 181.

Csillag, I., Jellinek, H. (1960): Regeneration of the wall of large veins with different grafts. *Acta chir. Acad. Sci. hung.* **1,** 4.

Csillag, I., Jellinek, H. (1961): A new method of treatment for injuries of the great veins. Their regeneration under different transplantation conditions. *Quart. Rev. Surg.* **18,** 111.

Földi, M., Jellinek, H., Rusznyák, I., Szabó, Gy. (1954): Vizsgálatok a nyirokcapillarisok működéséről (Investigations on the activity of lymphatic capillaries). *Osztályközlemények* **5,** 89.

Földi, M., Jellinek, H., Rusznyák, I., Szabó, Gy. (1955): Eiweißspeicherung in den Endothelzellen der Lymphkapillaren. *Acta med. Acad. Sci. hung.* **7,** 211.

Földi, M., Jellinek, H., Szabó, Gy. (1955): Untersuchungen über das Lymphsystem der Schilddrüse. *Acta med. Acad. Sci. hung.* **7,** 161.

Hüttner, I., Jellinek, H., Kerényi, T. (1968): Fibrin formations in vascular fibrinoid change in experimental hypertension. An electron microscopic study. *Exp. molec. Path.* **9,** 309.

Hüttner, I., Jellinek, H., Kerényi, T., Szemenyei, K. (1965): Savecseteléssel létrehozott fibrinoid és falnekrozis kialakulása (Fibrinoid necrosis of the vascular wall induced by painting with acid). *Morph. Ig. Orv. Szemle* **5,** 91.

Hüttner, I., Jellinek, H., Kerényi, T., Szemenyei, K. (1966a): Fibrinoid necrosis of the vascular wall induced by painting with acid. *Acta morph. Acad. Sci. hung.* **14,** 169.

Hüttner, I., Kerényi, T., Pogátsa, G., Gábor, Gy., Veress, B., Jellinek, H. (1966b): Coronarveränderungen nach Gabe von Noradrenalin und Isodihydroperparin. *Frankf. Z. Path.* **76,** 107.

Hüttner, I., Kerényi, T., Veress, B., Tóth, A., Konyár, Éva, Jellinek, H. (1967a): Über die Verteilung der alkalischen Phosphatase in der Gefässadventitia von Ratten bei experimenteller Hypertonie. *Acta Histochem. (Jena)* **26,** 21.

Hüttner, I., More, R. H. (1970): Ultrastructural evidence for specific endothelial permeability in experimental hypertension. *Fed. Proc.* **29,** Abstracts, p. 488.

Hüttner, I., More, R. H., Jellinek, H. (1970a): Vascular hyalinosis resulting from fibrinoid change. Fifty-Ninth Annual Meeting of the International Academy of Pathology, 11 March, 1970, Abstr.

Hüttner, I., More, R. H., Jellinek, H. (1970b): Vascular hyalinosis resulting from fibrinoid change. An electron microscopic study. *Lab. Invest.* **22,** 501.

Hüttner, I., More, R. H., Rona, G. (1970c): Fine structural evidence of specific mechanism for increased endothelial permeability in experimental hypertension. *Amer. J. Path.* **61**, 395.

Hüttner, I., More, R. H., Rona, G., Jellinek, H. (1969a): Diversity of fibrin ultrastructure in experimental vascular fibrinoid. *Lab. Invest.* **20**, 588 (Abstract).

Hüttner, I., More, R. H., Rona, G., Jellinek, H. (1970d): Mechanism of increased transport in arterial endothelium during experimental hypertension. 8th International Congress of the International Academy of Pathology, Mexico City.

Hüttner, I., Rona, G., Jellinek, H., More, R. H. (1969b): Atherosclerosis as a 'healing process' of fibrinoid vascular change. An ultrastructural study. 2nd International Symposium on Atherosclerosis. Nov. 25, Chicago, Abstr.

Hüttner, I., Rona, G., Jellinek, H., More, R. H. (1969c); Fibrine se présentant sous la forme particulière de cristeaux dans les lesions fibrinoides vasculaires. 24e Congrès de l'Association des Médicines de Laboratoire de la Provence de Quebec. Sherbrooke, Juin 18–19, Abstr.

Hüttner, I,. Rona, G., More, R. H. (1970e): Ultrastructural studies on myocardial fibrin deposition in experimental hypertension. 3rd Annual Meeting of the International Study Group for Research in Cardiac Metabolism. Stowe, Vermont. Abstr.

Hüttner, I., Rona, G., More, R. H. (1970f): Fibrin deposition within cardiac muscle cells in experimental malignant hypertension. An electron microscopic study. *Arch. Path.* **91**, 19.

Hüttner, I., Veress, B., Tóth, A., Konyár, Éva, Kerényi, T., Jellinek, H. (1967b): Die Anwendung der unspezifischen Esterasereaktion zur Untersuchung der Zellnekrose. *Acta Histochem.* **26**, 10.

Jellinek, H. (1959): Experimental data on the pathomorphology of venous wall regeneration. Thesis, Budapest.

Jellinek, H. (1964): Similarity of non-arteriosclerotic vascular changes of different origin. Thesis, Budapest.

Jellinek, H. (1967): Fibrinoid vascular changes showing the same morphologic pattern following induction by various experimental conditions. *Angiology* **18**, 547.

Jellinek, H. (1969): Plasma in vessel walls suspect as factor in atherosclerosis. *Medical Tribune* **2**.

Jellinek, H. (1970a): Failure of etiological differentiation of human diseases associated with fibrinoid necrosis. *Angiology* **21**, 691.

Jellinek, H. (1970b): The role of the elastic membrane in the development of the two forms of vascular fibrinoid: the subendothelial and media fibrinoid. *Angiology* **21**, 636.

Jellinek, H. (1970c): The pathogenesis of atherosclerosis in arterial hypertension. *Bull. int. Soc. Cardiol.* **2**, 4.

Jellinek, H., Csillag, I. (1959a): Entwicklung elastischer Fasern in der regenerierten Venenwand nach Ablösung des Transplantates. *Zbl. allg. Path. path. Anat.* **100**, 158.

Jellinek, H., Csillag, I. (1959b): Zur Regeneration des in der homoioplastisch transplantierten Venenwand herbeigeführten Defektes. *Zbl. allg. Path. path. Anat.* **100**, 163.

Jellinek, H., Csillag, I., Gergely, R. (1958): A comparison of the experimental results for gastric hemorrhage of arterial origin with resection and autopsy material. *Surg. Gynec. Obstet.* **107**, 495.

Jellinek, H., Csillag, I., Kádár, Anna (1960): Hazai műanyag ér-protézisek alkalmazásának eredményei kisérletekben (Experimental results of the application of plastic vascular prostheses in Hungary). *Orv. Hetil.* **101**, 950.

Jellinek, H., Csillag, I., Kádár, Anna (1961a): Die Verwendung von Kunststoffprothesen in der Gefässchirurgie und histologische Untersuchungen der Gefässregeneration. *Metabolismus Parietis Vasorum* Praha, Sept. 4–9, p. 102.

Jellinek, H., Csillag, I., Kádár Anna (1961b): Regeneration of vessel walls after the implantation of knitted synthetic tubes. *Acta chir. Acad. Sci. hung.* **2**, 1.

Jellinek, H., Csillag, I., Kádár Anna (1963): Feinstrukturelle Untersuchungen bei der Anwendung von Kunststoffgefässen. *Acta chir. Acad. Sci. hung.* **4**, 257.

Jellinek, H., Csillag, I., Novák, I. (1953): A new method of resorting defects in the wall of great abdominal veins. *Acta morph. Acad. Sci. hung.* **3**, 149.

Jellinek, H., Földi, M., Büky, B., Mészáros, S. (1961c): Some data concerning the problem of interconnections between intraadventitial spaces of the pulmonary arteries and the lymph vessels. *Acta morph. Acad. Sci. hung.* **11**, 41.

Jellinek, H., Földi, M., Kádár, Anna (1961d): Die histopathologischen Folgen der Lymphgefässverödung. *Metabolismus Parietis Vasorum* Praha, Sept. 4–9, p. 412.

Jellinek, H., Gábor, Gy., Solti, F., Veress, B. (1967a): The problem of the coronary changes due to disturbance of vascular wall permeability. *Angiology* **18**, 179.

Jellinek, H., Gábor, Gy., Solti, F., Veress, B. (1968): Az érfalátáramlás szerepe a coronaria-elváltozások kialakulásában (The problem of the coronary changes due to disturbance of vascular wall permeability). *Orv. Hetil.* **108**, 2.

Jellinek, H., Hüttner, I., Kádár, Anna, Kerényi, T., Konyár, Éva, Szemenyei, Klára, Veress, B. (1967b): New ideas and possibilities in the vessel wall pathology on the basis of our experiments (In Hungarian). *MTA V. Oszt. Közl.* **18**, 265.

Jellinek, H., Hüttner, I., Kádár, Anna, Kerényi, T., Veress, B. (1967c): Vergleichende histologische und elektronenmikroskopische Untersuchungen von Gefässveränderungen verschiedenen Ursprungs. *Verh. dtsch. path. Ges.* **51**, 243.

Jellinek, H., Hüttner, I., Kerényi, T., Gábor, Gy., Pogátsa, G. (1965a): Noradrenalinnal létrehozott fibrinoid érfalnecrosis kialakulása (Fibrinoid necrosis of the vascular wall induced by noradrenalin). *Morph. Ig. Orv. Szemle* **5**, 104.

Jellinek, H., Hüttner, I., Kerényi, T., Pogátsa, G. Gábor, Gy. (1966a): Fibrinoid necrosis of the vascular wall induced by noradrenaline. *Acta morph. Acad. Sci. hung.* **14**, 183.

Jellinek, H., Hüttner, I., Kerényi, T., Veress, B., Konyár, Éva, Szentágothai, Klára (1965b): Fibrinoid necrosis of small blood vessels. *Acta morph. Acad. Sci. hung.* Suppl. **13**, 63.

Jellinek, H., Nagy, Z., Hüttner, I., Bálint, A., Kóczé, A., Kerényi, T. (1969): Investigation of the permeability changes of the vascular wall in malignant hypertension by means of colloidal iron preparation. *Brit. J. exp. Path.* **50**, 13.

Jellinek, H., Szemenyei, Klára, Kerényi, T., Hüttner, I. (1965c): Muscularis típusú kisarteriák savecsetelés után észlelt elváltozása (Alteration of muscular-type small arteries induced by painting with acid). *Morph. Ig. Orv. Szemle* **5**, 88.

Jellinek, H., Veress, B., Bálint, A., Nagy, Z. (1970): Lymph vessels to rat aorta and their changes in experimental atherosclerosis. An electron microscopic study. *Exp. Molec. Path.* **13**, 370.

Jellinek, H., Veress, B., Hüttner, I., Kerényi, T. (1966b): Über die Morphologie der lymphstauungsbedingten Koronarveränderungen. *Frankf. Z. Path.* **75**, 331.

Kádár, Anna, Farkas, Judit, Jellinek, H. (1965a): A regenerálódó aorta intima proliferatiojának sejtes elemeire vonatkozó vizsgálatok (Investigations on the cellular elements of the intimal proliferation of the regenerating aorta). *Morph. Ig. Orv. Szemle* **5**, 294.

Kádár, Anna, Gorácz, Gy., Jellinek, H., Hüttner, I. (1961): Histochemische Untersuchungen bei Gefässveränderungen mit spezieller Berücksichtigung der Gefässnekrose. *Metabolismus Parietis Vasorum* Praha, Sept. 4–9, p. 251.

Kádár, Anna, Jellinek, H., Veress, B. (1969a): The ultrastructure of cell elements and fine fiber production of regenerating great vessels. Acta VI. Internationalis Angiologorum Congressus. Editorial Cientifico-Medica, Swets and Zeitlinger, Barcelona, p. 895.

Kádár, Anna, Konyár, Éva, Jellinek, H., Lajosi, F. (1965b): Lósavóval előidézett fibrinoid érfalnecrosis kialakulásának vizsgálata (Fibrinoid necrosis induced by horse serum). *Morph. Ig. Orv. Szemle* **5**, 201.

Kádár, Anna, Veress, B., Jellinek, H. (1967): The ultrastructure of cell elements and fine fiber production of regenerating great vessels. *VIth International Congress of Angiology. Sept. 12–16, Barcelona,* Abstr.

Kádár, Anna, Veress, B., Jellinek, H. (1969b): Ultrastructural elements in experimental intimal thickening. II. Study of the development of elastic elements in intimal proliferation. *Exp. Molec. Path.* **11**, 212.

Kádár, Anna, Veress, B., Jellinek, H. (1969c): Relationship of elastic fibre production with smooth muscle cells and pulsation effects in large vessels. *Acta morph. Acad. Sci. hung.* **17**, 187.

Kádár, Anna, Veress, B., Jellinek H. (1969d): Development of elastic fibre under functional strain. *Acta morph. Acad. Sci. hung.* **17** (Proc.).

Kerényi, T., Hüttner, I., Jellinek, H. (1965): Periodikus struktúra kialakulása subendothelialis fibrinoidban (Development of periodic structure in subendothelial fibrinoid). *Morph. Ig. Orv. Szemle* **5**, 195.

Kerényi, T., Hüttner, I., Jellinek, H. (1966a): Über die Entwicklung der periodischen Struktur im subendothelialen Fibrinoid. *Z. micr. anat. Forsch.* **74**, 121.

Kerényi, T., Jellinek, H. (1970): Adatok a kísérletes hypoxiás szervkárosodások histochemiájához és szubmikroszkópos morphologiájához (Histochemistry and submicroscopical morphology of experimental hypoxic lesions). *Magy. Path. Társ. Évkönyve.*

Kerényi, T. Jellinek, H. (1971a): Adatok a hypoxiás szervkárosodások hisztokémiájához és ultrastruktúrájához (Histochemistry and ultrastructure of hypoxic organ lesions). *Magy. Path. Társ. Évkönyve.*

Kerényi, T., Jellinek, H. (1971b): Die Wirkung von Solcoseryl auf die Aortenwand-Regeneration. *Arzneimittel-Forsch.* **21**, 474.

Kerényi, T., Jellinek, H., Hüttner, I., Gorácz, Gy., Konyár, Éva (1966b): Fibrinoid necrosis of the vascular wall in experimental malignant hypertension. *Acta morph. Acad. Sci. hung.* **14**, 175.

Kerényi, T., Kádár, Anna, Soltész, L. (1973): Műanyag érprotézisek acellularis neointimája emberi anyagon (Acellular neointima of plastic vascular prostheses in humans). *Morph. Ig. Orv. Szemle* (in press).

Kóczé, A., Bálint, A., Nagy, Z., Hintalan, J., Jellinek, H. (1970): Értágulat szerepe és jelentősége a kisarteria károsodásának létrejöttében patkányokon (Role and significance of vasodilation in the development of the small artery in rat). *Morph. Ig. Orv. Szemle* **10**, 4.

Konyár, Éva, Jellinek, H. (1973): Hypotensiv készítmények hatásának érzékelése patkány experimentalis perinephritises hypertoniában (Effect of hypotensive preparations in experimental perinephritic hypertension in rat). *Gyógyszerészet* (in press).

Konyár, Éva, Krasznai, I., Földes, J., Jellinek, H. (1971): Experimentalis perinephritises laesiok savanyú mucopolysaccharida synthesisének vizsgálata ^{35}S-sulfáttal (Investigation with ^{35}S-sulphate of AMS-synthesis in experimental perinephritic lesions). *Morph. Ig. Orv. Szemle* **11**, 3.

Nagy, L., Szemenyei, Klára (1965): Vascular changes in rats painted with HCl and fed with cholesterol. *Acta morph. Acad. Sci. hung.* Suppl. **13**, 67.

Nagy, Z., Bálint, A., Solti, F., Jellinek, H. (1970): Localis mechanicus nyirokpangás hatása permeabilitásra kutyák végtagjain (Effect of local mechanic lymph congestion on the permeability of the limbs of dogs). *Morph. Ig. Orv. Szemle* **10**, 4.

Nagy, Z., Hüttner, I., Bálint, A., Kóczé, A., Kerényi, T., Jellinek, H., (1968): Érpermeabilitás változás vizsgálata kolloidalis vaskészítményekkel kísérletes malignus hypertoniában (Investigation of the permeability changes of the vascular wall in malignant hypertension by means of colloidal iron preparations). *Morph. Ig. Orv. Szemle* **8**, 198.

Nagy, Z., Jellinek, H., Veress, B., Kóczé, A., Bálint, A., Solti, F. (1969:) Effect of experimental lymph congestion on coronary artery permeability in the dog. *Acta morph. Acad. Sci. hung.* **17**, 167.

Nagy, Z., Papp, M., Bálint, A. (1971): Pancreatic vascular injury in experimental pancreas necrosis. A light- and electron-microscopic study. *Acta morph. Acad. hung.* **19**, 175.

Oravecz, Gy., Madas, I., Nagy, Z. (1971): Piesoelektromos jelátalakító felhasználásával kialakított kisállat vérnyomásmérő készülék (Apparatus for measuring blood pressure in small animals making use of piezoelectric signal transformer). *Orvos és Technika* **2**, 27.

Papp, M., Jellinek, H. (1961): Wechselbeziehungen zwischen Erkrankungen der peripheren Venen und denen der Lymphgefässe. *Metabolismus Parietes Vasorum* Praha, Sept. 4–9, p. 408.

Papp, M., Jellinek, H. (1962): Über den Zusammenhang zwischen den Erkrankungen der peripheren Venen und Lymphgefässen. *Acta. med. Acad. Sci. hung.* **XVIII/4**, 435.

Sótonyi, P., Hüttner, I., Jellinek, H., Tóth, A., Makói, Zita (1965): Enzymhistochemische Untersuchungen an den Gefässwänden bei Versuchstieren. *Acta histochem. (Jena)* **21**, 213.

Szemenyei, Klára, Kóczé, A., Jellinek, H. (1968): Experimental injury of muscular-type blood vessels by chemical agents. *Acta morph. Acad. Sci. hung.* **16,** 157.

Szemenyei, Klára, Nagy, L., Jellinek, H., Csillag, I. (1961): Submikroskopische und histochemische Untersuchungen der Aortenwand-Regeneration bei experimenteller Nekrose. *Metabolismus Parietis Vasorum*, Praha, Sept. 4–9, p. 257.

Szinay, Gy., Jellinek, H. (1951): Die Sklerose der Gefässe des Myometriums und der Ovarien. *Acta. morph. Acad. Sci. hung.* **1,** 3.

Szinay, Gy., Jellinek, H., Szeker, J. (1963): Érelváltozások a hydronephroticus és pyelonephritises vesékben (Vascular changes in the hydronephrotic and pyelonephritic kidneys). *Morph. Ig. Orv. Szemle* **3,** 48.

Veress, B., Bálint, A., Kóczé, A., Nagy, Z., Jellinek, H. (1970): Increasing aortic permeability by atherogenic diet. *J. Atheroscler. Res.* **11,** 369.

Veress, B., Jellinek, H., Bálint, A., Nagy, Z. (1969a): Az aorta nyirokereinek elektronmikroszkópos vizsgálata atherogen étrenden tartott patkányokban (Electronmicroscopic examination of the lymphatic vessels of the aorta in rats kept on atherogenic diet). *Orv. Hetil.* **110,** 2987.

Veress, B., Jellinek, H., Hüttner, I., Kerényi, T., Solti, F., Iskum, M., Hartai, Anna, Nagy, Júlia (1966a): Über die Morphologie der lymphstauungsbedingten Koronarveränderungen. *Frankfurt. Z. Path.* **75,** 331.

Veress, B., Jellinek, H., Kóczé, A., Venesz, Ilona (1969b): The distribution of lipids in malignant hypertensive fibrinoid necrosis. *J. Atheroscler. Res.* **10,** 55.

Veress, B., Kádár, Anna, Bartos, G., Jellinek, H. (1970): Electronmicroscopic examination of the incorporation of synthetic vascular prosthesis. *Acta morph. Acad. Sci. hung.* **18,** 63.

Veress, B., Kádár, Anna, Jellinek, H. (1969c): Ultrastructural elements in experimental intimal thickening. I. Electron microscopic study of the development and cellular elements of intimal proliferation. *Exp. Molec. Path.* **11,** 200.

Veress, B., Kerényi, T., Hüttner, I., Jellinek, H. (1966b): The phases of muscle necrosis. *J. Path. Bact.* **92,** 511.

Veress, B., Kóczé, A., Jellinek, H. (1969d): Morphology of early large vessel lesions in experimental hypertension. *Brit. J. exp. Path.* **50,** 600.

GENERAL BIBLIOGRAPHY

Abramson, D. I. (1962): *Blood Vessels and Lymphatics*. Academic Press, New York.

Adams, C. W. M. (1964): Arteriosclerosis in man, other mammals and birds. *Biol. Rev.* **39**, 372.

Adams, C. W. M. (1967): *Vascular Histochemistry*. Lloyd-Luke, London.

Adams, C. W. M.. Bayliss, O. B. (1963): Histochemical observations on the liberalisation and origin of sphingomyelin, cerebroside and cholesterol in the normal and atherosclerotic human artery. *J. Path. Bact.* **85**, 113.

Adams, C. W. M., Bayliss, O. B., Orton, C. C. (1967): Plasma protein accumulation in arterial degeneration. *J. Atheroscler. Res.* **7**, 473.

Adams, C. W. M., Moym, R. S. (1966): Autoradiographic demonstration of cholesterol filtration and accumulation in atheromatous rabbit aorta. *Nature (Lond.)* **210**, 175.

Adams, C. W. M., Virág, S., Morgan, R. S., Orton, C. C. (1968): Dissociation of cholesterol and ^{125}I labelled plasma protein in flux in normal and atheromatous rabbit aorta. A quantitative histochemical study. *J. Atheroscler. Res.* **8**, 679.

Ahmed, N. M. (1967): Age and sex differences in the structure of the tunica media of the human aorta. *Acta anat. (Basel)* **66**, 45.

Alarcon-Segovia, D., Brown, A. D. (1964): Classification and etiologic aspects of necrotizing angiitides; an analytic approach to a confused subject with a critical review of the evidence for hypersensitivity in polyarteriitis nodosa. *Proc. Mayo Clin.* **391**, 205.

Albertini, A. (1943): Zum Begriff der Fibrinoid Degeneration. *Schweiz. Z. allg. Path.* **6**, 417.

(Alekseyeva) Алексеева, Ш. А. (1959): Симпозиум по проблеме атеросклероза. Тхезис, Ленинград, п. 4.

Alexander, A. F., Jensen, R. (1963): Normal structure of the bovine pulmonary vasculature. *Amer. J. vet. Res.* **27**, 1083.

Alksue, J. F. (1959): The passage of colloidal particles across the dermal capillary wall under the influence of histamine. *Anat. J. exp. Physiol.* **44**, 51.

Allison, P. R., Bleehan, N., Brown, W., Pickering, G. W., Robb-Smith, A. H. T., Russel, R. P. (1967): The production and resolution of hypertensive vascular lesions in the rabbit. *Clin. Sci.* **33**, 39.

Altmann, H. W., Lick, R., Stutz, E. (1962): Die Wirkung langfristiger Bestrahlung mit radioaktivem Strontium (Sr[90]) auf die Rattenniere. *Beitr. path. Anat.* **127**, 79.

Altschul, R. (1954): *Endothelium. Its Development, Morphology, Function and Pathology*. McMillan, New York, p. 123.

Altschul, R. (1957): Über eine eigenartige Reaktion der Endothelzellen. *Virchows Arch. path. Anat.* **330**, 357.

Altschul, R., Paul-Boemler, E. (1963): Endothelium in contracted arteries. *Virchows Arch. Path. Anat.* **336**, 383.

Anderson, M. S. (1963): Electron microscopy of the glomerulus and renal tubules in experimental hypertension. *Amer. J. Path.* **43**, 257.

Andres, K. H. (1963): Elektronenmikroskopische Untersuchungen über Endoneurium in Spinalganglien von Ratten nach Bestrahlung mit 185 MEU-Protonen. *Z. Zellforsch.* **61**, 23.

Andriewitsch, P. (1901): Zur Frage über die Veränderungen der Arterienwandungen bei ihrer Reizung von Seiten der Adventitia. Inaug. Diss, St. Petersburg.

(Anestyadi, Zota) Анестиади, В., Зота, Е. (1970): Атеросклерозиеластика артерии. Картя Молдовеняские, Китинев.

Anitschkow, N. (1913): Über die Veränderungen der Kaninchenaorta bei experimenteller Cholesteatose. *Beitr. Path. Anat.* **56,** 370.

Anitschkow, N. (1933): Experimental arteriosclerosis in animals. In, Cowdry, E. V. (Ed): *Arteriosclerosis.* MacMillan, New York, p. 271.

Arkin, A. (1930): A clinical and pathological study of periarteritis nodosa. *Amer. J. Path.* **6,** 401.

Arnold, J. (1873): Über Diapedesis. Eine experimentelle Studie. *Arch. Path. Anat.* **58,** 203.

Arturson, G., Kjellmer, I. (1964): Capillary permeability in skeletal muscle during rest and activity. *Acta physiol. scand.* **62,** 41.

Ascheim, E. (1964): Determination of vascular permeability. *Nature (Lond.)* **201,** 1201.

Aschoff, L. (1924): *Placed Particular Emphasis on the Thesis of Lipid Inhibition at the Sites of Degeneration.* Hoeder, New York, p. 131.

Ashford, T. P., Freiman, D. G. (1967): The role of the endothelium in the initial phases of thrombosis (an EM study.) *Amer. J. Path.* **297,** 257.

Ashford, T. P., Palmerio, C., Fine, J. (1966): Structural analogue in vascular muscle to the functional disorder in refractory traumatic shock and reversal by corticosteroid; electron microscopic evaluation. *Amer. J. Surg.* **164,** 575.

Ashworth, C. T., Haynes, D. M. (1948): Lesion in elastic arteries associated with hypertension. *Amer. J. Path.* **24,** 195.

Ashworth, C. T., Stenbridge, V. A., Sanders, E. (1960): Lipid absorption, transport and hepatic assimilation with electron microscopy. *Amer. J. Physiol.* **198,** 1326.

Asscher, A. W., Anson, S. G. (1963): A vascular permeability factor of renal origin. *Nature (Lond.)* **198,** 1097.

Auerbach, D. (1877): Über die Obliteration der Arterien nach Ligatur. Thesis, Bonn.

(Avtandilov) Автандилов, Т. Т. (1970): Динамика атеросклеротического процесса у человека. Академия медицинских Наук СССР, Медицина, Москва.

Bader, H. (1963): The anatomy and physiology of the vascular wall. In, Dow, P. (Ed.): *Handbook of Physiology.* Section 2, Circulation 2. American Physiological Society, Washington. D. C., p. 865.

Baggenstoss, A. H., Shick, R. M., Polley, H. F. (1951): The effect of cortisone on the lesions of periarteriitis nodosa. *Amer. J. Path.* **27,** 537.

Balis, J. V., Chan, A. S., Cohen, R. E. (1966): Lathyrogenic injury to foetal rat aorta and postnatal repair. *Exp. molec. Path.* **5,** 396.

Balis, J. V., Chan, A. S., Cohen, R. E. (1967): Morphogenesis of human aortic correlation. *Exp. molec. Path.* **6,** 25.

Balis, J. V., Haust, M. D., Morek, R. H. (1964): Electronmicroscopic studies in human atherosclerosis; cellular elements in aortic fatty streaks. *Exp. molec. Path.* **3,** 521.

Ball, J. (1954): Rheumatoid arthritis and polyarteritis nodosa. *Ann. rheum. Dis.* **13,** 277.

Baló, J. (1924): Periarteritis nodosa beim Hunde und vergleichende Untersuchungen über diese Erkrankungen beim Menschen und Hunde. *Virchows Arch. path. Anat.* **248,** 337.

Baló, J. (1958): Elastase és atherosclerosis (Elastase and atherosclerosis). *MTA Biol. és Orv. Oszt. Közl.* **9,** 425.

Baló, J., Banga, I. (1949a): Die Zerstörung der elastischen Fasern der Gefässwand. *Schweiz. Z. Path.* **12,** 350.

Baló, J., Banga, I. (1949b): Elastase and elastase inhibitor. *Nature (Lond.)* **164,** 491.

Baló, J., Banga, I. (1950): Elastolytic activity of pancreatic extracts. *Biochem. J.* **46,** 384.

Banga, I. (1966): *Structure and Function of Elastin and Collagen.* Akadémiai Kiadó, Budapest.

Banga, I., Loeven, W. A., Romhányi, Gy. (1965): Histochemical studies of elastic fibres by the use of elastolytic enzymes separated by chromatography on DEAE sephadex column. *Acta. morph. Acad. Sci. hung.* **13,** 385.

Banga, I., Schuler, D., László, J. (1954): Change of elastase inhibitor in the blood of ammonium hydroxide treated rabbits. *Acta physiol. Acad. Sci. hung.* **5,** 1.

Barajas, L. (1964): The innervation of the juxtaglomerular apparatus. An electron microscopic study of the innervation of the glomerular arterioles. *Lab. Invest.* **13,** 916.

Baráth, J. (1953): Az öregedés és a hypertoniás megbetegedések kapcsolata (The importance of presenile disturbances in the pathogenesis of hypertensive arterial diseases). *Orv. Hetil.* **40,** 1106.

Bartman, J. H. (1968): Ultrastructure of elastic tissue of the newborn rat aortic media. *J. Microscopie.* **7,** 355.

Bartos, G. (1968): Occurrence of specific tissue elements several years after alloplastic vascular repair. *Acta morph. Acad. Sci. hung.* **16,** 295.

Bartos, G., Kormos, V., Kustos, Gy., Szöllősy, L., Török, B., Tóth, I., Temes, Gy. (1965a): Problems of alloplastic vascular repair. I. Structure of vascular prostheses. *Acta chir. Acad. Sci. hung.* **6,** 109.

Bartos, G., Kormos, V., Szöllősy, L., Kustos, Gy., Török, B., Tóth, I., Pap, J. (1965b): Problems of alloplastic vascular repair. II. Porosity of synthetic vascular prostheses. *Acta. chir. Acad. Sci. hung.* **6,** 119.

Bartos, G., Kormos, V., Szöllősy, L., Török, B., Kustos, Gy. (1961): On a new alloplastic vascular prosthesis. *Zbl. Chir.* **86,** 1955.

Bartos, G., Kormos, V., Szöllősy, L., Török, B., Kustos, Gy. (1966): Über eine neue Gefässprothese. *Zbl. Chir.* **86,** 1995.

Bartos, G., Szöllősy, L. (1967): Problems of alloplastic vascular repair. III. Connection between the porosity and the degenerative changes of the neointima. *Acta morph. Acad. Sci. hung.* **15,** 245.

Baumgarten, P. (1876): Über die sogenannte Organisation des Thrombus. *Zbl. med. Wiss.* **14,** 593.

Baumgartner, H. R., Studer, A. (1963): Gezielte Überdehnung der Aorta abdominalis am normo- und hypercholesterinaemischen Kaninchen. *Path. et Microbiol. (Basel)* **26,** 129.

Bedford, G. R., Katritsky, A. R. (1963): Proton magnetic resonance spectra of degeneration products from elastin. *Nature (Lond.)* **200,** 652.

Bednar, B. (1965): Hypertonische Veränderungen der Lungengefässe. *Virchows Arch. path. Anat.* **340,** 35.

Bednar, B. (1970): Foixova-Alajouaniova angiohypertroficka myelomalacie. *Čs. Pat.* **6,** 11.

Bell, E. T. (1946) *Renal Diseases.* 1st ed. Lea and Febiger, Philadelphia, Pennsylvania.

Bell, E. T., Clawson, B. J. (1928): Primary (essential) hypertension; a study of four hundred and twenty cases. *Arch. Path.* **5,** 939.

Benacerraf, B., Potter, J. L., McCluskey, R. T., Miller, F. J. (1960): The pathologic effects of intravenously administered soluble antigen–antibody complexes. II. Acute glomerulonephritis in rats. *J. exp. Med.* **111,** 195.

Beneke, R. (1890): Die Ursachen der Thrombusorganisation. *Beitr. path. Anat.* **7,** 95.

Ben-Ishay, Z., Davies, A. M., Laufer, A. (1968): Fibrogenesis in the human myocardium. An electronmicroscopic study. *Exp. molec. Path.* **8,** 358.

Ben-Ishay, Z., Spiro, P., Wiener, J. (1966): The cellular pathology of experimental hypertension. III. Glomerular alterations. *Amer. J. Path.* **49,** 773.

Bennett, H. S. (1956): The concepts of membrane flour and membrane vesiculation as mechanisms for active transport and ion pumping. *J. biophys. biochem. Cytol.* **2,** Suppl, 99.

Bennett, H. S. (1963): Morphological aspects of extracellular polysaccharides. *J. Histochem. Cytochem.* **11,** 14.

Bennett, H. S., Luft, I. H., Hampton, I. C. (1959): Morphological classifications of vertebrate blood capillaries. *Amer. J. Physiol.* **196,** 381.

Benninghoff, A. (1930): Blutgefässe und Herz. In, *Handbuch der mikroskopischen Anatomie des Menschen.* Springer, Berlin, Vol I, pp. 1–232.

Bensch, K. G., Gordon, G. B., Miller, L. (1964): Fibrillar structures resembling leiomyofibrils in endothelial cells of mammalian pulmonary blood vessels. *Z. Zellforsch.* **63,** 759.

Berdjis, C. C. (1960): Cardiovascular system and radiation. Late effects of X-rays on the arteries of the adult rat. *Strahlentherapie* **112,** 595.

Beregi, E. (1959): Über die mit Pilocarpin und Kaltwasser herbeigeführte Anaphylaxie ähnliche Reaktion. *Acta microbiol. Acad. Sci. hung.* **6,** 35.

Beregi, E. (1967): Comparative morphological examinations of allergic reaction in young and old animals. Thesis, Budapest.

Beregi, E., Perényi, L., Simon, J. (1963): Immunofluorescence studies in experimental periarteritis nodosa in rabbits of different ages. *Gerontologia* **8**, 233.

Beregi, E., Simon, J. (1967): A comparative morphological examination of the earliest allergic lesions in old and young animals. *Gerontologia* **13**, 144.

Beregi, E., Simon, J., Földes, I. (1964): Anaphylaxia of rabbits and rats of different ages. *Gerontologia* **10**, 183.

Berki, E., Korányi, A., Major, E., Peres, T. (1969): Ultrastructural study of inorganic substances in atherosclerotic aorta tissue. *Calc. Tiss. Res.* **4**, 84.

Berlepsch, K. (1964): Diskussion zur Biochemie der Arterienwand. *Bibl. Card. Fasc.* **15**, 28.

Bescol-Liversac, J. (1963): Les mucopolysaccharides sulfates. Études dans leurs relations avec les structures tissulaires par l'emploi du ^{35}S-sulfate. Thèse Doctorat en Sciences Naturelles.

Biava, C. (1962): Smooth muscle cells in relation to elastogenesis. An electron microscopic study. *Anat. Rec.* **142**, 216.

Biava, C. (1964): Mallory alcoholic hyalin: A heteroformique lesion of hepatocellular ergastoplasm. *Lab. Invest.* **13**, 301.

Biava, C., Bencosme, S. (1962): Elastogenesis and smooth muscle cells. *Lab. Invest.* **11**, 675.

Biava, C., Brynjolfsson, G. (1967): Observations on early ultrastructural changes in renal arterioles of patients with essential hypertension. *Amer. J. Path.* **50**, 96.

Bierring, F., Kabayashi, T. (1963): Electron microscopy of the normal rabbit aorta. *Acta. path. microbiol. scand.* **57**, 154.

Biggs, M. W., Kritchevsky, D. (1961): Observations with radioactive hydrogen (^{3}H) in experimental atherosclerosis. *Circulation* **4**, 34.

Birmingham, A. T., Ernest, K., Newcombe, J. F. (1969): Antagonism of the response of human isolated arteries to noradrenaline. *Brit. J. Pharmacol.* **35**, 127.

Biron, P., Campeau, L., David, P. (1969): Fate of angiotensin I and II in the human pulmonary circulation. *Amer. J. Card.* **24**, 544.

Björkerud, S. (1969a): Reaction of the aortic wall of the rabbit after superficial, longitudinal, mechanical trauma. *Virchows Arch. path. Anat.* **347**, 197.

Björkerud, S. (1969b): Atherosclerosis initiated by mechanical trauma in normolipidemic rabbits. *J. Atheroscler. Res.* **9**, 209.

Blakemore, A. H., Voorhees, A. B., jr. (1954): Use of tubes constructed from 'N' cloth in bridging arterial defects—experimental and clinical. *Ann. Surg.* **140**, 324.

Bleyl, U. (1967): Fibrin stabilisierender Faktor in der menschlichen Aorta. *Virchows Arch. path. Anat.* **342**, 199.

Bleyl, U. (1969): *Arteriosklerose und Fibrininkorporation.* Springer, Berlin.

Block, E. H. (1963): A method for studying the dynamics quantitatively at the microscopic level *in situ* in living organs. *Angiology* **14**, 97.

Blumenthal, N. T. (1967): Hemodynamic factors in the etiology of arteriosclerosis. In, Cowdry': *Atherosclerosis.* Thomas, Springfield, p. 510.

Bohle, A., Kohler, M., Tomsche, V. (1953): Über das Verhalten der epitheloiden Zellen der Vasa afferentia einseitig nephrektomierter Ratten bei renaler Hypertonie durch Einkapselung einer Niere. *Beitr. path. Anat.* **113**, 414.

Bohr, D. F., Sobieski, J. (1968): A vasoactive factor in plasma. *Fed. Proc.* **27**, 1396.

Bolme, P., Fuxe, K. (1967): Identification of sympathetic cholinergic nerve terminals in arterioles of skeletal muscle. *Acta pharmacol. (Kbh.)* **25**, Suppl. 4, 79.

Borst, R. H., Marx, M., Smidt, W., Hermann, M. (1969): Elektronenmikroskopische und enzymhistochemische Befunde an ableitenden Lymphgefässen im Dünndarmmesenterium der Ratte. *Z. Zellforsch. Abt. Histochem.* **101**, 338.

Bosch, K. (1960): Kombinationsformen der Arteriitis. *Virchows Arch. path. Anat.* **333**, 142.

Böttcher, C. J. F. (1888): Untersuchungen über die histologischen Vorgänge und das Verhalten des Blutes in doppelt unterbundenen Gefässen. *Beitr. path. Anat.* **2**, 199.

Böttcher, C. J. F. (1964): Chemical constituents of human atherosclerotic lesion. *Proc. roy. Soc. Med.* **57**, 792.

Boyd, G. G. (1957): Cogan's syndrome: Report of 2 cases with signs and symptoms suggesting periarteritis nodosa. *Arch. Otolaryng.* **65**, 24.

Brandt, P. W., Pappas, G. D. (1960): An electron microscopic study of pinocytosis in amoeba. I. The surface attachment place. *J. biophys. biochem. Cytol.* **8,** 675.

Brånemark, P. J., Ekholm, R., Lindke, J. (1968): Colloidal carbon used for identification of vascular permeability. *Med. Exp.* **18,** 139.

Bredt, H. (1961): Morphologie und Pathogenese der Arteriosklerose. In, *Die Arteriosklerose.* Thieme, Stuttgart, pp. 6–50.

Bredt, H. (1969): Morphology. In, Schettler, F. G., Boyd, G. S. (Eds): *Atherosclerosis.* Elsevier, Amsterdam–London–New York, Vol. 1, p. 1.

Bretán, M., Oblatt, E., Róna, Gy., Kerényi, N. (1954): Veseelváltozások kisérleti úton létrehozott steroid (Cortison) diabetesben. Adatok az angiopathia diabetica pathogenesiséhez [Renal changes in experimental steroid (cortisone) diabetes. Pathogenesis of angiopathic diabetes]. *Magy. Belorv. Arch.* **7,** 23.

Brickner, R. M. (1927): The role of the capillaries and their endothelium in the distribution of colloidal carbon by the blood stream. *Bull. Johns Hopk. Hosp.* **40,** 90.

Bronte-Steward, B., Heptinstall, R. H. (1954): The relationship between experimental hypertension and cholesterol-induced atheroma in rabbits. *J. Path. Bact.* **68,** 407.

Brooks, R. E. (1969): Ruthenium red stainable surface layer on lung alveolar cells. EM interpretation. *Stain Technol.* **44,** 173.

Bruns, R. (1963): Transport of ferritin across the capillary wall: an electron microscopic study. *Anat. Rec.* **145,** 360.

Bruns, R., Palade, G. E. (1968): Studies on blood capillaries. II. Transport of ferritin molecules across the wall of muscle capillaries. *J. Cell. Biol.* **37,** 277.

Buck, R. C. (1955): Uptake of radioactive sulfate by arteries of normal and cholesterol-fed rabbits. *J. Histochem. Cytochem.* **3,** 435.

Buck, R. C. (1958): The fine structure of endothelium of large arteries. *J. biophys. biochem. Cytol.* **4,** 187.

Buck, R. C. (1961): Intimal thickening after ligature of arteries. An electron microscopic study. *Circulat. Res.* **9,** 418.

Buck, R. C. (1962): Lesions in the rabbit aorta produced by feeding a high cholesterol diet followed by a normal diet. An electron microscopic study. *Brit. J. exp. Pathol.* **43,** 236.

Buck, R. C. (1963): Histogenesis and morphology of arterial tissue. In, Sandler, M., Bonrue, G. H. (Eds): *Atherosclerosis and its Origin.* Academic Press, New York, Vol. 4.

Buckley, J. K., Ryan, G. B. (1969): Increased vascular permeability. The effect of histamine and serotonin on rat mesenteric blood vessels *in vivo. Amer. J. Path.* **55,** 329.

Buluk, K. Malofiejew, M. (1969): The pharmacological properties of fibrinogen degradation products. *Brit. J. Pharmacol.* **35,** 79.

Bunce, D. F. M. (1965): Structural differences between distended and collapsed arteries. *Angiology* **16,** 53.

Burdach, F. (1885): Über den Senftleben'schen Versuch die Bindegewebsbildung in totden doppelt unterbindenen Gefässen betreffend. *Virchows Arch. path. Anat.* **100,** 217.

Burri, P. H., Weibel, E. R. (1968): Beeinflussung einer spezifischen cytoplasmatischen Organelle von Endothelzellen durch Adrenalin. *Z. Zellforsch.* **88,** 426.

Byrom, F. B. (1954): The pathogenesis of hypertensive encephalopathy and its relation to the maligant phase of hypertension. Experimental evidence from the hypertensive rat. *Lancet* ii, 201–211.

Byrom, F. B. (1964): Angiotensin and renal vascular damage. *Brit. J. exp. Path.* **45,** 7.

Byrom, F. B., Dodson, L. F. (1948): The causation of acute arterial necrosis in hypertensive disease. *J. Path. Bact.* **60,** 357.

Cain, H., Fazekas, St. (1963): Studien über die Folgen einer vorübergehenden experimentellen Nierenischämie. *Virchows Arch. path. Anat.* **336,** 389.

Campbell, M. (1954): Development of atherosclerosis in dogs with hypercholesteremia and chronic hypertension. *Circulat. Res.* **2,** 243.

Campbell, R. S. F. (1965): Early atherosclerosis in the pig: a histological and histochemical study. *J. Atheroscler. Res.* **5,** 483.

Campbell, W. G., Santos-Buch, C. A. (1959): Widely distributed necrotizing arteritis induced in rabbits by experimental renal alterations. I. Comparison with the vascular lesions induced by injections of foreign serum. *Amer. J. Path.* **35,** 439.

Campbell, W. G., Santos-Buch, C. A. (1963): Widely distributed necrotising arteritis induced in rabbits by experimental renal alterations. III. Studies on activity and decay of necrotising factors. *Amer. J. Path.* **43**, 131.

Cappelli, B., Conti, G., Laszt, L., Mándi, B. (1968*a*): Action du facteur P sur les artères de l'embryon de poulet cultivée *in vitro*. *Angiologica* **5**, 28.

Cappelli, B., Conti, G., Laszt, L., Mándi, B. (1968*b*): Données histo-chimiques sur la paroi artérielle de l'embryon de poulet cultivée *in vitro*. *Angiologica* **5**, 41.

Carettero, O., Gross, F. (1967): Renin substrate in plasma under various experimental conditions in the rat. *Amer. J. Physiol.* **213**, 695.

Carlson, L. A., Fröberg, S. O. (1969): Effect of training with exercise on plasma and tissue lipid levels of ageing rats. *Gerontologia* **15**, 14.

Casley-Smith, J. R. (1964): An electron microscopic study of injured and abnormally permeable lymphatics. *Ann. N. Y. Acad. Sci.* **116**, 803.

Casley-Smith, J. R. (1965): Endothelial permeability. II. The passage of particles through the lymphatic endothelium of normal and injured rats. *Brit. J. exp. Path.* **46**, 35.

Casley-Smith, J. R., Reade, P. C. (1965): An electron microscopical study of the uptake of foreign particles by the levers of foetal and adult rats. *Brit. J. exp. Path.* **46**, 473.

Cavallero, C., Turolla, E. (1964): Morphologische Beobachtungen bei menschlicher und experimenteller Atherosklerose. In, *IVth Pathological Conference in Zurich*. Karger, Basel.

Cavallero, C., Turolla, E., Ricevuti, G. (1969): Lésion artérielles par choc orthostatique chez le lapin. *Arch. Mal. Cœur* Suppl. **1**, 10.

Cavallero, C., Turolla, E., Ricevuti, G. (1971*a*): Cell proliferation in the atherosclerotic plaques of cholesterol-fed rabbits. Part I. Colchicine and (^{3}H)thymidine studies. *Atherosclerosis*, **13**, 9.

Cavallero, C., Turolla, E., Ricevuti, G. (1971*b*): Cinetica della parete arteriosa nell'aterogenesi sperimentale. *Minerva Medica* **62**, 3410.

Cecio, A. (1967): Ultrastructural features of cytofilaments within mammalian endothelial cells. *Z. Zellforsch.* **83**, 40.

Cervos-Navarro, H. (1964): Die Bedeutung der EM für die Lehre vom Stoffaustausch zwischen dem Zentralnervensystem und dem übrigen Körper. *Dtsch. Z. Nervenheilk.* **186**, 206.

Chambers, R., Zweifach, H. W. (1940): Capillary endothelial cement in relation to permeability. *J. Cell. comp. Physiol.* **15**, 255.

Chambers, R., Zweifach, H. W. (1947): Intracellular cement and capillary permeability. *Physiol. Rev.* **27**, 436.

Chase, W. H. (1969): Distribution and fine structure of elastic fibres in mouse-lung. *Exp. Cell. Res.* **17**, 121.

Choi, J. H., More, R. H., Wyllie, J. C., Haust, M. D. (1968): Electron microscopic studies of fibrinoid. *Laval med.* **39**, 30.

Christensen, S. (1961): Plasma phospholipid and plasma protein transfer across the intimal surface on the normal and slightly atherosclerotic thoracic aorta of the cockerel. *J. Atheroscler.* **1**, 140.

Christensen, S. (1962): Transfer of plasma phospholipid across the aortic intimal surface of cholesterol-fed cockerels. *J. Atheroscler. Res.* **2**, 131.

Christensen, S. (1967): Intimal uptake of plasma lipoprotein and atherosclerosis. *Progr. Biochem. Pharmacol.* **4**, 244.

Churg, J. (1963*a*): Vascular lesions in anti-kidney serum nephritis. *Amer. J. Path.* **43**, 21/a.

Churg, J. (1963*b*): Renal and renoprival vascular disease in the rat. *Arch. Path.* **75**, 547.

Clarke, I. A. (1965*a*): The vasa vasorum of normal human lower limb arteries. *Acta Anat. (Basel)* **61**, 481.

Clarke, I. A. (1965*b*): An X-ray microscopic study of the postnatal development of the vasa vasorum in the human aorta. *J. Anat. (Lond.)* **99**, 877.

Clarke, I. A. (1965*c*): An X-ray microscopic study of the vasa vasorum of the normal human aortic arch. *Torax* **20**, 76.

165

Clarke, I. A., (1965*d*): An X-ray microscopic study of the postnatal development of the vasa vasorum in the pulmonary trunk and arteries. *Torax* **20**, 348.

Clementi, F., Palade, G. E. (1969): Intestinal capillaries. I. Permeability to peroxidase and ferritin. *J. Cell. Biol.* **41**, 33.

Cliff, W. I. (1967): The aortic tunica media in growing rats studied with the electron microscope. *Lab. Invest.* **17**, 599.

Cochrane, C. G., Weigle, W. O. (1958): The cutaneous reaction of soluble antigen–antibody complexes. *J. exp. Med.* **108**, 591.

Cochrane, C. G., Weigle, W. O., Dixon, F. J. (1959): The role of polymorphonuclear leukocytes in the initiation and cessation of the Arthus vasculitis. *J. exp. Med.* **110**, 481.

Cohen, S. G., Sapp, T. M. (1959): Histopathologic cardiovascular responses to passive sensitisation. *J. inf. Dis.* **105**, 124.

Cohnheim, J. (1867): Über Entzündung und Einterrung. *Arch. Anat. Physiol.* **40**, 1.

Cohnheim, J. (1873): *Neue Untersuchungen über die Entzündung.* Hirschwald, Berlin.

Comel, M., Laszt, L. (1968): Biochemie der Gefässwand. Teil I. In, *Internationales Symposium, Fribourg, 21–22, Juni 1968.* Karger, Basel–New York, 1969.

Congin, L., Baccino, F. M. (1964): Ultrastruttura dell'aorta normale e arteriosclerotica. *Arch. De Vecchi* **43**, 345.

Constantinides, P. (1961): Production of experimental atherosclerosis in animals. *J. Atheroscler. Res.* **1**, 374.

Constantinides, P. (1965): *Experimental Atherosclerosis.* Elsevier, Amsterdam–New York–London.

Constantinides, P. (1968): Lipid deposition in injured arteries. *Arch. Path.* **85**, 280.

Constantinides, P., Booth, J. Carlson, G. (1960): Production of advanced cholesterol atherosclerosis in the rabbit. *Arch. Path. (Chic.)* **80**, 712.

Constantinides, P., Gutmann-Auersperg, N., Hospes, D. (1958): Acceleration of intimal atherogenesis through prior medical injury. *Arch. Path.* **66**, 247.

Constantinides, P., Lawder, J. (1963): Experimental thrombosis and haemorrhage in atherosclerotic arteries. *Fed. Proc.* **22**, 251.

Constantinides, P., Robinson, M. (1969*a*): Ultrastructural injury of arterial endothelium. I. Effects of pH osmolarity anoxia and temperature. *Arch. Path. (Chic.)* **88**, 99.

Constantinides, P., Robinson, M.|(1969*b*): Ultrastructural injury of arterial endothelium. II. Effects of vasoactive amines. *Arch. Path. (Chic.)* **88**, 106.

Constantinides, P., Robinson, M. (1969*c*): Ultrastructural injury of arterial endothelium. III. Effekts of enzymes and surfactons. *Arch. Path. (Chic.)* **88**, 113.

Cooke, P. H., Smith, S. C. (1968): Smooth muscle cells: the source of foam cells in atherosclerotic white Carneau pigeons. *Exp. molec. Path.* **8**, 171.

Coret, I. A., Hughes, M. J. (1964): A further study of hypoxic smooth muscle. *Arch. int. Pharmacodyn.* **149**, 330.

Costa, V., Aresu, P. (1964): Observations ultrastructurels au microscope electronique sur la structure de la tunica media de l'aorte de rat normal. *Proc. IIIrd Conf. Electron Microscopy, Prague.* **B**, 107.

Cotran, R. S. (1965): The delayed and prolonged vascular leakage in inflammation. II. An electron microscopic study of the vascular response after thermal injury. *Amer. J. Pathol.* **46**, 589.

Cotran, R. S., Karnovsky, M. J. (1967): Vascular leakage induced by horseradish peroxidase in the rat. *Proc. Soc. exp. Biol. (N.Y.)* **126**, 557.

Cotran, R. S., Suter, E. R., Majno, G. (1967): The use of colloidal carbon as a tracer for vascular injury. *Vasc. Dis.* **4**, 107.

Coirtice, F. C., Garlick, D. G. (1962): The permeability of the capillary wall to the different plasma lipoproteins of the hypercholesterolaemic rabbit in relation to their size. *Quart. J. exp. Physiol.* **47**, 221.

Coirtice, F. C., Schmidt-Diedrichs, A. (1963): Long-term effects on injury of the wall of the carotid artery in normal and hyperlipaemic rabbits. *Brit. J. exp. Path.* **44**, 339.

Cox, G. E., Trueheart, R. E., Kaplan, J., Taylor, C. B. (1963): Atherosclerosis in rhesus monkeys. IV. Repair of arterial injury; an important secondary atherogenic factor. *Arch. Path. (Chic.)* **76**, 166.

Crane, W. A. J. (1962a): Sites of mucopolysaccharide synthesis in the lesions of experimental hypertension in rats. *J. Path. Bact.* **83**, 183.

Crane, W. A. J. (1962b): Sulphate utilisation and mucopolysaccharide synthesis by the mesenteric arteries of rats with experimental hypertension. *J. Path. Bact.* **84**, 113.

Crane, W. A. J., Dutta, L. P. (1963): The utilisation of tritiated thymidine for deoxyribonucleic acid synthesis by the lesions of experimental hypertension in rats. *J. Path. Bact.* **86**, 83.

Crane, W. A. J., Dutta, L. P. (1964): The influence of age on the uptake of ^{35}S-sulphate and ^{3}H thymidine by the mesenteric arteries of rats with regenerating adrenal glands. *J. Path. Bact.* **88**, 291.

Crane, W. A. J., Ingle, D. S. (1964): Tritiated thymidine uptake in rat hypertension. *Arch. Path.* **78**, 209.

Crawford, W. J. (1957): Cogan's syndrome associated with polyarteritis nodosa. *Med. J.* **60**, 835.

Creech, I., jr., Deterling, R. A., jr., Edwards, S., Julina, O. C., Linton, R. R., Schumacher, H., jr. (1957): Vascular prostheses. Report of the Committee for the Study of Vascular Prosthesis of the Society for Vascular Surgery. *Surgery* **41**, 62.

Cruickshank, B. (1954): The arteritis of rheumatoid arthritis. *Ann. rheum. Dis.* **13**, 136.

Curran, R. C. (1957): The elaboration of mucopolysaccharides by vascular endothelium. *J. Path. Bact.* **74**, 347.

Cutts, J. H. (1966): Vascular lesions resembling polyarteritis nodosa in rats undergoing prolonged stimulation with oestrogen. *Brit. J. exp. Path.* **47**, 401.

Dalldorf, F. G. (1963): Estrogenic hormones, urethra cornification and arteriosclerotic vascular disease in men. *Amer. J. clin. Path.* **42**, 64.

Daniel, P. M., Prichard, M. M. L., Ward-McQuaid, I. N. (1954): Removal of the clip on the renal artery in rabbits with experimental chronic hypertension. *Quart. J. exp. Physiol.* **39**, 101.

Daoud, A. S., Jarmolich, J., Fani, K., Zumbo, O. (1964a): Possible medial origin of intimal smooth muscle cells in pre-atheroma phase of arteriosclerosis. *Fed. Proc.* **23**, 195.

Daoud, A. S., Jarmolich, J., Zumbo, O., Fani, K., Florentin, R. (1964b): Preatheroma phase of coronary atherosclerosis in man. *Exp. molec. Path.* **3**, 475.

Daoud, A. S., Jones, R., Scott, R. F. (1968): Dietary-induced atherosclerosis in miniature swine. III. Lipid values: cholesterol, triglyceride and phospholipid and esterified fatty acid values in serum and in aortic intima-media tissue. *Exp. molec. Path.* **8**, 263.

Daugherty, R. M., Scott, J. B., jr., Haddy, F. J. (1967): Effects of generalized hypoxemia and hypercapnia on forelimb vascular resistance. *Amer. J. Physiol.* **213**, 1111.

Dauid, H., Hackensellner, A., Wolf, W. (1963): Submikroskopische Untersuchungen an der Neointima in Kunststoffprothesen beim Hund. *Frankfurt. Z. Path.* **72**, 548.

Dauid, H., Kunz. J. (1965): Strukturveränderungen der Media der Kaninchen-Aorta nach lokaler Bestrahlung (^{90}Sr–^{90}Y). *Z. Zellforsch.* **66**, 83.

David, J. N., Adams, C. W. M., Bayliss, O. B. (1963): Gradient in cholesterol concentration across human aortic wall. *Lancet* **ii**, 1254.

Davson, H., Oldendorf, W. H. (1967): Transport in the enteral venous system. *Proc. roy. Soc. Med.* **60**, 326.

Day, T. D. (1952): The permeability of interstitial connective tissue and the nature of the interfibrillary substance. *J. Physiol.* **117**, 1.

Dayton, S. (1961): Decline in rate of cholesterol synthesis during mutation of chicken aorta. *Proc. Soc. exp. Biol. (N. Y.)* **108**, 257.

DeBakey, M. E., Jordan, G. L., jr., Abbott, J. P., Halpert, B., O'Neal, R. M. (1964): The fate of dacron vascular grafts. *Arch. Surg. (Chic.)* **89**, 757.

DeDuve, C. (1963): The lysosome concept. In, *CIBA Foundation Symposium on Lysosomes*. Churchill, London, p. 1.

Dees, M. B. (1923): On the fenestrated membrane of Henle. *Anat. Rec.* **26**, 161.

DeFaria, J. L. (1961): Aortenmedionekrose mit sekundärer Arteriosklerose bei den kongenitalen zyanotischen Herzkrankheiten. *Beitr. path. Anat.* **125**, 129.

DeFaria, J. L. (1965a): Role of medial changes in the pathogenesis of the diffuse intimal thickening and in atherogenesis. *J. Atheroscler. Res.* **5**, 509.

DeFaria, J. L. (1965b): Über die Rolle der Mediaveränderungen für die Pathogenese der Intimasklerose sowie die Begrenzung der Arteriosklerose in der Aorta ascendens des Menschen. *Beitr. path. Anat.* **132**, 114.

Deming, Q. B., Mosbach, E. H., Bevans, M., Abell, L., Martin, E., Bunn, L., Halpern, E. (1957): Effect of desoxycorticosterone + NaCl-induced hypertension of dietary atherosclerosis and dietary hyperlipemia in the rat. *Fed. Proc.* **16**, 355.

Deming, Q. B., Mosbach, E. H. Bevans, M., Halpern, E., Koplan, R. (1958): Blood pressure, cholesterol content of serum and tissues and atherogenesis in the rat. *J. exp. Med.* **107**, 581.

DeSuto-Nagy, G. I., Waters, L. L. (1951): The effect of altered lipid metabolism on experimental lesions of the coronary arteries. *Circulation* **4**, 468.

Deterling, R. A., jr., Bhonslay, S. B. (1955): An evaluation of synthetic materials and fabrics suitable for blood vessel replacement. *Surgery* **38**, 71.

Devine, C. E. (1967): Electron microscope autoradiography of rat arteriolar axons after noradrenaline infusion. *Proc. Univ. Otago med. Sch.* **45**, 7.

Devine, C. E., Simpson, F. O. (1968a): The morphological basis for the sympathetic control of blood vessels. *N. Z. med. J.* **67**, 326.

Devine, C. E., Simpson, F. O. (1968b): Localisation of tritiated norepinephrine in vascular sympathetic axons of the rat intestine and mesentery by electron microscope radioautography. *J. Cell. Biol.* **38**, 183.

Dewey, M. M., Barr, L. (1962): Intercellular connection between smooth muscle cells: the nexus. *Science* **137**, 670.

Dietrich, K. (1930): Beiträge zur Pathologie der Arterien des Menschen. *Virchows Arch. path. Anat.* **274**, 452.

Dill, L. V., Isenhour, C. E. (1942): Occurrence of atheroma in aorta in rabbits with renal hypertension. *Arch. Path.* **33**, 655.

Dixon, K. C. (1961): Deposition of globular lipid in arterial cells in relation to anoxia. *Amer. J. Path.* **39**, 65.

Dixon, F. J., Vazquez, J. J., Weigle, W. O., Cochrane, C. G. (1958): Pathogenesis of serum thickness. *Arch. Path.* **65**, 18.

Dobrovolskaya-Zavadskaya, N. (1924): Action des foyers radioactifs sur les vaisseaux sanguins. *Lyon Chir.* **21**, 397.

Doerr, W. (1963): *Perfusionstheorie der Arteriosklerose.* Thieme, Stuttgart.

Downing, J. E., Vidone, R. A., Brandt, H. M., Liebow, A. A. (1963): The pathogenesis of vascular lesions in experimental hyperkinetic pulmonary hypertension. *Amer. J. Path.* **43**, 739.

Duff, G. L. (1932): Vital staining of the rabbit aorta in the study of atherosclerosis. *Amer. J. Path.* **8**, 218.

Duff, G. L., McMillan, G. C. (1951): The pathology of atherosclerosis. *Amer. J. Med.* **11**, 92.

Duff, G. L., McMillan, G. C., Lantsch, E. V. (1954): The uptake of colloidal thorium dioxide by the arterial lesions of cholesterol atherosclerosis in the rabbit. *Amer. J. Path.* **30**, 941.

Duff, G. L., McMillan, G. C., Ritchie, A. C. (1957): The morphology of early atherosclerotic lesions of the aorta demonstrated by the surface technique in rabbits fed cholesterol. *Amer. J. Path.* **33**, 845.

Duguid, J. B. (1949): Pathogenesis of atherosclerosis. *Lancet* ii, 925.

Duguid, J. B., Anderson, G. S. (1952): Pathogenesis of hyaline arteriosclerosis. *J. Path. Bact.* **64**, 519.

Duncan, L. E., jr. (1963): Mechanical factors in the localisation of atheroma. In, Jones, R. J. (Ed.): *Evolution of the Atherosclerotic Plaque.* Chicago University Press, Chicago, p. 171.

Duncan, L. E., jr., Buck, K. (1962): Comparison of rates at which albumin enters walls of small and large aorta. *Amer. J. Physiol.* **203**, 1167.

Duncan, L. E., jr., Buck, K., Lynch, A. (1963): Lipoprotein movement through canine aortic wall. *Science* **142**, 972.

Duncan, L. E., jr., Cornfield, J., Buck, K. (1959): Circulation of labelled albumin through the aortic wall of the dog. *Circulat. Res.* **7**, 370.

Duncan, L. E., jr., Cornfield, J., Buck, K. (1962): The effect of blood pressure on the passage of labelled plasma albumin into canine aortic wall. *J. clin. Invest.* **41**, 1537.

Dunihue, F. W. (1941): Effect of cellophane perinephritis on the granular cells of the juxtaglomerular apparatus. *Arch. Path.* **32**, 211.

Dustin, P., jr. (1962): Arteriolar hyalinosis. *Int. Rev. exp. Path.* **1**, 73.

Dutz, H., Voigt, K. (1957): Die Beeinflussbarkeit der experimentellen Hypertonie bei Ratten durch Serpasil und kochsalzreiche Nahrung. *Z. ges. exp. Med.* **129**, 305.

Dybrye, M. D. (1959): Studies on the metabolism of the mucopolysaccharides of human arterial tissue by means of ^{35}S with special reference to changes related to age. *J. Geront.* **14**, 32.

Dziewiatowski, D. D. (1951): Isolation of chondroitin sulfate ^{35}S from articular cartilage of rats. *J. biol. Chem.* **189**, 187.

Dziewiatowski, D. D., Benesch, R. (1949): On the possible utilization of sulfate sulfur on the suckling rat for the synthesis of chondroitin sulfate as indicated by the use of radioactive sulfur. *J. biol. Chem.* **178**, 931.

Eadles, C. H., jr., Phillip, G. E., Blanstein, A., Hsu, I. C., Solberg, V. B. (1965): Contrast of dose hypertension with renal hypertension in the etiology of coronary atherosclerosis in the adult male Wistar rat. *Angiologia* **2**, 61.

Efskind L. (1941): Die Regenerationsverhältnisse im Intimaepithel nach Gefäss-Sutur. *Acta. chir. scand.* **89**, 283.

Ehinger, B., Falek, B., Sporrang, B. (1966): Adrenergic fibres to the heart and to peripheral vessels. *Bibl. anat. (Basel)* **8**, 35.

Ehrenreich, T., Olmstead, E. V. (1951): Malignant hypertension following the administration of cortisone in periarteritis nodosa. *Arch. Path.* **52**, 145.

Ehrreich, S. J., Furchgott, R. F. (1968): Relaxation of mammalian smooth muscles by visible and ultraviolet radiation, *Nature (Lond.)* **218**, 682.

Eisenstein, R., Zervlois, L. (1963): An electron microscopic study of Vitamin-D induced aortic proliferation. *Lab. Invest.* **12**, 865.

Eisenstein, R., Zervlois, L. (1964): Vitamin-D induced aortic calcification. *Arch. Path.* **77**, 27.

El-Maghraby, M. A. H. A., Gardner, D. L. (1968): A comparative study in young male animals of 10 species of the distribution of alkaline phosphatase activity in small arteries. *Histochemie* **16**, 227.

Emmrich, R (1963): Beziehungen zwischen Gefässwand und Blutplasma kleinerer Arterien und der Arteriolen. In, *Gefässwand und Blutplasma.* Fischer, Jena.

Endes, P. (1963): Investigation of the granular cells of glomerular arterioles. Thesis, Budapest.

Endes, P., Takácsi-Nagy, L. (1952): Bioptische Untersuchungen der Niere bei essentieller Hypertonie. *Acta morph. Acad. Sci. hung.* **2**, 191.

Essbach, H. (1961): Pathologische Anatomie der kranken Gefässwand. In, *Gefässwand und Blutplasma.* Fischer, Jena.

Esterly, J. A., Glagov, S. (1963): Altered permeability of the renal artery of the hypertensive rat; an EM study. *Amer. J. Path.* **43**, 619.

Esterly, J. A., Glagov, S., Ferguson, D. J. (1968): Morphogenesis of intimal obliterative hyperplasia of small arteries in experimental pulmonary hypertension. An ultrastructural study of the role of smooth muscle cells. *Amer. J. Path.* **52**, 325.

Ewans, H. M. (1915): The macrophages of mammals. *Amer. J. Physiol.* **37**, 243.

Fabius, A. J. M. (1959): Failure to demonstrate precipitating antibodies against vessel extracts in patients with vascular disorders. *Vox Sang. (Basel)* **4**, 247.

Fabris, A. (1901): Experimentelle Untersuchungen über die Pathogenese der Aneurysmen. *Virchows Arch. path. Anat.* **165**, 439.

Fahimi, H. D., Drochmans, P. (1965): Essais de standardisation de la fixation du glutaraldehyde. I. Purification et détermination de la concentration du glutaraldehyde. *J. Microscopy* **4**, 725.

Fahr, T. (1925): Pathologische Anatomie des Morbus Brightii. In, Henke, F., Lubarsch, O., Rössle, R. (Eds): *Handbuch der speziellen pathologischen Anatomie und Histologie.* Springer, Berlin, Vol. 6, p. 156.

Fahr, T. (1934): Pathologische Anatomie des Morbus Brightii. In, Henke F., Lubarsch, O., Rössle, R. (Eds): *Handbuch der speziellen pathologischen Anatomie und Histologie.* Springer, Berlin, Vol. 6, p. 807.

Fahr, T. (1941): Maligne Nephrosklerose und Periarteriitis nodosa. *Dtsch. med. Wschr.* **67,** 1223.

Fahrenbach, W. H., Saudberg, L. B., Greany, E. G. (1965): Ultrastructural studies on early elastogenesis. *Anat. Rec.* **155,** 563.

Farquhar, M. G., Palade, G. E. (1960): Segregation of ferritin in glomerular protein absorption droplets. *J. biophys. biochem. Cytol.* **7,** 297.

Farquhar, M. G., Palade, G. E. (1963): Functional complexes in various epithelia. *J. Cell. Biol.* **17,** 375.

Fawcett, D. W. (1959): The fine structure of capillaries, arterioles and small arteries. In, Reynolds, S. R. M., Zweifach, B. W. (Eds): *The Microcirculation.* Illinois Press, Urbana, Vol. III, p. 1.

Fawcett, D. W. (1965): Surface specializations of absorbing cells. *J. Histochem. Cytochem.* **13,** 75.

Fawcett, D. W., Wittenberg, I. (1962): Structural specialization of endothelial cell junctions. *Anat. Rec.* **142,** 231.

Fekete, Á. (1970a): Permanent hypertension induced by ligation of one renal artery in the dog. *Acta med. Acad. Sci. hung.* **27,** 191.

Fekete, Á. (1970b): Egyoldali arteria renalis lekötés útján kutyában létrehozott tartós hypertonia. (Permanent hypertension induced by ligation of one renal artery in the dog.) *Kísérl. Orvostud.* **22,** 132.

Felt, V. (1960): The role of the blood vessel wall in the pathogenesis of atherosclerosis. *Rev. Czech. Med.* **6,** 126.

Fennel, R. H., Reddy, C. R. R. M., Vasquez, J. J. (1961): Progressive splenic sclerosis and malignant hypertension. Immunohistochemical study of renal lesions. *Arch. Path.* **72,** 209.

Fennel, R. H., jr., Santamaria, A. (1962): Anaphylaxis in the rat immunohistochemical studies of the liver. *Amer. J. Path.* **41/5,** 521.

Fernando, N. V. P., Movat, H. Z. (1963): Fibrillogenesis on regenerating tendon. *Lab. Invest.* **12,** 214.

Fessler, J. H. (1960): A structural function of mucopolysaccharide in connective tissue. *Biochem. J.* **76,** 124.

Finkbiner, R. B., Decker, S. P. (1963): Ulceration and perforation of the intestine due to necrotizing arteriolitis. *New Engl. J. Med.* **268,** 14.

Finlayson, R., Symmers, C., Fiemos, R. N. T. W. (1962): Atherosclerosis: a comparative study. *Brit. med. J.* **1,** 501.

Fishberg, A. M. (1925): Anatomic findings in essential hypertension. *Arch. intern. Med.* **35,** 650.

Fishberg, A. M. (1954): *Hypertension and Nephritis.* 5th ed. Lea and Febiger, Philadelphia, p. 283.

Fischer, E. R. (1957): Polyarteritis nodosa associated with rheumatoid arthritis: Report of a case with comments relative to the concept of rheumatoid, heart disease. *Amer. J. clin. Path.* **27,** 191.

Fischer, E. R., Creed, D. L., Baird, W. F. (1958): Effect of renal hypertension on cholesterol atherosclerosis in the rabbit. *Lab. Invest.* **7,** 231.

Fischer, E. R., Hellstrom, H. R. (1961): Cogan's syndrome and systemic vascular disease. Analysis of pathologic features with reference to its relationship to thromboangiitis obliterans (Buerger). *Arch. Path.* **72,** 572.

Fischer, E. R., Perez-Stable, E., Pardo, V. (1966): Ultrastructular studies in hypertension: I. Comparison of renal vascular and juxtaglomerural cell alterations in essential and renal hypertension in man. *Lab. Invest.* **15,** 1409.

Fischer, E. R., Perez-Stable, E., Pardo, V. (1967): Ultrastructural studies in hypertension. In, Bajusz, E., Jasmin, G. (Eds): *Methods and Achievements in Experimental Pathology.* 4th ed. Karger, Basel–New York, p. 237.

Fischer, H. (1965): Die Struktur der Arterienwand mit besonderer Berücksichtigung der Einwirkung des hydrostatischen Drucks. *Angiologica* **2,** 285.

Fishman N. H. (1968): Mechanical injury to the coronary arteries during operative cannulation. *Amer. Heart J.* **75,** 26.

Florentin, R. A., Nam, S. C. (1968): Dietary-induced atherosclerosis in miniature swine. I. Gross and light microscopy observations: time of development and morphologic characteristics of lesions. *Exp. molec. Path.* **8,** 263.

170

Florentin, R. A., Nam, S. C., Lee, K. T., Thomas W. A. (1969): Increased ^{3}H-thymidine incorporation into endothelial cells of swine fed cholesterol for 3 days. *Exp. molec. Path.* **10**, 250.

Florey, F. S. (1966): The endothelial cell. *Brit. med. J.* **2**, 487.

Florey, F. S. (1967): The uptake of particulate matter by endothelial cells. *Proc. roy. Soc. B.* **166**, 375.

Florey, F. S. (1970): The permeability of arterial endothelium to horseradish peroxidase. *Proc. roy. Soc. B.* **174**, 435.

Florey, H. W. (1964): The transport of materials across the capillary wall. *Quart. J. exp. Physiol.* **49**, 117.

Florey, H. W., Geer, S. J., Kiser, J., Poole, J. C. F., Telander, R., Werthessen, N. T. (1962): The development of the pseudointima living fabric grafts of the aorta. *Brit. J. exp. Path.* **43**, 655.

Florey, H. W., Geer, S. J., Poole, J. C. F., Werthessen, N. T. (1961): The pseudointima living fabric grafts of the aorta. *Brit. J. exp. Path.* **42**, 236.

Florey, H. W., Poole, J. C. F., Meck, G. A. (1959): Endothelial cells and cement lines. *J. Path. Bact.* **77**, 625.

Földi, M., Kovács, A., Takács, L., Koltay, E. (1954a): Káliumkiválasztás hypoxaemiában (Potassium excretion in hypoxaemia). *Magy. Belorv. Arch.* **7**, 179.

Földi, M., Romhányi, Gy., Rusznyák, I., Soltik, F., Szabó, Gy. (1954b): Über die Insuffizienz der Lymphstörung im Herzen. *Acta med. Acad. Sci. hung.* **6**, 61.

Formahides, cit. Solowjev, A. (1929): Experimentelle Untersuchungen über die Heilungsvorgänge in der Arterienwand. *Beitr. path. Anat.* **83**, 485.

Forman, D. T., Choi, S. S., Taylor, C. B. (1968): Sulfate content of aortic wall in experimentally induced atherosclerosis. *Arch. Path.* **85**, 80.

Forssmann, W. G. (1969): A method for *in vivo* diffusion tracer studies combining perfusion fixation with intravenous tracer injection. *Histochemie* **20**, 277.

Fox, L. M., Fries, C. C., Wesslousti, S. A. (1963): Reaction of the aortic wall to specific injurants. In, *Fundamentals of Vascular Grafting.* McGraw-Hill, New York–Toronto–London, p. 106.

Freed, S. C., Proctor, J. (1968): Blood pressure response to 1-norepinephrine in rats treated with inhibitors of protein synthesis. *Angiology* **19**, 549.

French, J. E. (1966): Atherosclerosis in relation to the structure and function of the arterial intima, with special reference to the endothelium. *Int. Rev. exp. Path.* **5**, 253.

French, J. E., Jennings, M. A., Florey, H. W. (1965): Morphological studies on atherosclerosis in swine. *Ann. N. Y. Acad. Sci.* **127**, 780.

French, J. E., Jennings, M. A., Poole, J. C. F., Robinson, D. S., Florey, H. W. (1963): Intimal changes in the arteries of ageing swine. *Proc. roy. Soc. B.* **158**, 24.

Friederics, H. H. R. (1969): On the diaphragm across fenestral of capillary endothelium. *J. Ultrastruct. Res.* **27**, 373.

Friedman, B., Jarman, J., Klemperer, P. (1941): Sustained hypertension following experimental unilateral renal injuries. Effects of nephrectomy. *Amer. J. med. Sci.* **202**, 20.

Friedman, M., Byers, S. O. (1962): Excess lipid leakage: a property of very young vascular endothelium. *Brit. J. exp. Path.* **43**, 363.

Friedman, M., Byers, S. O. (1963): Endothelial permeability in atherosclerosis. *Arch. Path.* **76**, 99.

Friedman, M., Byers, S. O., St. Georges, S. (1966): Site of origin of the luminal foam cells of atherosclerosis. *Amer. J. clin. Path.* **45**, 238.

Fuchs, A., Weibel, E. R. (1966): Morphometrische Untersuchung der Verteilung einer spezifischen cytoplasmatischen Organelle in Endothelzellen der Ratte. *Z. Zellforsch.* **73**, 1.

Fuchs, M., Claus, F. (1967): Blutgefässveränderungen bei anaphylaktischem Oedem. *Beitr. path. Anat.* **135**, 297.

Fuchs, U. (1970): Die Arteriosklerose des Menschen. Elektronenmikroskopische Befunde. *Zbl. allg. Path. path. Anat.* **113**, 501.

Fuchs, U., Scharnweber, W. (1968): Elektronenmikroskopische Untersuchungen an Skelettmuskelkapillaren des Menschen bei Arteriosklerose und Diabetes mellitus. *Virchows Arch. path. Anat.* **343**, 276.

171

Gage, H. A., Fazekas, G., Riley, E. E. (1967): Freezing injury to large blood vessels in dogs. With comments on the effect of experimental freezing of bile ducts. *Surgery* **61**, 748.

Garbarsch, C., Matthiessen, M. E. Helin, P., Lorenzen, I. (1969): Arteriosclerosis and hypoxia. *J. Atheroscler. Res.* **9**, 283.

Gardner, D. L. (1960): The relationship between intermittent hypotension and the prevention by hydralazine of acute vascular disease in rats with steroid hypertension. *Brit. J. exp. Path.* **41**, 60.

Gardner, D. L. (1962a): Arteriolar necrosis and the prenecrotic phase of experimental hypertension. *Quart. J. exp. Phys.* **48**, 156.

Gardner, D. L. (1962b): The influence of intermittent Bretylium Tosylate (Darenthin) on the development of vascular disease in rats with hypertension caused by sodium retention. *Brit. J. exp. Path.* **43**, 88.

Gardner, D. L. (1962c): Arterial necrosis caused by methoxamine: A comparison between acute experimental hypertensive arterial disease in the rat and lesions caused by sympathomimetic amine. *Brit. J. exp. Path.* **43**, 213.

Gardner, D. L. (1963): Arteriolar necrosis and the prenecrotic phase of experimental hypertension. *Quart. J. exp. Phys.* **2**, 156.

Gardner, D. L. (1964): Aspects of arteriolar behaviour in experimental hypertension. In, *Biological Aspects of Occlusive-Vascular Disease*. Chalmers and Gresham, Edinburgh, p. 375.

Gardner, D. L. (1965): *Pathology of Connective Tissue Disease*. Edward Arnold, London.

Gardner, D. L. (1970): Immunological responses to vascular injury in severe hypertension. *Brit. med. J.* **1**, 602.

Gardner, D. L., Brooks, P. W. (1962): Prevention of vascular necrosis in rats with adrenal-regeneration hypertension by incomplete control of raised blood pressure *Brit. J. exp. Path.* **43**, 276.

Gardner, D. L., Brooks, P. W. (1963): Arteriolar necrosis in adrenal-regeneration hypertension influence of preventive treatment with hydralazine on tissue electrolytes. *Brit. J. exp. Path.* **44**, 31.

Gardner, D. L., Cuthbert, Judit (1967): A histochemical study of enzyme activity in normal and hypertensive rat visceral arterioles. *Brit. J. exp. Path.* **48**, 427.

Gardner, D. L., Honoré, L. H. (1964): Vascular response to polypeptides in adrenal-regeneration hypertension. *Arch. int. Pharmacodyn.* **150**, 492.

Gardner, D. L., Laing, C. P. (1965): Measurement of enzyme activity of isolated small arteries in early rat hypertension. *J. Path. Bact.* **90**, 399.

Gardner, D. L., Matthews, M. A. (1969): Ultrastructure of the wall of small arteries in early experimental hypertension. *J. Pathol.* **97**, 51.

Gardner, D. L., Wuagliata, F., Drossman, M., Kalish, M., Schimmer, B. (1970): Attempted prevention of arteriolar lesions in accelerated rat hypertension by immunosuppression. *Brit. J. exp. Path.* **51**, 242.

Gárdos, Gy. (1968): Ion transport, mint a sejtmembran specificus funkciója (Ion transport as a specific function of the cell membrane). *MTA Biol. Oszt. Közl.* **11**, 179.

Garrett, L., Carrier, O., jr., Douglas, B. H. (1967): Effect of reserpine on blood pressure and vascular electrolytes in hypertension. *Europ. J. Pharmacol.* **2**, 236.

Gaunt, R., Antochak, N., Miller, G. J., Renzi, A. A. (1955): Effect of reserpine (Serpasil) and hydralazine (Apresoline) on experimental steroid hypertension. *Amer. J. Physiol.* **182**, 63.

Gedigk, P., Fischer, R. (1959): Über die Entstehung von Lipopigmenten in Muskelfasern. Untersuchungen beim experimentellen Vitamin E-Mangel der Ratte und an Organen des Menschen. *Virchows Arch. path. Anat.* **332**, 431.

Gedigk, P., Wessel, W. (1964): Elektronenmikroskopische Untersuchungen des Vitamin E-Mangel-Pigmentes im Myometrium der Ratte. *Virchows Arch. path. Anat.* **337**, 367.

Geer, J. C. (1965a): Fine structure of human aortic intimal thickening and fatty streaks. *Lab. Invest.* **14**, 1764.

Geer, J. C. (1965b): Fine structure of canine experimental atherosclerosis. *Amer. J. Path* **47**, 21.

Geer, J. C., Catsulis, C., McGill, H. C., jr., Strong, J. P. (1968): Fine structure of the baboon aortic fatty streak. *Amer. J. Path.* **52**, 265.

Geer, J. C., Guidry, M. A. (1964): Cholesterol ester composition and morphology of human normal intima and fatty streaks. *Exp. molec. Path.* **3,** 485.

Geer, J. C., McGill, H. C., Strong, J. P. (1961): The fine structure of human atherosclerotic lesions. *Amer. J. Path.* **38,** 263.

Geer, J. C., Skelton, F. R., McGill, H. C. (1958): Observations with the electron microscope of arterial lesions in hypertensive rats. *Fed. Proc.* **17,** 438.

Gekle, D., Bruchhause, V. H., Fuchs, G. (1966): Über die Grösse der Porenäquinolente in isolierten Basalmembranen der Rattennierenrinde. *Pflügers Arch. ges. Physiol.* **289,** 180.

Germuth, F. G., jr., Flanagan, C., Montenegro, M. R. (1957): The relationships between the chemical nature of the antigen, antigen dosage, rate of antibody synthesis and the occurrence of arteritis and glomerulonephritis in experimental hypersensitivity. *Bull. Johns Hopk. Hosp.* **101,** 149.

Gerő, S. (1962): Az atherosclerosis kutatás fő kérdései. I. A lipoid anyagok szerepe az atherosclerosis kórtanában (Main problems of atherosclerosis research. I. Role of lipoid substances in the pathology of atherosclerosis). Thesis, Budapest.

Gerő, S. (1969): Allergy and anti-immune factors. In, Schettler F. G., Boyd, G. S. (Eds): *Atherosclerosis.* Elsevier, Amsterdam—London—New York, p. 455.

Gerő, S., Gergely, J., Jakab, L., Székely, J., Virág, S. (1961a): Comparative immunoelectrophoretic studies on homogenates of aorta, pulmonary arteries and inferior vena cava of atherosclerotic individuals. *J. Atheroscler. Res.* **1,** 88.

Gerő, S., Gergely, J., Dévényi, L., Jakab, L., Székely, J., Virág, S. (1961b): Role of intimal mucoid substrates in the pathogenesis of atherosclerosis. I. Complex formation *in vitro* between mucopolysaccharides from atherosclerotic aortic intimas and plasma lipoprotein and fibrinogen. *J. Atheroscler. Res.* **1,** 67.

Gerő, S., Gergely, J., Farkas, K., Dévényi, T., Kocsár, L., Jakab, L., Székely, J., Virág, S. (1962): Szöveti és vér mucopolysaccharida változások cholesterinnel etetett állatokon (Changes in tissue and blood mucopolysaccharides in animals fed cholesterol). *Orv. Hetil.* **103,** 1015.

Gerő, S., Székely, J. (1968): Allergiás és autoimmun tényezők szerepe arteriosclerosisban (Role of allergic and autoimmune factors in arteriosclerosis). *Orvosképzés* **5,** 322.

Gey, K. F., Burkard, W. P., Pletscher, A. (1965): Variation of the norepinephrine metabolism of the rat heart with age. *Gerontologia* **11,** 1.

Ghani, A. R., Still, W. J. S. (1967): The role of blood borne cells in organization of mural thrombi in Dacron aortic prosthesis in canines. *Amer. J. Path.* **50,** 6.

Ghidoni, J. J., Liotta, D., Hall, C. W., Adams, J. G., Lechter, A., Barrionneva, M., O'Neal, R. M., DeBakey, M. E. (1968): Healing of pseudointimas in velour-lined, impermeable arterial prostheses. *Amer. J. Path.* **53,** 375.

Giacomelli, F., Wiener, J., Spiro, D. (1969): Ultrastructure and permeability of cerebral vessels in experimental hypertension. *Amer. J. Path.* **55,** 33/a.

Giese, J. (1961): Deposition of serum proteins in vascular walls during acute hypertension. *Acta path. microbiol. scand.* **33,** 167.

Giese, J. (1964): Acute hypertensive vascular disease. 2. Studies on vascular reaction and permeability changes by means of vital microscopy and colloidal tracer technique. *Acta path. microbiol. scand.* **62,** 497.

Giese, J. (1966): *The Pathogenesis of Hypertensive Vascular Disease.* Munksgaard, Copenhagen, p. 1.

Gitlin, D., Craig, J. M., Janeway, C. A. (1957): Studies on the nature of fibrinoid in the collagen diseases. *Amer. J. Path.* **33,** 55.

Godfraind, T., Kaba, A., Polster, P. (1968): Differences in sensitivity of arterial smooth muscles to inhibition of their contractile response to depolarisation by potassium. *Arch. int. Pharmacodyn.* **172,** 236.

Gofmann, J. W., Young, W. (1965): The filtration concept of atherosclerosis and serum lipids in the diagnosis of atherosclerosis. In, Sandler, M., Bourne, G. H. E. (Eds): *Atherosclerosis and its Origin.* Academic Press, New York, p. 197.

Gold, H. (1962): Atherosclerosis in the a rat. Effect of X-ray and high fat diet. *Proc. Soc. exp. diet. Med.* **111,** 593.

Goldberger, E. (1959): Etiology and pathogenesis of syndromes associated with periarteritis nodosa lesions. A unified theory. *Amer. J. Cardiol.* **3,** 656.

Goldblatt, H. (1957): Pathogenesis of malignant hypertension. *Circulation* **16**, 697·

Goodman, H. M. (1968): Proposed mode of action of histamine. *Nature* **219**, 1053.

Gorácz, Gy. (1963): Cardiac and vascular changes in experimental hypertension. Thesis, Budapest.

Gostimirovich, D. (1968): Estrogen effects on the aortic wall in young immature rabbits. *Virchows Arch. path. Anat.* **343**, 258.

Gottlieb, H., Lalich, J. J. (1954): Occurrence of atherosclerosis in aorta of swine. *Amer. J. Path.* **30**, 851.

Gottlob, R., Zinner, G. (1962): Über die Regeneration geschädigter Endothelien nach hartem und weichem Trauma. *Virchows Arch. path. Anat.* **336**, 16.

Gozman, J. W., Young, W. (1963): The filtration concept of atherosclerosis and serum lipids in the diagnosis of atherosclerosis. In, Sandler, M., Bourne, G. H. E. (Eds): *Atherosclerosis and its Origin.* Academic Press, New York, p. 197.

Graham, R. C., Karnovsky, M. J. (1966): Glomerular permeability ultrastructural cytochemical studies using peroxidases as protein tracers. *J. exp. Med. Path.* **124**, 1123.

Greenlee, Th., K., Ross, R., Harmann, J. L. (1966): The fine structure of elastic fibers. *J. Cell. Biol.* **30**, 59.

Gresham, G. A., Howard, A. N., King, A. J. (1962): A comparative histopathological study of the early atherosclerotic lesion. *Brit. J. exp. Path.* **43**, 21.

Gresham, G. A., Howard, A. N., McQueen, J. (1965): Atherosclerosis in primates. *Brit. J. exp. Path.* **46**, 94.

Griesemer, E. C., Coret, I. A. (1960): Recovery responses of hypoxic arterial smooth muscle. *J. Pharmacol. exp. Ther.* **130**, 294.

Grollman, A., Ashworth, C., Suki, W. (1963): Atherosclerosis in the chicken. *Arch. Path.* **75**, 618.

Groniowski, I., Biezyskowa, W., Walski, M. (1969): Electron microscope studies on the surface coat of the hyaline. *J. Cell. Biol.* **40**, 585.

Gross, F. (1958): Renin und Hypertension, physiologische oder pathologische Wirkstoffe? *Klin. Wschr.* **36**, 693.

Grotte, G. (1956): Passage of dextran molecules across the blood—lymph barrier. *Acta chir. scand.* **24**, 5.

Gruber, G. B. (1925): Zur Frage der Periarteritis nodosa mit besonderer Berücksichtigung der Gallenblasen- und Nierenbeteiligung. *Virchows Arch. path. Anat.* **258**, 441.

Grundmann, E., Amlie, J. G. (1961): Zur pathologischen Anatomie der Makroglobulinämie Waldenström. *Frankfurt. Z. Path.* **71**, 443.

Gumenyuk, L. I. (1960): A comparative study of the changes occurring in the small arteries in various forms of experimentally induced hypertension. *Arch. Path.* **22**, 68.

Günn, F. L., Shelbrune, J. D., Benjamin, F. T. (1968): Disorders of cell volume regulation. I. Effects of inhibition of plasma membrane adenosine triphosphatase with ouabain. *Amer. J. Path.* **53**, 1041.

Gupta, P. P., Tandon, H. D., Ramalingaswami, U. (1969): Spontaneous vascular lesions in indian pigs. *J. Path. Bact.* **99**, 19.

Gutstein, W. H., Lataillade, J. N., Lewis, L. (1962): The role of neuroexcitation in arteriosclerosis. In, *Metabolismus Parietis Vasorum* Praha, Acad. Press, p. 307.

Gutstein, W. H., Lazzarini-Robertson, A., jr., LaTaillade, J. N. (1963): The role of local arterial irritability in the development of arterio-atherosclerosis. *Amer. J. Path.* **42**, 61.

Hackel, W. (1930): Untersuchungen über die vitale Durchtränkung der Kaninchenaorta mit Trypanblue. *Z. ges. exper. Med.* **72**, 762.

Hackensellner, H. A., David, H., Uerlings, I. (1965): Licht- und elektronenmikroskopische Untersuchungen an doppelt ligierten Arterien (A. carotis des Kaninchens). *Acta biol. med. germ.* **14**, 34.

Hackensellner, H. A., Töpelmann, I. (1965): Das Flächenbild des Endothels der doppelt ligierten Arteria carotis des Kaninchens. *Acta morph. Acad. Sci. hung.* **13**, 359.

Hager, H. (1961): Elektronenmikroskopische Untersuchungen über die Feinstruktur der Blutgefässe und perivaskulären Räume im Säugetiergehirn. *Acta neuropath. Berl.* **1**, 9.

Haining, R., Kimball, T. S. (1934): Polyarteritis nodosa. *Amer. J. Path.* **10,** 349.

Hall, C. E. (1949): Electron microscopy of fibrinogen and fibrin. *J. biol. Chem.* **179,** 857.

Hall, C. E., Slayter, H. S. (1959): The fibrinogen molecule: its size, shape and mode of polymerisation. *J. biophys. biochem. Cytol.* **5,** 11.

Halpert, B., O'Neal, R. (1966): Vasa vasorum of dacron prosthesis in canine aorta. *Arch. Path.* **81,** 412.

Ham, K. N. (1962): The fine structure of normal rat aorta. *Austr. J. exp. Biol. med. Sci.* **40,** 341.

Ham, K. N., Hurley, J. V. (1965): Acute inflammation: an electron microscope study of turpentine induced pleurity in the rat. *J. Path. Bact.* **90,** 365.

Hama, K. (1960): The fine structure of some blood vessels of the earthworm, *Esenia foetide. J. biophys. biochem. Cytol.* **7,** 717.

Hamoir, G. (1969): The muscle proteins of the vascular wall. *Angiologica* **6,** 190.

Hampton, J. C. (1958): An electron microscope study of the hepatic uptake and excretion of submicroscopic particles injected into the blood stream and into bile duct. *Acta anat. (Basel)* **32,** 262.

Harington, M., Kincaid-Smith, P., McMichael, S. (1959): Results of treatment in malignant hypertension. *Brit. med. J.* **11,** 969.

Harman, D. (1962): Atherosclerosis inhibiting effect of an antihistamine drug chlorphenylamine. *Circulat. Res.* **11,** 277.

Harms, D. (1967): Über den Verschluss der Ductes arteriosi von *Gallus domesticus.* *Z. Zellforsch.* **81,** 433.

Hartmann, H. A., Miller, E. C., Miller, J. A. (1959): Periarteritis in rats given single injection of 4'-fluoro-10-methyl-1,2-benzanthracene. *Proc. Soc. exp. Biol. (N. Y.)* **101,** 626.

Hasleton, P. S., Health, D., Brewer, D. B. (1968): Hypertensive pulmonary vascular disease in states of chronic hypoxia. *J. Path. Bact.* **95,** 431.

Hass, G. M., Landerholm, W., Hemmens, A. (1966): Production of calcific atheroarteriosclerosis and thromboarteritis with nicotine, vitamin-D and dietary cholesterol. *Amer. J. Path.* **49,** 739.

Hass, G. M., Trueheart, R. E., Hemmens, B. S. (1961): Experimental athero-arteriosclerosis due to calcific medial degeneration and hypercholesteremia. *Amer. J. Path.* **38,** 289.

Hass, G. M., Trueheart, R. E., Taylor, C. B., Stumpe, M. (1958): An experimental histologic study of hypervitaminosis D. *Amer. J. Path.* **34,** 395.

Hassler, O. (1962): The windows of the internal elastic lamella of the cerebral arteries. *Virchows Arch. path. Anat.* **335,** 127.

Hassler, O. (1970): The origin of the cells constituting arterial intima thickening. An expérimental autoradiographic study with the use of H³ thymidine. *Lab. Invest.* **22,** 286.

Hatt, P. Y., Berjal, G., Bonnet, M., Jovannot, P. (1968): L'artériographie hypertensive expérimentale chez le rat. In, *Colloques Internationaux du Centre National de la Recherche Scientifique,* No. 169. Cent. National de la Recherche Scientifique, Paris, p. 871.

Hatt, P. Y., Berjal, G., Bonvalet, J. P. (1966): Structures artérielle et artériolaires au cours de l'hypertension expérimentale du rat. Étude au microscope électronique. In, *1. Réunion de Club International sur l'Hypertension Artérielle.* Expérience Scientifique Française, Paris, vol. 1, p. 460.

Hauss, W. H. (1970): Die unspezifische Mesenchymreaktion—gesätzmässig erste krankhafte Veränderung bei der Arteriosklerose. *Sandorama* **II,** 21.

Haust, M. D., Balis, J. U., More, R. H. (1962): Electron microscopic study of intimal lipid accumulations in human aorta and their pathogenesis. *Circulat. Res.* **26,** 656.

Haust, M. D., More, R. H. (1957): Morphologic evidence and significance of permeation in the genesis of arteriosclerosis. *Circulation* **16,** 496.

Haust, M. D., More, R. H. (1963): Significance of the smooth muscle cell in atherogenesis. In, Jones, R. J. (Ed.): *Evolution of the Athero-Sclerotic Plaque.* Univ. of Chicago Press, Chicago and London, Vol. I, p. 51.

Haust, M. D., More, R. H. (1966): Morphological evidence of different modes of secretion of connective tissue precursors by fibroblasts and by smooth muscle cells. *Amer. J. Path.* **48,** 15/a.

175

Haust, M. D., More, R. H., Bencosme, S. A., Balis, J. U. (1965a): Elastogenesis in human aorta. An electron microscopic study. *Exp. molec. Path.* **4**, 508.

Haust, M. D., More, R. H., Bencosme, S. A., Balis, J. U. (1967): Electron microscopic studies in human atherosclerosis. Extracellular elements in aortic dots and streaks. *Exp. molec. Path.* **6**, 300.

Haust, M. D., More, R. H., Movat, H. Z. (1960): The role of smooth muscle cells in the fibrogenesis of arteriosclerosis. *Amer. J. Path.* **37**, 377.

Haust, M. D., Wyllie, J. C., More, R. H. (1964): Atherogenesis and plasma constituents. I. Demonstration of fibrin in the white plaque by the fluorescent antibody technique. *Amer. J. Path.* **44**, 265.

Haust, M. D., Wyllie, J. C., More, R. H. (1965b): Electron microscopy of fibrin in human atherosclerotic lesions. Immunohistochemical and morphologic identification. *Exp. molec. Path.* **4**, 205.

Hawn, C. Z., Jeneway, C. A. (1947): Histological and serological sequences in experimental hypersensitivity. *J. exp. Med.* **85**, 571.

Hayes, J. R. (1967): Histological changes in constricted arteries and arterioles. *J. Anat. (Lond).* **101**, 343.

Heberer, G. (1966): Haemodynamisch-bedingte Gefässwandschäden. In, Heberer, G., Rau, G., Leder, H. N. (Eds): *Aorta und grosse Arterien.* Springer, Berlin–Heidelberg–New York, p. 81.

Heinlein, H., Volland, W., Vogel, K. (1961): Beitrag zur Nosologie und Pathogenese der Periarteritis nodosa mit Wiedergabe sechs eigener Fälle. *Z. Kreisl.-Forsch.* **50**, 849

Heptinstall, R. H., Porter, K. A. (1957): The effects of a brief period of high blood pressure on cholesterol-induced atheroma in rabbits. *Brit. exp. Path.* **38**, 55.

Herberston, B. M., Kellaway, T. D. (1960): Arterial necrosis in the rat produced by methoxamine. *J. Path. Bact.* **80**, 87.

Herxheimer, G. (1923): cit. Zollinger (1959) *Zbl. path. Beiheft* **33**, 111.

Hess, R., Pearse, A. G. E. (1958): The histochemistry of indoxylesterase of rat kidney with special reference to its cathepsin-like activity. *Brit. J. exper. Path.* **39**, 292.

Hess, R., Stäubli, W. (1963a): The development of aortic lipoidosis in the rat (A correlation histochemical and electron microscopic study). *Amer. J. Path.* **43**, 301.

Hess, R., Stäubli, W. (1963b): Vergleichende histochemische und elektronemikroskopische Untersuchungen von Aortaveränderungen bei experimenteller Lipoidose. *Verh. dtsch. Ges. Path.* **47**, 369.

Hess, R., Stäubli, W. (1969): Ultrastructure of vascular changes. In, Schettler, F. G. Boyd, G. S. (Eds): *Atherosclerosis.* Elsevier, Amsterdam–London–New York, Vol. 2, p. 49.

Hinke, J. A. M., Willson, M. L., Burnham, S. C. (1964): Calcium and contractility of arterial smooth muscle. *Amer. J. Physiol.* **206**, 211.

Hirano, A., Zimmerman, H. M., Levine, S. (1965): The fine structure of arterial fluid accumulation. IX. Edema following silver nitrate implantation. *Amer. J. Path.* **47**, 531.

Hiraoka, M., Yamagishi, S., Sano, T. (1968): Role of calcium ions in the contraction of vascular smooth muscle. *Amer. J. Physiol.* **214**, 1084.

Hirst, A. E., Gore, I. (1962): Study of permeability of the human aorta. *Circulation* **26**, 657.

Hoak, J. C., Warner, E. D., Connor, W. E. (1969): New concept of Levarterenol-induced acute myocardinal necrosis. *Arch. Path.* **87**, 332.

Hoff, H. F. (1968): An electron microscopic study of the rabbit aortic intima after occlusion by brief exposure to a single ligature. *Brit. J. exp. Path.* **49**, 1.

Hoff, H. F., Gottlob, R. (1967): Regeneration von Arterien und Venen nach weichem Trauma; elektronenmikroskopische Untersuchungen. *Klin. Med.* **22**, 419.

Hoff, H. F., Gottlob, R. (1969): Studies on the pathogenesis of atherosclerosis with experimental model systems. *Virchows Arch. path. Anat.* **347**, 1.

Hoff, H. F., Graf, J. (1966): An electron microscopic study of phosphatase activity on the endothelial cells of rabbit aorta. *J. Histochem. Cytochem.* **14**, 719.

Hogan, M. J., Feeney, L. (1963a): The ultrastructure of the retinal blood vessels. I. The large vessels. *J. Ultrastruct. Res.* **9**, 10.

Hogan, M. J., Feeney, L. (1963b): The structure of the retinal vessels. II. The small vessels. *J. Ultrastruct. Res.* **9**, 29.

176

Hoggan, G., Hoggan, E. (1883): The lymphatics of the wall of the larger blood vessels and lymphatics. *J. Anat. (Lond.)* **17**, 1.

Höglund, S., Levin, O. (1965): Electron microscopic studies of some proteins from normal human serum. *J. mol. Biol.* **12**, 866.

Hollander, W. (1967): Recent advances in experimental and molecular pathology. Influx, synthesis and transport of arterial lipoproteins in atherosclerosis. *Exp. molec. Path.* **7**, 248.

Holle, G. (1967): *Lehrbuch der allgemeinen Pathologie.* Fischer, Jena, p. 270.

Holt, S. J. (1958): Studies of the enzyme cytochemistry. V. An appraisal of indigogenic reactions for esterase localization. *Proc. roy. Soc. Med.* **148**, 520.

Honoré, L. H., Gardner, D. L. (1962): Altered vascular reactivity of rats with adrenal regeneration hypertension. *Experientia (Basel)* **18**, 419.

Howard, R. O., Richardson, D. W., Smith, M. H., Patterson, J. L. (1965): Oxygen consumption of arterioles and venules as studied in the Cartesian diver. *Circulat. Res.* **16**, 187.

Hruza, Z., Zweifach, B. W. (1967): Effect of age on vascular reactivity to catecholamines in rats. *J. Geront.* **22**, 469.

Huber, J. (1960): Experimentelle Untersuchungen zur Frage der kontralateralen renalen Fixierung bei einseitigem Nierendrosselungshochdruck. *Z. ges. exp. Med.* **133**, 285.

Huezer, W. C. (1944/45): Arteriosclerosis. *Arch. Path.* **38**, 162.

Hurley, I. V., Ryan, B. (1967): A delayed increase in venular permeability following intrapleural injections in the rat. *J. Path. Bact.* **93**, 87.

Hurley, I. V., Spector, W. G. (1965): A topographical study of increased vascular permeability in acute turpentine induced pleuritis. *J. Path. Bact.* **89**, 245.

Husni, E. A., Manion, W. C. (1967): Atrophy of the arterial wall incident to localized chronic hypotension. *Surgery*, **61**, 611.

Imai, H., Lee, K. T., Pastori, S., Paulilio, E., Florentin, R., Thomas, W. A. (1966): Atherosclerosis in rabbits. Architectural and subcellular alterations of smooth muscle cells of aortas in response to hyperlipemia. *Exp. molec. Path.* **8**, 273.

Imai, H., Thomas, W. A. (1968): Cerebral atherosclerosis in swine. Role of necrosis in progression of diet-induced lesions from proliferative to atheromatous stage. *Expmolec. Path.* **8**, 330.

Irey, M. S., Manion, W. C., Taylor, H. B. (1970): Vascular lesions in women taking oral contraceptives. *Arch. Path.* **89**, 1.

Ishii, S. Matano, S. (1968): Electron microscopic observations on phosphatase activities of the chorioid plexus in rat brain. II. On the structural localisation of β-glycerophosphatase of the alkali pH. *Okajimas Folia anot. jap.* **44**, 149.

Ishizaka, K., Campbell, D. H. (1958): Biological activity of soluble antigen–antibody complexes. I. Skin reactive properties. *Proc. Soc. exp. Biol. (N. Y.)* **97**, 635.

Iwanaga, Y., Tamimura, A., Kitsukawa, H., Tanigawa, J., Aihara, M., Kawashima, T., Mae, A., Nahashima, T. (1969): The role of endothelial cells in the pathogenesis of atherosclerosis. *Acta path. jap.* **19**, 161.

Jackson, J. G., Puchtler, H., Sweat, F. (1968): Investigation of staining, polarization and fluorescence microscopic properties of pseudo-elastic fibres on the renal arterial system. *J. roy. Microscopical Soc.* **88**, 473.

Jacobsen, N. O., Jorgensen, F., Thomsen, A. C. (1966): An electron microscopic study of small arteries and arterioles in the normal human kidney. *Néphron* **3**, 17.

Jaffe, R. H., Willis, D., Bachem, A. (1929): Über nach elektrischen Gefässwandschädigungen auftretende Heilungsvorgänge. *Zbl. allg. Path.* **44**, 1241.

Jakab, L., Seregélyi, Éva (1970): Effect of glucosamine and of its derivatives on $^{35}S_4$-incorporation into dog aorta. *Acta med. Acad. Sci. hung.* **27**, 129.

Jancso, M. (1947): Histamine as a physiologic activator of the reticuloendothelial system. *Nature* **160**, 227.

Janssen, W., Michot, F. (1960): Über die Pathomorphose der Periarteriitis nodosa nach Behandlung mit Corticosteroiden. *Path. et Microbiol. (Basel)* **23**, 511.

Jarmolich, J., Daoud, A. S., Landau, J., Fritz, K. E., McElvence, E. (1968): Aortic media explants. Cell proliferation and production of mucopolysaccharides, collagen and elastic tissue. *Exp. Molec. Path.* **9**, 171.

Jäger, E. (1932): Zur pathologischen Anatomie der Thromboangiitis obliterans bei juveniler Extremitätengangrän. *Virchows Arch. path. Anat.* **284**, 526.

Jennings, M. A., Broch, L. G., Florey, H. W. (1966): A comparison of connective tissue lining aortic grafts with extravascular connective tissue. *Proc. roy. Soc. B.* **165**, 206.

Jennings, M. A., Florey, H. W., Stehbens, W. E., French, J. E. (1961): Intimal changes in the arteries of a pig. *J. Path. Anat.* **81**, 49.

Jennings, M. A., Marchesi, V. T., Florey, H. (1962): The transport of particles across the walls of small blood vessels. *Proc. roy. Soc. Med.* **156**, 14.

Jobst, K. (1954): Beiträge zur submikroskopischen Struktur der fibrinoiden Degeneration. *Acta morph. Acad. Sci. hung.* **4**, 333.

Joiner, D. W., Puchtler, H., Sweat, F. (1968): Staining of immature collagen by resorcin-fuchsin in infant kidneys. *J. roy. Microscopical Soc.* **88**, 461.

Jones, T. C., Zook, B. C. (1965): Aging changes in the vascular system of animals. *Ann. N. Y. Acad. Sci.* **127**, 671.

Jordan, G. L., Stump, M. M., DeBakey, M. E., Halpert, B. (1962): Endothelial lining of dacron prostheses of porcine thoracic aortas. *Proc. Soc. exp. Biol. (N. Y.)* **110**, 340.

Jores, L. (1898): Über die Neubildung elastischer Fasern in der Intima bei Endarteritis. *Z. Beitr. path. Anat.* **24**, 458.

Jores, L. (1924): Arterien. In, Henke, F., Lubarsch, O. (Eds): *Handbuch der speziellen pathologischen Anatomie und Histologie.* Vol. II. *Herz und Gefässe.* Springer, Berlin, p. 608.

Jorgen, J. (1967): An *in vitro* method for the study of cholesterol uptake at the endothelial cell surface on the rabbit aorta. *Biochem. biophys. Acta. (Amst.)* **135**, 532.

Jorgensen, F., Thorsen, A. Chr. (1968): Dimensions of some wall components of small arteries and arterioles in the normal human kidney. *Acta path. microbiol. scand.* **76**, 501.

Junge-Hülsing, G., Wirth, W., Matthes, K., König, F. (1963): Über die Veränderungen des Bindegewebsstoffwechsels bei der Arteriosklerose und bei anderen Gefässerkrankungen. In, *Gefässwand und Blutplasma.* Fischer, Jena, p. 28.

Jurukova, Z., Rohr, H. P. (1968): Beitrag zur Bildung bindegewebiger Matrix in platten Muskelzellen. Elektronenmikroskopisch-autoradiographische Untersuchungen mit ^{35}S-Sulfat an platten Muskelzellen nach Doppelligatur der Arteria carotis. *Path. Europ.* **3**, 551.

Kagan, A., Livsic, A. M., Sternby, N., Vickert, A. M. (1968): Coronary artery thrombosis and the acute attack of coronary heart disease. *Lancet* **ii**, 1199.

Kahn, S. G., Slocum, A. (1967): Enzyme activities in aortas of chickens fed atherogenic diets. *Amer. J. Physiol.* **213**, 367.

Kalliomäki, J. L., Kasanen, A. (1969): A new combination of hypertensive drugs (reserpine, dihydralazine, furosemide and triamterene) for the treatment of arterial hypertension without risk of hypopotassaemia. *Curr. ther. Res.* **11**, 344.

Kanisawa, M., Schroeder, H. A. (1969): Renal arteriolar changes in hypertensive rats given cadmium in drinking water. *Exp. molec. Path.* **10**, 81.

Kao, V. C., Wissler, R. W. (1965): A study of the immunohistochemical localisation of serum lipoproteins and other plasma proteins in human atherosclerotic lesions. *Exp. molec. Path.* **4**, 465.

Karrer, H. E. (1960a): The striated musculature of blood vessels. II. Cell interconnections and cell surface. *J. biophys. biochem. Cytol.* **8**, 135.

Karrer, H. E. (1960b): EM study of developing chick embryo aorta. *J. Ultrastruct. Res.* **4**, 420.

Karrer, H. E. (1961): An electron microscopic study of the aorta in young and in aging mice. *J. Ultrastruct. Res.* **5**, 1.

Karnovsky, M. J. (1965): A formaldehyde-glutaraldehyde fixative of high osmolality for use in electron microscopy. *J. Cell. Biol.* **27**, 137/a (Abstract).

Karnovsky, M. J. (1967): The ultrastructural basis of capillary permeability studied with peroxidase as a tracer. *J. Cell. Biol.* **35**, 213.

Kasai, T., Pollak, O. J. (1964): Smooth muscle cells in aortic cultures of untreated and cholesterol-fed rabbits. *Z. Zellforsch.* **62**, 743.

Katz, Y .J., Patek, P. R., Bernick, S. (1962): Effect of angiotensin on juxtaglomerular cells and vessels of the kidney. *Circ. Res.* **11**, 955.

Kaye, G. I., Cole, J. D., Donn, A. (1965): Electron microscopy: sodium localisation on normal and abnormal treated transporting cell. *Science* **150**, 1167.

Keech, M. K. (1960): Electron microscope study of the normal rat aorta. *J. biophys. biochem. Cytol.* **7**, 533.

Kellaway, T. D., Herbertson, B. M., Mortimer, T. F. (1962): Arterial lesions induced in rabbits by soluble foreign protein and by methoxamine. *J. Path. Bact.* **84**, 45.

Kelly, F. B., jr., Taylor, C. B., Hass, G. M. (1952): Experimental atherosclerosis localization of lipids in experimental arterial lesion of rabbits with hypercholesteremia. *Arch. Path.* **53**, 419.

Kemnitz, P., Willgeroth, Ch. (1969): Coarctatio aortae abdominalis vom Takayashu-Typ bei einem 15-jährigen Mädchen. *Zbl. allg. Path. path. Anat.* **112**, 505.

Kemper, J. W., Baggenstoss, A. H., Slocumb C. H. (1957): The relationship of therapy with cortisone to the incidence of vascular lesions in rheumatoid arthritis. *Ann. Intern. Med.* **46**, 831.

Kent, S. P., (1967): Diffusion of plasma proteins into cells: a manifestation of cell injury in human skeletal myocardial ischemia. *Amer. J. Path.* **50**, 623.

Kent, S. P. (1969): Diffusion of plasma proteins into cells: a manifestation of cell injury in rabbit muscle exposed to lecithinase C. *Arch. Path.* **88**, 407.

Keynan, A., Auiram, A., Czaczkes, J. W., Ullmann, T. D. (1969): Reversal of excessive hypertension in patients with terminal renal failure by intermittent hemodialysis and bilateral nephrectomy. *Israel J. med. Sci.* **5**, 400.

Kirck, J. E. (1962): The diaphorase and cytochrome reductase activities of arterial tissue in individuals of various ages. *J. Geront.* **17**, 276.

Kirck, J. E. (1964): Comparison of enzyme activities of arterial samples from sexually mature men and women. *Clin. Chem.* **10**, 184.

Kirck, J. E., Laursen, T. J. S. (1955a): Dehydrogenase activities of human aortic tissue determined with a quantitative tetrazolium technique. *J. Geront.* **10**, 18.

Kirck, J. E., Laursen, T. J. S. (1955b): Diffusion coefficients of various solutes for human aortic tissue with special reference to variations in tissue permeability with age. *J. Geront.* **10**, 288.

Kirck, J. E., Ritz, E. (1967): The glyceraldehyde-3-phosphate and glycerophosphate dehydrogenase activities of arterial tissue in individuals of various ages. *J. Geront.* **22**, 427.

Kirkpatrick, J. B. (1967): Pathogenesis of foam cell lesions in irradiated arteries. *Amer. J. Path.* **50**, 291.

Kjeldsen, K. (1969): *Smoking and Atherosclerosis*. Munksgaard, Copenhagen, p. 145.

Kjeldsen, K., Wanstrup, J., Astrup, P. (1968): Enhancing influence of arterial hypoxia on the development of atheromatosis in cholesterol-fed rabbits. *J. Atheroscler. Res.* **8**, 835.

Kline, J. K. (1960): Myocardial alterations associated with pheochromocytomas. *Amer. J. Path.* **38**, 539.

Klinge, F. (1930): Die Eiweissüberempfindlichkeit (Gewebsanaphylaxie) der Gelenke. Experimentelle pathologisch-anatomische Studie zur Pathogenese des Gelenk-Rheumatismus. *Beitr. path. Anat.* **83**, 185.

Kluge, T. (1969): The permeability of mesothelium to horseradish peroxidase. A light and electron microscopic study with special reference to the morphology of pericardial mast cells. *Acta path. microbiol. scand.* **75**, 257.

Kluge, T., Hovig, T. (1968): Pericardial absorption of exogenous peroxidase in rats. *Acta path. microbiol. scand.* **73**, 521.

Knieriem, H. J. (1967): Electron microscopic study of bovine atherosclerotic lesion. *Amer. J. Path.* **50**, 1035.

Knold, P., Gerbert, G., Brecht, K. (1968): The antagonism of polonium and catecholamines on the vascular tone of isolated arterial segments. *Experientia (Basel)* **24**, 692.

Kobayashi, S. (1968a): Some observations on the pinocytosis and fenestrations of the capillary endothelium. *J. Electron Microscopy* **17**, 272.

Kobayashi, S. (1968b): Some observations on the capillary vehicles and the pores. *J. Electron Microscopy* **17**, 322.

Kobernick, S. D., More, R. H. (1959): The pathogenesis of lesions in rabbits by administration of foreign serum proteins. I. The effects of cold, ACTH and cortisone on lesions of heart, kidneys and arteries. *Lab. Invest.* **81**, 777.

Kocsár, L., Jakab, L., Gergely, J., Gerő, S., Székely, J. (1961): Radioaktív kén beépülésének változásai nyúl aortájába és egyéb szöveteibe a) cholesterinetetés; b) különböző antigénekkel való immunizálás hatására [Changes of the incorporation of radioactive sulphur into the aorta and other tissues of the rabbit after (a) cholesterin feeding; (b) immunization with various antigens]. *Kísérl. Orvostud.* **13**, 52.

12*

Kojimahara, M. (1967): Healing and exacerbation of arterial lesions in rats with experimental hypertension with special reference to effect of anti-hypertensive drugs on arterial lesions. *Gumma J. med. Sci.* **16**, 1.

Koletsky, S. (1955): Necrotizing vascular disease in rat. I. Observation on pathogenesis. *Arch. Path.* **59**, 312.

Koletsky, S. (1957): Necrotizing vascular disease in rat. II. Role of sodium chloride. *Arch. Path.* **63**, 405.

Koletsky, S. (1959): Role of salt and renal mass in experimental hypertension. *Arch. Path.* **68**, 11.

Koletsky, S., Resnick, H., Behrin, D. (1959): Mesenteric artery electrolytes in experimental hypertension. *Proc. Soc. exp. Biol. (N. Y.)* **102**, 12.

Koletsky, S., Rivera-Velez, J. M., Pritchard, W. H. (1964): Experimental renal hypertension. Origin of high blood pressure and vascular disease. *Arch. Path.* **78**, 24.

Koletsky, S., Roland, C., Rivera-Velez, J. M. (1968): Rapid acceleration of atherosclerosis in hypertensive rats on high fat diet. *Exp. molec. Path.* **9**, 322.

Koc, V. C. H., Wissler R. W. (1965): A study of the immunohistochemical localization of serum lipoproteins and other plasma proteins in human atherosclerotic lesions. *Exp. Mol. Path.* **4**, 465.

Könn, G., Berg, P. (1965): Tierexperimentelle chronische pulmonale Hypertonie nach rezidivierender Mikrolungenembolie und ihre Rückwirkung auf Herz und Arterien. *Beitr. path. Anat.* **132**, 86.

Köppel, G. (1967): Elektronenmikroskopische Untersuchungen zur Gestalt und zum makromolekulären Band des Fibrinogenmoleküls und der Fibrinfasern. *Z. Zellforsch.* **77**, 443.

Korb, G. (1965): Elektronmikroskopische Untersuchungen zur Aludrin (Isoproterenolsulfat)-Schädigung des Herzmuskels. *Virchows Arch. path. Anat.* **339**, 136.

Kosan, R. L., Burton, A. C. (1966): Oxygen consumption of arterial smooth muscle as a function of active tone and passive stretch. *Circulat. Res.* **18**, 79.

Koszewski, B. J. (1958): Brachial arteritis or aortic arch arteritis. A new inflammatory arterial disease (pulseless disease). *Angiology* **9**, 180.

Koszewski, B. J., Hubbard, T. F. (1957): Pulseless disease due to brachial arteritis. *Circulation* **15**, 406.

Kowalewski, K. (1954): Uptake of radiosulphate by mucopolysaccharides of aorta in cholesterol fed cockerels. *Proc. Soc. exp. Biol. (N. Y.)* **101**, 536.

Kretschmann, H. J. (1963): Fluoreszenz-polarisationsmikroskopische Analyse der Ultrastruktur von Elastikalamellen und Elastikafasern. *Z. Zellforsch.* **60**, 7.

Krompecher, I. (1928): Die Entwicklung der elastischen Elemente der Arterienwand. *Z. Anat. Entwickl.-Gesch.* **85**, 704.

Krompecher, I. (1966): *Form und Funktion in der Biologie.* Akademische Verlagsgesellschaft, Leipzig.

Kunz, J., Fuhrmann, I., Hackensellner, H. A. (1968): Zur Frage der Synthese sulfatierter Mukopolysaccharide durch das Endothel grosser Gefässe des Kaninchens. *Experimentelle Path.* **2**, 285.

Kunz, J., Hecht, A., Hegewald, H. (1965): Morphologische und fermenthistochemische Untersuchungen der Aorta des Kaninchens nach lokaler Einwirkung von $Sr^{90} - Y^{90}$ Betastrahlen. *Frankfurt. Z. Path.* **74**, 293.

Kunz, J., Kienz, D., Klein, O. (1967a): Zur Wirkung von Hydrocortisonacetat auf den Zellstoffwechsel bei der experimentellen Intimaproliferation der Rattenaorta. *Virchows Arch. path. Anat.* **342**, 353.

Kunz, J., Kienz, D., Klein, O. (1967b): Autoradiographische Untersuchungen zur Synthese in DNS Kollagen und Mucopolysacchariden bei der experimentellen Proliferation der Aortaintima. *Virchows Arch. path. Anat.* **342**, 345.

Kussmaul, A., Maier, R. (1866): Über eine bisher nicht beschriebene eigentümliche Arterienerkrankung (Periarteritis nodosa), die mit Morbus Brightii und rapid fortschreitender allgemeiner Muskellähmung einhergeht. *Dtsch. Arch. Klin. Med.* **1**, 484.

Kühl, I. (1956): Über allergisch-hyperergische Erscheinungen bei Mäusen nach β-Naphthylaminbehandlung, gekennzeichnet durch Periarteritis nodosa, Aktivierung des retikuloendothelialen Systems, Plasmazellhyperplasie und Paraproteinose der Organe. *Virchows Arch. path. Anat.* **328**, 49.

Ladányi, P., Lelkes, Gy. (1968): Study of experimental fibrillogenesis in tunica muscularis of the rat ureter. *Acta morph. Acad. Sci. hung.* **16**, 147.

Laitinen, E. (1963): Changes in the elemental structure of the aorta in human and experimental atherosclerosis. *Acta path. microbiol. scand.* Suppl. **167**, 1.

Lalich, J. J. (1969): Coronary artery hyalinosis in rats fed allylamine. *Exp. molec. Path.* **10**, 14.

Landis, E. M., Pappenheimer, J. R. (1963): Exchange of substances through the capillary walls. In, Hamilton, W. F., Dow, P. (Eds): *Handbook of Physiology*, Chapter 29, Section 2; *Circulation 2*. American Physiological Society, Washington, D. C., p. 961.

Lang, J. (1965): Mikroskopische Anatomie der Arterien. In, *Int. Symp. Morph. and Histochem. of the Vascular Wall*. Fribourg. Part I. *Angiologica* **2**, 225.

Lang, J., Nordwig, A. (1966): Über die Membrana elastica interna von Arterien muskulären Typs. *Z. Zellforsch.* **73**, 313.

Lange, F. (1924): Studien zur Pathologie der Arterien, insbesondere zur Lehre von der Arteriosklerose. *Virchows Arch. path. Anat.* **248**, 463.

Langen, C. D. (1953): The pressure gradient in the arterial wall and the problem of arteriosclerosis. *Cardiologia* **22**, 315.

Lansing, A. J., Rosenthal, F. B., Dempsey, E. W., Alex, A. M. (1952): The structure and chemical characterization of elastic fiber as revealed by elastase and by electronmicroscopy. *Anat. Res.* **114**, 557.

Laperrouza, C. A. (1962): Zwei Fälle von Ceroidpigmentbildung des Mesenterialfettes und der glatten Muskulatur mit schwerer pseudoperniziöser Anämie bei Parkinsonismus. *Virchows Arch. path. Anat.* **335**, 544.

Laszt, L. (1964): Zur Biochemie der Arterienmuskulatur. *Biol. cardiol.* **15**, 3.

Laurent, T. C. (1966): *In vitro* studies on the transport of macromolecules through connective tissue. *Fed. Proc.* **2**, 1128.

Laurent, T. C., Persson, H. (1964): The interaction between polysaccharides and other macromolecules. VII. The effects of various polymers on the sedimentation rates of serum albumin and alpha-cystallin. *Biochim. biophys. Acta (Amst.)* **83**, 141.

Lautsch, E. V., McMillan, G. C. (1953): Technics for the study of the normal and atherosclerotic arterial intima from its endothelial surface. *Lab. Invest.* **2**, 397.

Layton, L. L. (1951): The anabolic metabolism of radioactive sulfate by animal tissues *in vitro* and *in vivo. Cancer* **4**, 198.

Leary, T. (1941): The genesis of atherosclerosis. *Arch. Path.* **32**, 507.

Lee, F. C. (1922): On the lymphatic vessels in the wall of the thoracic aorta of the rat. *Anat. Rec.* **23**, 343.

Lelkes, Gy., Guba, F. (1962): Electron microscopic study of elastic fibre development. *Acta morph. Acad. Sci. hung.* Suppl. **19**, 65.

Lelkes, Gy., Karmazsin, L. (1965): Development of elastic elements in tissue cultures. *Acta morph. Acad. Sci. hung.* **5**, 149.

Lendrum, A. C. (1963): The hypertensive diabetic kidney as a model of the so-called 'collagen diseases'. *Canad. med. Ass.* **88**, 442.

Lendrum, A. C. (1967): Deposition of plastic substances in vessel walls. *Path. Microbiol.* **30**, 681.

Letterer, E. (1956): Die allergisch-hyperergische Entzündung. In, Büchner, F., Letter-er, E., Roujet, F. (Eds): *Handbuch der allgemeine Pathologie und pathologischen Anatomie*, Springer, Berlin–Göttingen–Heidelberg, VII/1, 4970.

Likar, I. N., Likar, L. J., Robinson, R. W. (1968): Bovine arterial disease. 3. Elastic tissue and mural acid mucopolysaccharides in bovine coronary arteries without gross lesions. *J. Atheroscler. Res.* **8**, 643.

Likar, I. N., Likar, L. J., Robinson, R. W., Gouvelis, A. (1969): Microthrombi and intimal thickening in bovine coronary arteries. *Arch. Path.* **87**, 146.

Lindner, J. (1965): Autoradiographische Methoden. *Acta. histochem. (Jena)* **5**, 200.

Lindsay, S., Chaikoff, I. L. (1965): Arteriosclerosis in cat; naturally occurring lesion in aorta and coronary arteries. *Arch. Path.* **60**, 29.

Lindsay, S., Chaikoff, I. L. (1966): Naturally occurring arteriosclerosis in nonhuman primates. *J. Atheroscler. Res.* **6**, 36.

Lindsay, S., Kohn, H. I., Dakin, R. L., Jew, J. (1962): Aortic arteriosclerosis in the dog after localized aortic X-irradiation. *Circulat. Res.* **10**, 51.

Linzbach, I. A. (1957): Die Bedeutung der Gefässwandfaktoren für die Entstehung der Arteriosklerose. *Verh. dtsch. Ges. Path.* **41,** 24.

Löhlein, M. (1917): Über Schrumpfnieren. *Beitr. path. Anat.* **63,** 570.

Lojda, Z. (1962): Topochemistry of enzymes in the vascular wall. *Metabolismus Parietis Vasorum* Praha, p. 232.

Lojda, Z. (1965): Histochemistry of the vascular wall. In, *Int. Symposium Morph. Histochem. Vasc. Wall.* Fribourg, Part II, *II,* 364.

Loomeijer, F. J., Van der Veen, K. J. (1962): Incorporation of (1-^{14}C)-acetate into various lipids by rat aorta *in vitro. J. Atheroscler. Res.* **2,** 478.

Loomis, D. (1946): Hypertension and necrotizing arteritis in rat following renal infarction. *Arch. Path.* **41,** 231.

Lorenzen, I. (1963): *Experimental Arteriosclerosis. Biochemical and Morphological Changes Induced by Adrenaline and Thyroxine.* Munksgaard, Copenhagen.

Lőrincz, J., Gorácz, Gy. (1954): New method of inducing experimental hypertension in the rat. *Acta physiol. Acad. Sci. hung.* **5,** 489.

Lőrincz, J., Gorácz, Gy. (1965): Experimental malignant hypertension. *Acta morph. Acad. Sci. hung.* **5,** 11.

Loth, H. (1965): Coarctatio aortae (Aortenisthmus-Stenose) mit Aneurysmabildung und peripherer Arteriosklerose. *Beitr. path. Anat.* **132,** 265.

Loustalot, P. (1960): Shut-term atheromatosis in the rat (A quantitative method). *Helv. Physiol. Acta.* **18,** 343.

Luciano, L., Junger, E., Reale, E. (1968): Glykogen in glatten Muskelzellen der Gefässwand von Säugetieren. Elektronenmikroskopische und spektrophotometrische Untersuchungen. *Histochemie* **15,** 219.

Luft, J. H. (1961): Improvement in epoxy resin embedding methods. *J. Cell. Biol.* **9,** 409.

Luft, J. H. (1964a): Fine structure of the diaphragm across capillary 'pores' in mouse intestine. *Anat. Rec.* **148,** 307.

Luft, J. H. (1964b): EM of cell extravenous coats as revealed by ruthenium red staining. *J. Cell. Biol.* **23,** 109.

Luft, J. H., (1965a): Fine structure of capillaries: the endocapillary layer. *Anat. Rec.* **151,** 380.

Luft, J. H. (1965b): The fine structure of hyaline cartilage matrix following ruthenium red fixative and staining. *J. Cell. Biol.* **27,** 118.

Luft, J. H. (1966): Fine structure of capillary and endocapillary layers as revealed by ruthenium red. *Fed. Proc.* **25,** 1773.

Lusztig, G. (1970): A hízósejtek histochemiai vizsgálata az aorta adventitiában kisérletes hypercholesterinaemia kapcsán (Histochemical examination of mast cells in the adventitia of the aorta in experimental hypercholesterinaemia). *Morph. Ig. Orv. Szemle* **10,** 4.

Lusztig, G., Jósa, L., Góg, B., Franczen, Margit (1968): Az aortafal rétegeinek MPS-i atherosclerosisban (Mucopolysaccharides of the aortic wall layers in atherosclerosis). *Kisérl. Orvostud.* **20,** 48.

Magyar, I., Róna, Gy., Vágó, E. (1954): Hyperglykaemia és arteriosclerosis (Hyperglycaemia and arteriosclerosis). *Magy. Belorv. Arch.* **7,** 116.

Mairano, C., Giugiaro, H. (1954): Azione di fermenti fibrinolitici di origine pancraeatica sul processo di quarigione delle arteriotomie su vasi di piccolo calibri. Richerche istologische sperimentali. *Minerva cardioangiol.* **2,** 300.

Majno, G. (1968): Endothelium, pericytes and smooth muscle: three contractile cells abstracted. *Amer. J. Path.* **52,** 61.

Majno, G., Palade, G. E. (1961): Studies on inflammation. I. The effect on histamine and serotonin on vascular permeability: an electron microscopic study. *J. biophys. biochem. Cytol.* **11,** 571.

Majno, G., Shea, S. M., Leventhal, M. (1969): Endothelial contraction induced by histamine-type mediators. An electron microscopic study. *J. Cell. Biol.* **42,** 647.

Makoff, G. M. (1899): Über die Bedeutung der traumatischen Verletzung von Arterien (Quetschung-Dehnung) für die Entwicklung der wahren Aneurysmen und der Arteriosklerose. *Beitr. path. Anat.* **25,** 431.

Malyschew, B. F. (1929): Über die Reaktion des Endothels der Arteria carotis des Kaninchens bei doppelter Unterbindung. *Virchows Arch. path. Anat.* **272,** 727.

182

Mancini, R. E., Vilar, O. M., Dellacha, O. W., Davidson, J. C., Alvarez, G. B. (1962): Extravascular distribution of fluorescent albumin, globulin and fibrinogen in connective tissue structures. *J. Histochem. Cytochem.* **10**, 194.

Maner, J. M. (1959): Morphologic and histological changes in postpartum uterine blood vessels. *Arch. Path.* **67**, 175.

Marchand, F. (1904): Über Arteriosklerose (Atherosklerose). *Wschr. dtsch. Ges. inn. Med.* **21**, 21.

Marchesi, V. T. (1962): The passage of colloidal carbon through inflammal endothelium. *Proc. roy. Soc. Med.* **156**, 550.

Marchetti, G., Merlo, L., Noseda, V. (1968): Myocardial uptake of fatty acids and carbohydrates after beta-adrenergic blockade. *Amer. J. Card.* **22**, 370.

Marine, D., Baumann, E. J. (1945): Periarteritis nodosa-like lesions in rats fed thiouracil. *Arch. Path.* **39**, 325.

Marshall, J. M., Tachmias, V. T. (1965): Cell surface and pinocytosis. *J. Histochem. Cytochem.* **13**, 92.

Marshall, J. R., O'Neal, M. (1966): The lipophage in hyperlipemic rats. An electron microscopical study. *Exp. Molec. Path.* **5**, 1.

Marshall, J. R., O'Neal, M., DeBakey, M. E. (1966): The ultrastructure of uncomplicated human atheroma in surgically resected aortas. *J. Atheroscler. Res.* **6**, 120.

Martinez, A. (1964): Elektronenmikroskopische Untersuchungen der Arteriosklerose der Menschen. *Virchows Arch. path. Anat.* **307**, 291.

Martinez, N. S., Dahl, E. V., Grindlay, J. H. (1957): Early tissue response to polyvinyl sponge aortic grafts. *Surgery* **42**, 1002.

Masson, G. M. C. (1967): Studies on the role of renin in hypertension In, Bajusz, E., Jasmin, G. (Eds): *Methods and Achievements in "Experimental Pathology"*, 3. Karger, Basel, p. 122.

Masson, G. M. C., Corcoran, A. C., Page, I. H. (1959): High arterial pressure as a primary cause of hypertensive vascular lesions. *Cleveland Clin. Quart.* **26**, 24.

Masson, G. M. C., Hazard, J. B., Corcoran, A. C., Page, I. H. (1950): Experimental vascular disease due to desoxycorticosterone and anterior pituitary factors. II. Comparison of pathologic changes. *Arch. Path.* **49**, 641.

Masson, G. M. C., McCormack, L. J., Dustan, H. P., Corcoran, A. C. (1958): Hypertensive vascular disease as a consequence of increased arterial pressure. Quantitative study in rats with hydralazine treated renal hypertension. *Amer. J. Path.* **34**, 817.

Matthews, M. A., Gardner, D. L. (1966): The fine structure of the mesenteric arteries of the rat. *Angiology* **17**, 902.

Maximov, A. A., Bloom, W. (1957): The blood vascular system. In, *A Textbook of Histology*. Saunders, Philadelphia–London, p. 228.

Mayersbach, H. (1956): Der Wandbau der Gefässübergangsstrecken zwischen Arterien rein elastischen und rein muskulösen Typs. *Anat. Am.* **102**, 333.

Maynard, E. A., Schultz, R. L., Pease, D. C. (1957): Electron microscopy of the vascular bed of rat cerebral cortex. *Amer. J. Anat.* **100**, 409.

McCombs, H. L., Zook, B. C., McGandy, R. B. (1969): Fine structure of spontaneous atherosclerosis of the aorta in the squirrel monkey. *Amer. J. Path.* **55**, 235.

McCormack, L. S., Beland, J. E., Schneckloth, R. E., Corcoran, A. C. (1958): Effects of antihypertensive treatment on the evolution of the renal lesions in malignant nephrosclerosis. *Amer. J. Path.* **34**, 1011.

McCully, K. S. (1969): Vascular pathology of homocysteinemia. Implications for the pathogenesis of arteriosclerosis. *Amer. J. Path.* **56**, 111.

McFortane, R. G. (1964): The development of ideas on fibrinolysis. *Brit. med. Bull.* **20**, 173.

McGee, W. G., Ashworth, C. T. (1963): Fine structure of chronic hypertensive arteriopathy in the human kidney. *Amer. J. Path.* **43**, 273.

McGill, H. C., jr., Geer, J. C. (1963): The human lesion, fine structure. In, Jones, R. J. (Ed.): *Evolution of Atherosclerotic Plaques*. Univ. of Chicago Press, Chicago, p. 65.

McGill, G. C., jr., Geer, J. C., Holman, R. L. (1971): Sites of vascular vulnerability in dogs, demonstrated by Evans blue. *Arch. Path.* **64**, 303.

McGee, W. G., Ashworth, C. T. (1963): Fine structure of chronic hypertensive arteriopathy in the human kidney. *Amer. J. Path.* **43**, 273.

McGill, H. C., jr., Frank, M. H., Geer, J. C. (1961): Aortic lesions in hypertensive monkeys. *Arch. Path.* **71**, 96.

McGill, H. C., jr., Strong, J. P., Holman, R. L., Werthessen, N. T. (1960): Arterial lesions in the Kenya Baboon. *Circulat. Res.* **8**, 670.

McKenzie, D. C., Drewenthal, J. (1960): Endothelial growth in nylon vascular grafts. *Brit. J. Surg.* **48**, 212.

McKinney, B. (1962): The pathogenesis of hyaline arteriosclerosis. *J. Path. Bact.* **83**, 449.

McQueen, E. G., Hodge, J. V. (1961): Modification of secondary lesions in renal hypertensive rats by control of the blood pressure with reserpine. *Quart. J. Med.* **30**, 213.

Meachim, G., Roy, S. (1967): Intracytoplasmic filaments in the cells of adult human cuticular cartilage. *Ann. rheum. Dis.* **26**, 50.

Meckel, H. (1903): Die Beteiligung der Gefässwand an der Thrombenorganisation mit besonderer Berücksichtigung des Endothels. In, *Eine experimentelle Studie zugleich als Beitrag zur Endothelfrage. s. phys. med. Soz. (Erlangen)* B. **34**, 92.

Mehrotra, R. M. L. (1953): An experimental study of the changes which occur in ligated arteries and veins. *J. Path. Bact.* **65**, 307.

Meijne, N. G. (1959): Endothelial growth after use of vascular nylon transplants. *Ned. T. Geneesk.* **4**, 1772.

Mellander, S., Indransson, B. (1968): Control of resistance, exchange and capacitance functions in the peripheral circulation. *Pharmacol. Rev.* **20**, 117.

Mellors, R. C., Brzosko, W. (1962): Studies in molecular pathology. I. Localization and pathogenic role of heterologous immune complexes. *J. exp. Med.* **115**, 891.

Mellors, R. C., Ortega, L. G. (1956): Analytical pathology. III. New observation on the pathogenesis of glomerulonephritis, lipid nephrosis, periarteritis nodosa and secondary amyloidosis in man. *Amer. J. Path.* **32**, 455.

Meyer, W. W. (1949): Die Bedeutung der Eiweissablagerungen in der Histogenese arteriosklerotischer Intimaveränderungen der Aorta. *Virchows Arch. path. Anat.* **316**, 268.

Meyer, W. W. (1958): Die Lebenshandlungen der Struktur von Arterien und Venen. *Verh. dtsch. Ges. Kreisl.-Forsch.* **24**, 15.

Meyer, W. W. (1964): Über die rhythmische Lokalization der atherosklerotischen Herde im zervikalen Abschnitt der Zerrebralarterie. *Beitr. path. Anat.* **130**, 24.

Middleton, C. C., Clarkson, T. B., Lofland, H. B., Puchard, R. W. (1964): Atherosclerosis in the squirrel monkey. *Arch. Path.* **78**, 16.

Miescher, P. A., Müller-Eberhand, J. (1968–1969): *Textbook of Immunopathology.* Vols I–II. Grune and Stratton, New York–London.

Miller, E. J., Martin, G. R., Piex, K. A. (1964): The utilization of lysine in the biosynthesis of elastin crosslinks. *Biochem. biophys, Res. Commun.* **17**, 248.

Mogilnitzky, B. N., Podljaschuk, L. D. (1929): Zur Frage über die Wirkung der Röntgenstrahlen auf das zentrale Nervensystem. *Fortschr. Roentgenstr.* **40**, 1096.

Mollo, F., Stramignoni, A. (1965): Cytoplasmic fibrillar ultrastructure in human lymph node cells. In, *Atti del V. Congresso Italiano di Microscopia Elettronica.* Abstr. Bologna, p. 97.

Molteni, A., Browine, A. C., Skelton, F. R. (1967): Electrolyte metabolism, renal vasopressor concentration and adrenal cortical hormone biosynthesis in methylandrostenediol hypertension. *Circulation* **36**, 189.

Mond, E., Mack, J. (1959): Report of myocardial injury in a patient receiving levarterenol. *Amer. Heart. J.* **60**, 134.

Montgomery, P. O. B., Muirhead, E. E. (1953): Similarities between the lesions in human malignant hypertension and in the hypertensive state of the nephrectomized dog. *Amer. J. Path.* **29**, 1147.

Montgomery, P. O. B., Muirhead, E. E. (1954): A characterization of hyaline arteriolar sclerosis by histochemical procedures. *Amer. J. Path.* **30**, 521.

Moon, H. D. (1957): Coronary arteries in fetuses, infants and juveniles. *Circulation* **16**, 263.

Moore-Jones, D. H., Michell, P., jr. (1966): Radioautographic localization of hydralazine-1-^{14}C in arterial walls. *Proc. Soc. exp. Biol. (N. Y.)* **122**, 576.

Moore, D. H., Ruska, H. (1957): The fine structure of capillaries and small arteries. *J. biophys. biochem. Cytol.* **3**, 457.

More, R. H., Haust, M. D. (1957): Encrustation and permeation of blood proteins in the genesis ɨ arteriosclerosis. *Amer. J. Path.* **33**, 593. Abstract.

More, R. H., Haust, M. D. (1961): Atherogenesis and plasma constituents. *Amer. J. Path.* **38**, 527.

More, R. H., McLean, C. R. (1949): Lesions of hypersensitivity induced in rabbits by massive injections of horse serum. *Amer. J. Path.* **25**, 413.

More, R. H., Movat, H. Z. (1959): Character and significance of the cellulose response in the collagen diseases and experimental hypersensitivity. *Lab. Invest.* **8**, 873.

Morehead, R. P., Little, J. M. (1945): Changes in the blood vessels of apparently healthy mongrel dogs. *Amer. J. Path.* **21**, 339.

Morgan, A. D. (1956): *The Pathogenesis of Coronary Occlusion.* Thomas, Springfield, p. 111.

Morris, B., Sass, M. B. (1966): The formation of lymph in the ovary. *Proc. roy. Soc. Med.* **164**, 577.

Moses, C. (1954): Development of atherosclerosis in dogs with hypercholesterolemic and chronic hypertension. *Circulat. Res.* **2**, 243.

Moskowitz, R. W., Baggenstoss, A. H., Slocumb, Ch. H. (1963): Histopathologic classification of periarteritis nodosa: a study of 56 cases confirmed at necropsy. *Proc. Mayo Clin.* **38**, 345.

Moss, A. J., Samuelson, P., Angell, C., Minken, S. L. (1968): Polarographic evaluation of transmural oxygen availability in intact muscular arteries. *J. Atheroscler. Res.* **8**, 803.

Movat, H. Z., Fernando, N. V. P. (1962): The fine structure of connective tissue. 1. The fibroblast. *Exp. molec. Path.* **1**, 509.

Movat, H. Z., Fernando, N. V. P. (1963*a*): Acute inflammation. The earliest fine structural changes at the blood tissue barrier. *Lab. Invest.* **12**, 895.

Movat, H. Z., Fernando, N. V. P. (1963*b*): The fine structure of the terminal vascular bed. I. Small arteries with an internal elastic lamina. *Exp. molec. Path.* **2**, 549.

Movat, H. Z., Fernando, N. V. P. (1963*c*): Allergic inflammation. *Amer. J. Path.* **42**, 41.

Movat, H. Z., Fernando, N. V. P. (1963*d*): Allergic inflammation. I. The earliest fine structural changes at the blood-tissue barrier during antigen–antibody interaction. *Amer. J. Path.* **62**, 41.

Movat, H. Z., Fernando, N. V. P. (1964*a*): The fine structure of the terminal vascular bed. II. The smallest arterial vessels. Terminal arterioles and metarterioles. *Exp. molec. Path.* **3**, 1.

Movat, H. Z., Fernando, N. V. P. (1964*b*): The fine structure of the terminal vascular bed. III. The capillaries. *Exp. molec. Path.* **3**, 87.

Movat, H. Z., Fernando, N. V. P. (1964*c*): The fine structure of the terminal vascular bed. IV. The venules and their perivascular cells (pericytes, adventitial cells). *Exp. molec. Path.* **3**, 98.

Movat, H. Z., Haust, M. D., More, R. H. (1959): The morphologic elements in the early lesions of atherosclerosis. *Amer. J. Path.* **35**, 93.

Movat, H. Z., More, R. H. (1957): The nature and origin of fibrin. *Amer. J. clin. Path.* **28**, 331.

Movat, H. Z., More, R. H., Haust, M. D. (1958): The diffuse intimal thickening of the human aorta with aging. *Amer. J. Path.* **34**, 1023.

Muirhead, E. E., Grollman, A. (1951*a*): A case of acute renal insufficiency in man manifesting in the arterial necrosis observed in dogs following bilateral nephrectomy. *Amer. J. Med.* **10**, 780.

Muirhead, E. E., Grollman, A. (1951): Acute renal insufficiency in man manifesting the arterial necrosis, observed in dogs following bilateral nephrectomy. *Amer. J. Med.* **10**, 780.

Muirhead, E. E., Turner, L. B., Grollman, A. (1951): Hypertensive cardiovascular disease. Vascular lesions of dogs maintained for extended periods following bilateral nephrectomy or ureteral ligation. *Arch. Path.* **51**, 575.

Muirhead, E. E., Turner, L. B., Grollman, A. (1951*b*): Hypertensive cardiovascular disease. Nature and pathogenesis of the arteriolar sclerosis induced by bilateral nephrectomy as revealed by a study of its tinctorial characteristics. *Arch. Path.* **52**, 266.

185

Müller, E., Locwenich, V. (1961): Das elektrohistochemische Verhalten der normalen und arteriosklerotisch veränderten Aorta-Intima. *Frankfurt. Z. Path.* **71,** 221.

Müller, E., Neumann, U. (1959): Untersuchungen über Elastase-Aktivität der Gefässintima im Bereiche arteriosklerotischer Herde. *Frankfurt. Z. Path.* **70,** 174.

Murakami, M., Sekimoto, H., Yasuda, Y., Masuda, S., Matsumoto, K., Shinagawa, T., Ikejima, K., Motoda, K., Yamada, T., Nagai, T., Yasumura, A., Kohayakawa, T., Tatsuguchi, M. (1964): cit.: Kojimahara. *Jap. J. Geriat.* **1,** 36.

Mustard, J. F. (1967): Recent advances in molecular pathology: a review. Platelet aggregation, vascular injury and atherosclerosis. *Exp. molec. Path.* **7,** 366.

Myers, D. B., Highton, Th. C., Rayus, D. G. (1969): Acid mucopolysaccharides closely associated with collagen fibrils in normal Ammon synovium. *J. Ultrastruct. Res.* **28,** 203.

Nagy, Gy., Gál, Gy. (1960): Adatok az essentialis pulmonalis hypertonia pathologiájához (Data on the pathology of essential pulmonal hypertension). *Magy. Belorv. Arch.* **13,** 142.

Nakajima, A., Horn, L. (1967): Electrical activity of single vascular smooth muscle fibers. *Amer. J. Physiol.* **213,** 25.

Nakashima, T. (1967): Early pattern of coronary atherosclerosis. In, *The 17th General Assembly of the Japan Medical Congress.* Suppl. **4,** 186.

Nakatani, M., Sasaki, T., Miyazaki, T., Nakamura, M. (1967a): Synthesis of phospholipids in arterial walls. I. Incorporation of ^{32}P into phospholipids of aortas and coronary arteries of various animals. *J. Atheroscler. Res.* **7,** 747.

Nakatani, M., Sasaki, T., Miyazaki, T., Nakamura, M. (1967b): Synthesis of phospholipids in arterial walls. II. Effects of age and the addition of adrenalin and acetylcholine on the incorporation of ^{32}P into phospholipids of rat aortas. *J. Atheroscler. Res.* **7,** 759.

Nam, S. C., Lee, K. T., Boylan, J., Thomas, W. A. (1965): Dietary lipid and thrombosis: study of 'trigger' mechanism for thrombosis in stock fed rats. *Exp. molec. Path.* **4,** 232.

Neufeld, H. N., Wagenwoort, C. A., Edwards, J. E. (1962): Coronary arteries in fetuses, infants, juveniles and young adults. *Lab. Invest.* **11,** 837.

Neumann, E. (1896): Zur Kenntnis der fibrinoiden Degeneration des Bindegewebs bei Entzündungen. *Virchows Arch. path. Anat.* **144,** 201.

Newman, H. A., McCandless, E. L., Zilversmit, D. B. (1961): The synthesis of ^{14}C-lipids in rabbit atheromatous lesions. *J. biol. Chem.* **236,** 1264.

Newman, H. A., Zilversmit, D. B. (1962): Quantitative aspects of cholesterol flux in rabbit atheromatous lesions. *J. biol. Chem.* **237,** 2078.

Newman, H. A., Zilversmit, D. B., (1964): Accumulation of lipid and unlipid constituents in rabbit atheroma. *J. Atheroscler. Res.* **4,** 261.

Nikulin, A., Lapp, H. (1965a): Elektronenmikroskopische Befunde an der terminalen Lungenstrombahn des Kaninchens nach Histamin-Liberation. *Frankfurt. Z. Path.* **74,** 381.

Nikulin, A., Schiemer, G. H. (1965b): Interferenzmikroskopische Untersuchung von Endothelzellen nach akuter Histamin-Liberation durch Polymycin B. *Frankfurt. Z. Path.* **74,** 400.

Nikulin, A., Walther, D. (1964): Der Einfluss von Histamin und Histamin-befreienden Substanzen auf die Blutgefässe während der postischämischen Erholungsphase. *Frankfurt. Z. Path.* **73,** 418.

Nowak, A., Kokot, F., Czekala, Z., Dosiak, J., Kuska, J. (1969): Fibrillolytic and renin activity in renal vein blood of patients with renovascular hypertension. *Thrombos. Diathes. haemorrh. (Stutt.)* **21,** 12.

Ogston, A. G., Sherman, F. F. (1961): Effect of hyaluronic acid upon diffusion of solutes and flow of solvent. *J. Physiol.* **156,** 67.

Ohta, G., Cohen, S., Singer, S. J. (1959): Demonstration of gamma globulin in vascular lesions of experimental necrotizing arteritis in the rat. *Proc. Soc. exp. Biol. (N. Y.)* **102,** 187.

Oka, M., Angrist, A. (1965): Histoenzymatic studies of arteries in high roll hypertension. *Lab. Invest.* **13,** 1604.

Oka, M., Angrist, A. (1967): Histoenzymatic studies of vessels in hypertensive rats. *Lab. Invest.* **16,** 25.

Oka, M., Brodie, S. S., Angrist, (1968): Sex-dependent vascular changes in young adults, aged and hypertensive rats. *Amer. J. Path.* **53**, 127.
Okamoto, K. (1969): Spontaneous hypertension in rats. *Int. Rev. exp. Path.* **7**, 227.
Okuneff, N. (1926): Über die vitale Farbstoffimbibition der Aortenwand. *Arch. Path.* **259**, 685.
Olah, I. (1968): A basalis membran (The basal membrane). *MTA Biol. Oszt. Közl.* **11**, 357.
Olsen, F. (1968): Penetration of circulating fluorescent protein into walls of arterioles and venules in rats with intermittent acute angiotensin-hypertension. *Acta. path. microbiol. scand.* **74**, 325.
Olsen, F. (1969a): Rate and ways of resolution of hypertensive vascular disease. *Acta path. microbiol. scand.* **77**, 39.
Olsen, F. (1969b): Arteriolar permeability and destruction of elastic membrane in hypertension. *Acta path. microbiol. scand.* **75**, 527.
Olsen, T. (1969c): Diabetic glomerulosclerosis: a comparison between human and experimental lesions. *Int. Rev. exp. Path.* **7**, 271.
Omae, T., Masson, G. M. C., Pagei, I. H. (1961): Release of pressor substances from renal grafts originating from rats with renal hypertension. *Circulat. Res.* **9**, 441.
O'Neil, R. M., Jordan, G. L., jr., Rabin, E. R., DeBakey, M. E., Halpert, B. (1964): Cells grown on isolated intravascular dacron hub. An electron microscopic study. *Exp. molec. Path.* **3**, 403.
Onoyama, K., Tanaka, K. (1969): Fibrinolytic activity of the arterial wall. *Thrombos. Diathes. haemorrh. (Stutt.)* **21**, 1.
Ooneda, G., Ooyama, Y., Matsuyama, K. (1965): Electron microscopic studies on the morphogenesis of fibrinoid degeneration in mesenteric arteries of hypertensive rats. *Angiology* **16**, 8.
Ooneda, G., Yoshida, Y., Takatama, M., Sekiguchi, M., Kato, M. (1962): Effect of epsilon-aminocaproic acid as an antifibrinolytic agent on arterial lesions in hypertensive rats with surgically constricted renal arteries. *Keio J. Med.* **11**, 157.
Opatowski, I. (1967): Elastic deformations of arteries. *J. appl. Physiol.* **23**, 772.
Opie, E. L., Lynch, C. J., Tershakovec, M. (1970): Sclerosis of the mesenteric arteries of rats. Its relation to longevity and inheritance. *Arch. Path.* **89**, 306.
O'Steen, W. K., Hall, E. C., Hall, O. S. (1967): Hypertension induced with hormones and 5-hydroxytryptophan. *Arch. Path.* **84**, 168.
Packham, M. A., Rowsell, H. C., Jorgensen, L. (1967): Localized protein accumulation in the wall of aorta. *Exp. molec. Path.* **7**, 214.
Paegle, D. R. (1969): Ultrastructure of calcium deposits in arteriosclerotic human aorta. *J. Ultrastruct. Res.* **26**, 412.
Page, I. H. (1954): The Lewis A. Connor Memorial Lecture. Atherosclerosis. An Introduction. *Circulation* **10**, 1.
Paik, W. Ch., Lalich, J. J. (1970): Factors which contribute to aortic fibrous repair in rats fed β-aminopropionitrile. *Lab. Invest.* **1**, 28.
Palade, G. E. (1953): The fine structure of blood capillaries. *J. appl. Physiol.* **24**, 1424.
Palade, G. E. (1961): Blood capillaries of the heart and other organs. *Circulation* **24**, 368.
Papacharalampous, N. X. (1964): Altersbedingte histologische und histochemische Veränderungen der Koronargefässe. *Virchows Arch. path. Anat.* **338**, 187.
Papamiltiades, M. (1952): Les lymphatiques de l'artère pulmonaire de l'homme. *Acta Anat. (Basel)* **16**, 116.
Pappenheimer, J. R. (1953): Passage of molecules through capillary walls. *Physiol. Rev.* **33**, 348.
Pardo, V., Perez-Stable, E., Fischer, E. R. (1968): Ultrastructural studies in hypertension. III. Gouty nephropathy. *Lab. Invest.* **18**, 143.
Parker, F. (1958): An electron microscopic study of coronary arteries. *Amer. J. Anat.* **103**, 247.
Parker, F. (1960): An electron microscopic study of experimental atherosclerosis. *Amer. J. Path.* **36**, 19.
Parker, F., Odland, G. F. (1966a): A correlative histochemical, biochemical and electron microscopic study of experimental atherosclerosis in the rabbit aorta with special reference to the myo-intimal cell. *Amer. J. Path.* **48**, 197.

Parker, F., Odland, G. F. (1966b): A light microscopic, histochemical and electron microscopic study of experimental atherosclerosis in rabbit coronary artery and a comparison with rabbit aorta atherosclerosis. *Amer. J. Path.* **48,** 451.

Parker, F., Odland, G. F., Ormsby, J. W., Williams, R. H. (1963): Some ultrastructural observations in the developing experimental atherosclerotic plaque in rabbit coronary artery and aorta. In, Jones, R. J. (Ed): *Evolution of the Atherosclerotic Plaque.* The Univ. of Chicago Press, Chicago, Vol. 1, p. 35.

Paronetto, F. (1965): Immunohistochemical observations on the vascular necrosis and renal glomerular lesions of malignant nephrosclerosis. *Amer. J. Path.* **46,** 901.

Paronetto, F., Strauss, L. (1962): Immunocytochemical observations in periarteritis nodosa. *Ann. intern. Med.* **56,** 289.

Partridge, S. M. (1966): Biosynthesis and nature of elastin structures. *Fed. Proc.* **25,** 1023.

Partridge, S. M., Elsden, D. F., Thomas, J. (1963): Constitution of the cross-linkages in elastin. *Nature* **197,** 1297.

Patek, P. R., Bernick, S., Ershoff, B. H., Wells, A. (1963a): Induction of atherosclerosis by cholesterol feeding in the hypophysectomized rat. *Amer. J. Path.* **42,** 137.

Patek, P. R., Bernick, S., McCallum, D. K. (1963b): Production of arterial lesions by a humoral factor in parabiotic rats. *Circulat. Res.* **12,** 291.

Paule, W. J. (1963): Electronmicroscopy of the newborn rat aorta. *J. Ultrastruct. Res.* **8,** 219.

Pease, D. C. (1966): Polysaccharides associated with the exterior surface epithelial cells of the kidney, intestine, brain. *Anat. Rec.* **154,** 400.

Pease, D. C., Molinari, S. (1960): EM of muscular arteries: Pial vessels of the cat and monkey. *J. Ultrastruct. Res.* **3,** 447.

Pease, D. C., Paule, W. J. (1960): Electron microscopy of elastic arteries, the thoracic aorta of the rat. *J. Ultrastruct. Res.* **3,** 469.

Pekelharing, C. A. (1890): Über Endothel-Wucherung in Arterien. *Beitr. path. Anat.* **8,** 245.

Petroff, J. L. (1922): Über die Vitalfärbung der Gefässwandungen. *Beitr. path. Anat.* **71,** 115.

Petry, G., Heberer, G. (1957): Die Neubildung der Gefässwand auf der Grundlage synthetischer Arterioprothesen. *Langenbecks Arch. Klin. Chir.* **286,** 249.

Petzold, H. (1959): Histochemie der pathologisch veränderten Gefässwand. In, *Gefässwand und Blutplasma.* Symposion an der Med. klin. d. Med. Akad., Magdeburg, 2–3 Okt., 1959, Fischer, Jena.

Phelan, E. L., Wong, L. C. K. (1968): Sodium, potassium and water in the tissues of rats with genetic hypertension and constricted renal artery hypertension. *Clin. Sci.* **35,** 487.

Pick, E. (1885): Über die Rolle des Endotheliums bei der Endarteritis post ligaturam. *Z. Heilk.* **6,** 459.

Pickering, G. W. (1945): The role of the kidney in acute and chronic hypertension following renal artery constriction in the rabbit. *Clin. Sci.* **5,** 229.

Pillai, P. A. (1964): A banded structure in the connective tissue of nerve. *J. Ultrastruct. Res.* **11,** 455.

Pogátsa, G., Gábor, Gy. (1963): Beiträge zum Mechanismus der Myokardschädigung durch Noradrenalin. *Acta Sec. Conv. Med. Int. Hung. Cardiologia* **7,** 346.

Pollak, O. J. (1969): *Monographs on Atherosclerosis. Tissue Cultures.* Karger, Basel.

Poole, J. C. F., Sanders, A. G., Florey, H. W. (1958): The regeneration of aortic endothelium. *J. Path. Bact.* **75,** 133.

Poole, J. C. F., Florey, H. W. (1958): Changes in the endothelium of the aorta and the behaviour of macrophages in experimental atheroma of rabbits. *J. Path. Bact.* **75,** 245.

Poole, J. C. F., Sanders, A. G., Florey, H. W. (1959): Further observations on the regeneration of aortic endothelium in the rabbit. *J. Path. Bact.* **77,** 637.

Prichard, R. W., Clarkson, T. B., Goodman, H. O., Lofland, H. B. (1964): Aortic atherosclerosis in pigeons and its complications. *Arch. Path.* **77,** 244.

Prior, J. T., Harmann, W. H. (1956): The effect of hypercholesterolemia upon intimal repair of the aorta of the rabbit following experimental trauma. *Amer. J. Path.* **32,** 417.

188

Prior, J. T., Jones, D. B. (1952): Structural alterations within the aortic intima in infancy and childhood. *Amer. J. Path.* **28**, 937.

Prose, P. H., Lee, L., Balk, S. D. (1965): Electron microscopic study of the phagocytic fibrin-clearing mechanism. *Amer. J. Path.* **47**, 403.

Puchtler, H., Sweat, F., Terry, M. S., Conner, H. M. (1969): Investigation of staining, polarization and fluorescence-microscopic properties of myoendothelial cells. *J. Microscopy* **89**, 95.

Pugh, R. C. B., Pickering, A. W., Blacket, R. B. (1952): The production of vascular lesions and cardiac hypertrophy by infusions of renin and noradrenaline in the rabbit. *Clin. Sci.* **11**, 241.

Putte, van der, S. C. J. (1969): The early development of the vasa sanguinea vasorum of the human descending aorta. *Angiologica* **6**, 54.

Raab, F. (1879): Über die Entwicklung der Narbe im Blutgefässe nach der Unterbindung. *Arch. Klin. Chir.* **23**, 156.

Raab, W., Bajusz, E., Kimura, H., Herrlich, H. G. (1968): Isolation stress, myocardial electrolytes and epinephrine cardiotoxicity in rats. *Proc. Soc. exp. Biol (N.Y.)* **127**, 142.

Radnai, B. (1969): Comparative morphology of small vessel lesions in rheumatoid arthritis and periarteritis nodosa. *Acta morph. Acad. Sci. hung.* **17**, 69.

Rajka, Ö., Korossy, S., Backhaus, R., Radnai, B., Gózony, M. (1959): Adatok a staphylogen sensibilisatiohoz. Nyulak kisérleti sensibilitatioja komplex staphylococcus-antigennel (Staphylogenic sensitization. Experimental sensitization of rabbits with complex staphylococcus antigen). *MTA V. Oszt. Közl.* **10**, 298.

Randerath, E. (1954): Die Bedeutung der allergischen Pathogenese bei der Arteriitis. Pathologisch-anatomisches Referat. *Verh. dtsch. Ges. inn. Med.* **60**, 359.

Rannie, J. (1963): Observations on the oxytalan fibre of the periodontal membrane. *Trans. Europ. Orthodonic. Soc.* **24**, 127.

Ranz, H. (1959): Experimentelle Untersuchungen zur Aetiologie der Periarteriitis. *Verh. dtsch. Ges. Path.* **43**, 247.

Reale, E., Ruska, H. (1965): Die Feinstruktur der Gefässwände. Int. Symp. Morphology, Histochemistry, Vascular Wall. Freiburg. *Angiologica* **2**, 314.

Renaud, S., Allard, C. (1963): Hypertension, thrombosis and atherosclerosis in the rat. *Canad. med. Ass. J.* **88**, 1275.

Rényi-Vámos, F. (1960): *Das innere Lymphgefäßsystem der Organe.* Akadémiai Kiadó, Budapest.

Restrepo, C., Tejeda, C., Correa, P. (1969): Nonsyphilitic aortitis. *Arch. Path.* **87**, 1.

Rhodin, J. A. (1962a): Fine structure of vascular wall in mammals. With special reference to smooth muscle component. *Physiol. Rev.* **42**, Suppl. 5, 48.

Rhodin, J. A. (1962b): The diaphragm of capillary endothelial fenestrations. *J. Ultrastruct. Res.* **6**, 171.

Rhodin, J. A. (1967): The ultrastructure of mammalien arterioles and precapillary sphincters. *J. Ultrastruct. Res.* **18**, 181.

Rhodin, J. A., Dalhamm, T. (1955): Electron microscopy of collagen and elastin in lamina propria of the tracheal mucosa of rat. *Exp. Cell. Res.* **9**, 371.

Rich, A. R. (1942): The role of hypersensitivity in periarteritis nodosa: as indicated by seven cases developing during serum sickness and sulfonamide therapy. *Bull. Johns Hopk. Hosp.* **71**, 123.

Rich, A. R., Gregory, J. E. (1943): The experimental demonstration that periarteritis nodosa is a manifestation of hypersensitivity. *Bull. Johns Hopk. Hosp.* **72**, 65.

Rinehart, J. F., Greenberg, L. D. (1951): Pathogenesis of experimental arteriosclerosis in pepidocine deficiency. *Arch. Path.* **51**, 12.

Robert, B., Robut, A. M. (1969): Mechanismes immunologiques dans l'atherosclerose. *Méd. et Hyg. (Genève)* **27**, 822.

Robert, L., Oudea, P., Parlebas, J., Zweibaum, A., Robert, B. (1965a): Immunochemistry of structural proteins and glycoproteins. In, *Structure and Function of Connective and Skeletal Tissues, NATO Symposium.* Butterworths, London, p. 406.

Robert, L., Stein, F., Pezess, M. P., Poullain, N. (1965b): Études immunochimiques sur l'élastine. Mechanisme autoimmunitaire de l'atheromatose, colloque sur l'atheromathose, Bordeaux. *Rev. Atherosclérose* **65/b**, 123.

Robert, L., Pareebas, J., Poullain, N., Robert, B. (1963): Données nouvelles sur l'immunochimie des proteines fibreuses du tissu conjonctif. In, Peeters, H. (Ed.): *Protides of the Biological Fluids.* Vol. 11. Elsevier, Amsterdam, p. 109.

Robert, L., Robert, B., Moczar, M., Moczar, E. (1967): Constituants macromoléculaires de la paroi artérielle: antigenicité et rôle dans l'atherosclerose. In, Scebat, L., Lenegre, J. (Eds): *Symposium sur l'Atheromatose du CNRS. Paris.* Abstr.

Roberts, J. C., Strauss, R. (1965): *Comparative Atherosclerosis.* Harper (Hoeber), New York.

Rodbard, S., Lehoczky, J. M., Terner, J. Y., Candlers, E. (1962): Mechanical factors affecting conversion of arterial smooth muscle into fibroblast or cartilage. *Metabolismus Parietis Vasorum* Praha, p. 696.

Rodgers, J. C., Puchtler, H., Gropp, S. (1967): Transition from elastin to collagen in internal elastic membranes. *Arch. Path.* **83,** 557.

Rojo-Ortega, J. M., Genest, J. (1968): A method for production of experimental hypertension in rats. *Canad. J. Physiol. Pharmacol.* **46,** 883.

Rokitansky, C. (1846): A manual of pathological anatomy. In, *Handbuch der pathologischen Anatomie.* Braunmüller, Vienna.

Romhányi, Gy. (1962): A polarizációs mikroszkópia szerepe a szubmikroszkopikus szerkezet-kutatásban (Role of polarization microscopy in submicroscopic structure research). *Morph. Ig. Orv. Szemle* **2,** 161.

Romhányi, Gy. (1965): On the submicroscopic structure of the elastic fibres in the bovine ligamentum nuchae as revealed by the polarization microscope. *Acta morph. Acad. Sci. hung.* **13,** 397.

Romhányi, Gy. (1966): Ultrastructure of the intercellular structure of connective tissue on the basis of polarization optical examination of topooptical reactions. Thesis, Pécs.

Rosnowski, A. (1968): Badania doswiadczalne elastoplazji (Experimental research of elastoplasy). *Poznanskie Towarystwo Przbyjaciol Nauk, Wydzial Lekarski, Prace Komisji Medycyny Doświadczalnej,* **38,** 145.

Ross, R., Bornstein, L. P. (1969): The elastic fiber, I. The separation and partial characterization of its macromolecular components. *J. Cell. Biol.* **40,** 366.

Ross, R., Bornstein, L. P. (1970): Studies of the components of the elastic fiber. In, Balázs, E. A. (Ed.): *Chemistry and Molecular Biology of the Intercellular Matrix.* Vol. I, Academic Press, New York–London, p. 641.

Ross, R., Sanberg, L. B. (1967): Further observations of the components of the elastic fiber. *J. Cell. Biol.* **35,** 118A (Abstract).

Rossmann, P., Vavra, I. (1967): Histology of vasonconstriction and vasodilatation of muscular arteries by the freeze-drying method. *Cor. Vasc.* **9,** 77.

Rowley, D. A. (1963): Mast cell damage and vascular injury in the rat: an electron microscopic study of a reaction produced by thorotrast. *Brit. J. exp. Path.* **44,** 284.

Roy, S. (1968): Ultrastructure of articular cartilage in experimental hemarthrosis. *Arch. Path.* **86,** 69.

Rudolph, G. (1964): Histochemische Untersuchung zum Stoffwechsel des bradytrophen Gewebs. *Verh. dtsch. Ges. Path.* **48,** 325.

Rusznyák, I., Földi, M., Szabó, Gy. (1960): *Physiologie und Pathophysiologie des Lymphkreislaufes.* Akadémiai Kiadó, Budapest.

Ryden, B. E., Vikgren, P., Melmed, R., Hood, B. (1967): Smooth muscle constrictor activity in hypertensive syndromes. *Acta med. scand.* **181,** 681.

Sabesin, S. M. (1964): Electron microscopy of hypersensitivity reactions. Intravascular antigen–antibody precipitation in acute anaphylactic shock. *Amer. J. Path.* **44,** 889.

Salgado, E. D. (1970): Medial aortic lesions in rats with metacorticoid hypertension. *Amer. J. Path.* **58,** 305.

Samson, P. C., Herrick, J. B. (1932): Tissue changes following continuous intravenous injection of epinephrine hydrochloride into dogs. *Arch. Path.* **13,** 745.

Santos-Buch, C. A. (1966): Extension of ATP-ase activity from pinocytotic vesicles of abating endothelium and smooth muscle to the internal elastic membrane of the major arterial circle of the iris of rabbit. *Nature* **211,** 600.

Saphir, O., Telischi, M., Ohringer, L. (1962): Rabbit sulfa drug hypersensitivity and lesions resembling early arteriosclerosis. *Arch. Path.* **73,** 414.

190

Sawyer, R. N., Valmond, I. (1961): Evidence of active ion transport across large canine blood vessel wall. *Nature* **189,** 470.

Schaeffer, J. P., Radosh, H. E. (1924): On the obliteration of the lumen of blood vessels. IV. The origin and nature of the mass which comes to occupy the lumen of an artery segment between two ligatures. *Amer. J. Anat.* **33,** 219.

Schallock, G. (1962): On the morphology of atherosclerosis. *J. Atheroscler. Res.* **2,** 25.

Schatzmann, H. J. (1962): Lipoprotein nature of red cell adenosine triphosphatase. *Nature* **196,** 677.

Schenk, E. A., Garman, E., Felgenbaum, A. S. (1966): Spontaneous aortic lesions in rabbits. I. Morphologic characteristics. *Circulat. Res.* **19,** 80.

Schettler, F. G., Boyd, G. S. (1969): *Atherosclerosis.* Elsevier, Amsterdam–London–New York.

Schilling, cit. Solovev (1925): Verh. Dtsch. Path. Ges. 20. Tagung, Würzburg.

Schlichter, J. G., Harris, R. (1949): The vascularization of the aorta. II. Comparative study of the aortic vascularization of several species in health and disease. *Amer. J. med. Sci.* **218,** 610.

Schlichter, J. G., Katz, L. N., Meyer, J. (1949): The occurrence of atheromatous lesions after cauterization of the aorta followed by cholesterol administration. *Amer. J. med. Sci.* **218,** 603.

Schmid, F. R., Cooper, N. S., Morris, Z., Currier, E. (1961): Arteritis in rheumatoid arthritis. *Amer. J. Med.* **30,** 56.

Schmidt, C. F. (1962): Second annual supplement on hypertension. *Circulat. Res.* **11,** 2.

Schmidt-Diedrichs, A., Courtice, F. C. (1963): The removal of various lipoproteins from doubly-ligated segments of artery and vein in the rabbit. *Brit. J. exp. Path.* **44,** 345.

Schneeberger-Keeley, E. E., Karnovsky, M. J. (1968): The ultrastructural basis of alveolar capillary membrane permeability to peroxidase used as a tracer. *J. Cell. Biol.* **37,** 781.

Schoefl., G. I. (1963): Studies on inflammation. III. Growing capillaries: their structure and permeability. *Virchows Arch. path. Anat.* **337,** 97.

Schoefl, G. I. (1964): Electron microscopic observations on the regeneration of blood vessels after injury. *Ann. N. Y. Acad. Sci.* **116,** 789.

Schoefl, G. I., French, J. E. (1968): Vascular permeability to particulate fat morphological observations on vessels of lactatory mammary gland and of lung. *Proc. roy. Soc. M ed.* **169,** 153.

Schoffeniels, E. (1969): Ionic composition of the arterial wall. *Angiologica* **6,** 65.

Schürmann, P. McMahon, H. E. (1933): Die maligne Nephrosklerose, zugleich ein Beitrag zur Frage der Bedeutung der Blutgewebsschranke. *Virchows Arch. Path. Anat.* **291,** 47.

Schwarz, W. (1964): Elektronenmikroskopische Untersuchungen über die Bildung der elastischen Formen in der Gewebsstruktur. *Z. Zellforsch. Abt. Histochem.* **63,** 636.

Scott, J. B., Daugherty, R. M., Overbeck, H. W., Haddy, F. J. (1968): Vascular effects of ions. *Fed. Proc.* **27,** 1403.

Scott, R. F., Florentin, R. A., Daoud, A. S. (1966): Coronary arteries of children and young adults. A comparison of lipids and anatomic features in New Yorkers and East Africans. *Exp. molec. Path.* **5,** 12.

Scott, R. F., Jones, R., Daoud, A. S., Zumbo, O., Coulston, F., Thomas, W. A. (1967a): Experimental atherosclerosis in rhesus monkeys. II. Cellular elements of proliferative lesions and possible role of cytoplasmic degeneration in pathogenesis as studied by electron microscopy. *Exp. molec. Path.* **7,** 34.

Scott, R. F., Morrison, E. S., Jarmolych, J., Nam, S. C., Kroms, M., Coulston, F. (1967b): Experimental atherosclerosis in rhesus monkeys. I. Gross and light microscopy features and lipid values in serum and aorta. *Exp. molec. Path.* **7,** 11.

Scott, R. F., Morrison, E. S., Thomas, W. A., Jones, R., Nam, S. C. (1964): Short-term feeding of unsaturated versus saturated fat in the production of atherosclerosis in the rat. *Exp. molec. Path.* **3,** 421.

Seeliger, H., Schopper, H. (1969): Die arterielle Verschlusskrankheit der Fingerarterien (Morphologie und Pathogenese). *Virchows Arch. path. Anat.* **347,** 327.

Seifert, G., Dreesbach, H. A. (1966): Die calciphylaktische Arteriopathie. *Frankfurt. Z. Path.* **75**, 342.

Seifert, K. (1962): Elektronmikroskopische Untersuchungen der Aorta des Hausschweines. *Z. Zellforsch.* **58**, 331.

Seifert, K. (1963a): Elektronenmikroskopische Untersuchungen der Aorta des Kaninchens. *Z. Zellforsch.* **60**, 293.

Seifert, K. (1963b): Über experimentelle Atheromatose der Kaninchenaorta. Licht- und elektronenmikroskopische Untersuchungen. *Z. Zellforsch.* **61**, 276.

Seifter, J., Baeder, D. H., Beckfield, W. J., Shama, G. P., Ehrich, W. E. (1953): Effect of hyaluronidase on experimental hypercholesterolemia in rabbits and rats and atheromatosis in rabbits. *Proc. Soc. exp. Biol. (N. Y.)* **83**, 468.

Selye, H. (1970): *Experimental Cardiovascular Diseases.* Vols I–II. Springer, New York–Berlin.

Selye, H., Hall, C. E., Rowley, E. M. (1943): Malignant hypertension produced by treatment with desoxycorticosterone acetate and sodium chloride. *Canad. med. Ass. J.* **49**, 88.

Selye, H., Pentz, E. (1943): Pathogenetical correlations between periarteriitis nodosa, renal hypertension and rheumatic lesions. *Canad. med. Ass. J.* **48–49**, 264.

Senftleben, H. (1879): Über den Verschluss der Blutgefässe nach der Unterbindung. *Virchows Arch. path. Anat.* **77**, 421.

Setti, G. C. (1965): Lymphatic system of the heart, pericardium and large vessels. *Riv. Pat. Clin.* **20**, 357.

(Shakhlamov) Шахламов, В. А. (1969): Аденозинтрифосфатзная активности ендотелиалных клеток функционалных (истиных кровеносных капиларов). *Вестник Академии Медицинских Наук.* **9**, 80.

Shapiro, J., Glasgow, J. L., Perkins, W. H., Hosvey, C. (1962): Effect of cyanide and fluoride, an *in vitro* incorporation of ^{3}H-cholesterol into rabbit artery. *Proc. Soc. exp. Biol. (N. Y.)* **109**, 675.

Shea, S. M., Karnovsky, M. J., Bossert, V. H. (1969): Vesicular transport across endothelium: simulation of a diffusion model. *J. theor. Biol.* **24**, 30.

Sheehan, J. F. (1944): Foam cell plaques in the intima of irradiated small arteries (one hundred to five hundred microns in external diameters). *Arch. Path.* **37**, 297.

Sheehan, H. L., Davis, J. C. (1959): Experimental hydronephrosis. *Arch. Path.* **68**, 185.

Shibata, S., Briggs, A. H. (1967): Mechanical activity of vascular smooth muscle under anoxia. *Amer. J. Physiol.* **212**, 981.

Shimamoto, T. (1963): The relationship of edematous reaction in arteries to atherosclerosis and thrombosis. *J. Atheroscler. Res.* **3**, 87.

Shimamoto, T. (1969a): Experimental study on atherosclerosis, an attempt at its prevention and treatment. *Acta path. jap.* **19**, 15.

Shimamoto, T. (1969b): Atherogenesis, thrombogenesis and pyridinolcarbamate treatment. In, Shimamoto, T., Numano, F. (Eds): *Atherogenesis.* Excerpta Med. Found, Amsterdam, p. 5.

Shimamoto, T., Namaro, F., Fujeta, F. (1966): Atherosclerosis-inhibiting effect of antibradychinin. *Amer. Heart J.* **71**, 216.

Shimamoto, T., Yamashita, Y., Sunaga, T. (1969a): Scanning electron microscopic observation of endothelial surface of heart and blood vessels. *Proc. Jap. Acad.* **45**, 507.

Shimamoto, T., Yamashita, Y., Numano, F., Sunaga, T. (1969b): The endothelial cell damages of pre-atheromatous and atheromatous lesions observed by scanning electron microscope. *Proc. Jap. Acad.* **45**, 761.

Shirley, H. H., Wolfram, C. G., Wasserman, K., Mayerson, H. S. (1957): Capillary permeability to macromolecules: stretched pore phenomenon. *Amer. J. Physiol.* **190**, 189.

Shoenberg, C. F. (1969): A study of myosin filaments in extract and homogenates of vertebrate smooth muscle. *Angiologica* **6**, 233.

Siew, S., Wagner, B. (1968): Application on the ruthenium red technique in the electron microscopy of the cardiovascular tissue. In, *IV. European Regional Conference in Electron Microscopy.* Tipog. Polyglotta Vaticana, Rome, p. 62.

Silberberg, M., Silberberg, R., Hasler, M. (1966): Fine structure of articular cartilage in mice receiving cortisone acetate. *Arch. Path.* **82**, 569.

Silva, D. G. (1969): Further ultrastructural studies on the temporomandibular point of the guinea pig. *J. Ultrastruct. Res.* **26**, 148.

Silva, D. G., Hart, J. A. (1967): Ultrastructural observations on the mandibular condyle of the guinea pig. *J. Ultrastruct. Res.* **20**, 227.

Silver, M. D., Wigle, E. D., Trimble, A. S., Bigelow, W. G. (1969): Iatrogenic coronary ostial stenosis. *Arch. Path.* **88**, 73.

Simms, H. S., Berg, B. N. (1957): Longevity and the onset of lesions in male rats. *J. Geront.* **12**, 244.

Simon, R. C., Still, W. J., O'Neal, R. M. (1961): The circulating lipophage in experimental atherosclerosis. *J. Atheroscler. Res.* **1**, 395.

Simpson, C. F., Harms, R. H. (1966): Pathology of aortic atherosclerosis and dissecting aneurysm of turkeys induced by diethylstilbestrol. *Exp. molec. Path.* **5**, 183.

Simpson, C. F., Harms, R. H. (1968): The nature of the atherosclerotic plaque of the aorta of turkeys. *J. Atheroscler. Res.* **8**, 143.

Simpson, C. F., Jones, J. E., Harms, R. H. (1967): Ultrastructure of aortic tissue in copper-deficient and control chick embryos. *J. Nutr.* **91**, 283.

Sinapius, D. (1964): Zur Morphologie der Fettresorption bei Atherosklerose der Coronaarterien. *Virchows Arch. path. Anat.* **338**, 150.

Sinapius, D. (1968): Die Entstehung subendothelialer Lipophagenherde bei Coronarsklerose. *Virchows Arch. path. Anat.* **345**, 169.

Sinapius, D., Gunkel, R. D. (1964): Ceroid bei Lipoidose und Atherosklerose der Aorta. Morphologie und Histochemie. *Frankfurt. Z. Path.* **73**, 485.

Skjorten, F. (1968): On the nature of hyaline microthrombi. A light microscopical immunofluorescent and ultrastructural study. *Acta path. microbiol. scand.* **73**, 489.

Slocumb, C. H., Polley, H. F., Ward, L. E., Hench, P. S. (1957): Diagnosis, treatment and prevention of chronic hypercortisonism in patients with rheumatoid arthritis. *Ann. intern. Med.* **46**, 86.

Sminkova, P. (1903): Ein Beitrag zur Genese der Arteriosklerose. *Beitr. Path. Anat.* **34**, 242.

Smirnova-Zamkova, A. J. (1951): cit. Zlateva. *Klin. med. Kiev.* **1**, 43.

Sobel, H. (1968): Aging of connective tissue and molecular transport. *Gerontology* **14**, 235.

Sokoloff, A. (1893): Über die Bedingungen der Bindegewebsneubildung in der Intima doppelt unterbundener Arterien. *Beitr. path. Anat.* **14**, 11.

Sokoloff, L., Bunim, J. J. (1957): Vascular lesions in rheumatoid arthritis. *J. Chron. Dis.* **5**, 668.

Somlyo, A. P., Somlyo, A. V. (1968): Vascular smooth muscle. I. Normal structure, pathology, biochemistry and biophysics. *Pharmacol. Rev.* **20**, 197.

Sótonyi, P. (1969): Personal communication.

Soustek, Z. (1956): Zur Morphologie der Quellungsnekrose (sogenannte fibrinoide Nekrose) der fibrinösen Durchtränkung und der fibrinoiden Infiltration der Arteriolen. *Zbl. allg. Path.* **95**, 509.

Spiro, D., Lattes, R. G., Wiener, J. (1965): The cellular pathology of experimental hypertension. I. Hyperplastic arteriosclerosis. *Amer. J. Path.* **47**, 19.

Solovev, A. (1929): Experimentelle Untersuchungen über die Heilungsvorgänge in der Arterienwand. *Beitr. path. Anat.* **83**, 485.

Solovev, A. (1930): Experimentelle Untersuchungen über die Bedeutung in lokaler Schädigung für die Lipoidablagerung in der Arterienwand. *Z. Ges. exp. Med.* **69**, 94.

Solovev, A. (1932): Über experimentell hervorgerufene Elasticarisse der Arterien und deren Bedeutung für die Lipoidablagerung. *Virchows Arch. path. Anat.* **283**, 213.

Stallabrass, P. (1963): Observations on the muscular coat of the human umbilical blood vessels. *J. Obstet. Gynaec. Brit. Cwlth* **70**, 1042.

Starling, E. H. (1895–1896): On the absorption of fluids from the connective tissue spaces. *J. Physiol.* **19**, 312.

Staubesand, J. (1963): Electronenmikroskopische Untersuchungen über die Passage von Metalsolen durch mesotheliale Membranen. II. Mitteilung zur Histologie des Herzbeutels. *Z. Zellforsch.* **58**, 915.

Stearner, S. P., Sanderson, M. H. (1969): Early vascular injury in the X-irradiated chick embryo: an electron microscopic study. *J. Path. Bact.* **99**, 213.

Stefanescu-Gavat, V., Hagi-Paraschiu, A. (1967): L'activité des ATP-ases dans divers types d'artéres. *Ann. histochem. (Jena)* **12**, 213.

Stefanini, M., Mednicoff, I. B. (1954): Demonstration of antivessel agents in serum of patients with anaphylactoid purpura and periarteritis nodosa. *J. clin. Invest.* **33**, 967.

Stehbens, W. E. (1962): The production of sulphated mucopolysaccharides by endothelium. *J. Path. Bact.* **83**, 337.

Stehbens, W. E. (1963): The renal artery in normal and cholesterol-fed rabbits. *Amer. J. Path.* **43**, 969.

Stehbens, W. E. (1965a): Endothelial vesicles and protein transport. *Nature* **207**, 197.

Stehbens, W. E. (1965b): Intimal proliferation and spontaneous lipid deposition in the cerebral arteries of sheep and steers. *J. Atheroscler. Res.* **5**, 556.

Stehbens, W. E., Florey, H. W. (1960): The behavior of intravenously injected particles observed in chambers in rabbits' hearts. *Quart. J. exp. Physiol.* **45**, 252.

Stehbens, W. E., Silver, H. D. (1966): Arterial lesions induced by methyl cellulose. *Amer. J. Path.* **48**, 483.

Stein, Y., Stein, O. (1962): Incorporation of fatty acids into lipoids of aortic slices of rabbits, dogs, rats and baboons. *J. Atheroscler. Res.* **2**, 400.

Sternby, N. H., Vanecek, R. (1965): Correlation of type and extent of atherosclerosis in aorta and coronary arteries obtained of autopsy. The search for predictors of coronary stenosis and myocardial infarction. *Bull. Wld Hlth Org.* **33**, 741.

Steward, G. T. (1962): Pulsation of lipids, lipoproteins and fibrinogen against excised segments of rabbit aorta. *Brit. J. exp. Path.* **43**, 345.

Still, W. J. S. (1963): An electron microscope study of cholesterol atherosclerosis in the rabbit. *Exp. molec. Path.* **2**, 491.

Still, W. J. S. (1964): Pathogenesis of experimental atherosclerosis. *Arch. Path.* **78**, 601.

Still, W. J. S. (1967): The early effect of hypertension on the aortic intima of the rat. *Amer. J. Path.* **51**, 721.

Still, W. J. S. (1968): The pathogenesis of the intimal thickenings produced by hypertension in large arteries in the rat. *Lab. Invest.* **19**, 84.

Still, W. J. S., Dennison, S. M. (1967): Reaction of the arterial intima of the rabbit to trauma and hyperlipemia. *Exp. molec. Path.* **6**, 245.

Still, W. J. S., Dennison, S. M. (1969): The pathogenesis of the glomerular changes in steroid induced hypertension in the rat. *Lab. Invest.* **20**, 249.

Still, W. J. S., Ghoni, A. R., Dennison, S. M. (1967): The organization of isolated mural thrombi in aortic grafts. *Amer. J. Path.* **51**, 1013.

Still, W. J. S., Hill, K. R. (1959): The pathogenesis of hyaline arteriolar sclerosis. *Arch. Path.* **68**, 42.

Still, W. J. S., Mariott, P. R. (1964): Comparative morphology of the early atherosclerosis lesion in non cholesterol atherosclerosis in the rabbit. An electron microscopic study. *J. Atheroscler. Res.* **4**, 373.

Still, W. J. S., O'Neal, R. M. (1961): Experimental atherosclerosis in the rat. The pathogenesis of the early lesion. *Fed. Proc.* **20**, 94.

Still, W. J. S., O'Neal, R. M. (1962): Electron microscopic study of experimental atherosclerosis in the rat. *Amer. J. Path.* **40**, 21.

Still, W. J. S., Prosser, P. R. (1964): The reaction of aortic endothelium of the rabbit to hyperlipemia and colloidal thorin. *J. Atheroscler. Res.* **4**, 517.

Stoeckenius, W. (1969): An electron microscope study of myelin figures. *J. biophys. biochem. Cytol.* **5**, 491.

Stolpmann, H. J. (1967): Elektronenmikroskopische Untersuchung des Hyalins der Pleura und Milzkapsel. *Frankfurt. Z. Path.* **77**, 213.

Sout, C. (1969): Coronary thrombosis without coronary atherosclerosis. *Amer. J. Card.* **24**, 564.

Straus, W. (1957): Use of horseradish peroxidase as a marker protein for studies of phagolysosomes, permeability and immunology. In, Bajusz, E., Jasmin, G. (Eds): *Methods and Achievements in 'Experimental Pathology'.* 4th ed. Karger, Basel– New York.

194

Stump, M. M., Jordan, G. L., DeBakey, M. E., Halpert, B. (1963): Gelatin impregnated dacron prosthesis implanted into porcine thoracic aorta. *Amer. J. Path.* **43**, 361.

Sun, C. N., Ghidoni, J. J. (1969): Membrane-bound microtubular and crystalline structure in endothelial cells of normal canine aorta. *Experientia (Basel)* **25**, 301.

Sunaga, T., Yamashita, Y., Shimamoto, T. (1969a): The intercellular bridge of vascular endothelium. The presence of two types of bridges of endothelial surface. *Proc. Jap. Acad.* **45**, 627.

Sunaga, T., Yamashita, Y., Shimamoto, T. (1969b): Epinephrine effect on arterial endothelial cells observed by scanning electron microscope. *Proc. Jap. Acad.* **45**, 808.

Suter, E. R., Majno, G. (1965): Passage of lipid across vascular endothelium in newborn rats. An electron microscopic study. *J. Cell. Biol.* **27**, 163.

Suzuki, M., Greenberg, S. D., Adams, J. G., O'Neal, R. M. (1964): Experimental atherosclerosis in the dog. A morphological study. *Exp. molec. path.* **3**, 455.

Suzuki, M., O'Neal, R. M. (1967): Circulating lipophages, serum lipids and atherosclerosis in rats. *Arch. Path.* **83**, 169.

Svenkerud, R., Kirkesaether, T., Arskog, R. (1962): Spontaneous atherosclerosis and other sclerogenic changes in the canine vascular system. *Arch. path. microbiol. scand.* **154**, 93.

Symmers, W. St. C. (1962): The occurrence of angiitis and of other generalized diseases of connective tissues as a consequence of the administration of drugs. *Proc. roy. Soc. Med.* **55**, 20.

Szabó, Z. (1962): A só és vízháztartás változásának és pathogenetikai szerepének néhány kérdése hypertonia betegségben (Changes in the salt and water equilibrium and their pathogenetic role in hypertension). *Orvosképzés* **37**, 463.

Szakács, J. E., Cannon, A. (1958): Norepinephrine myocarditis. *Amer. J. clin. Path.* **30**, 425.

Szigeti, I. (1964): Immunization and autoimmunization pathogenesis of human and experimental atherosclerosis. Thesis, Budapest.

Szilagyi, D. E. (1963): An elastic-dacron arterial prosthesis. In, Woorlowski, S. A. (Ed.): *Fundamentals of Vascular Grafting.* McGraw-Hill, New York, p. 138.

Szilagyi, D. E., Elliott, J. P., Smith, R. F. (1965): Long term behavior of a dacron arterial substitute. Clinical roentgenologic and histologic correlations. *Amer. Surg.* **162**, 453.

Szilagyi, D. E., Pfeifer, J. R., DeRusso, F. J. (1964): Long-term evaluation of elastic arterial substitutes. *Surgery* **55**, 165.

Szilagyi, D. E., Whitecomb, J. G., Shonnard, C. P. (1954): Replacement of long and narrow arterial segments. II. Experimental studies with an elastic ('Helanca') seamless woven nylon prosthesis. *Arch. Surg.* **74**, 944.

Szilagyi, T., Miltényi, L., Lévai, G., Benkő, K. (1967): Intravascularis praecipitatum képződés a tengerimalac anaphylaxiás shockjában (Intravascular precipitate formation in anaphylactic shock in guinea pig). *Kísérl. Orvostud.* **19**, 1.

Szinay, Gy. (1968): Adatok a kollagén-betegségek morphologiájához (Data on the morphology of collagen diseases). Thesis, Budapest.

Szöllősy, L., Bartos, G., Hüber, H. (1958): Gefäßsubstitutionsversuche an mit autoplastischen Geweben gefutterten Kunstsenffröhren. *Bruns' Beitr. klin. Chir.* **197**, 295.

Takagi, K. (1969a): Electron microscopical and biochemical studies of the elastogenesis in embryonic chick aorta. I. Fine structure of developing embryonic chick aorta *Kumamoto med. J.* **22**, 1.

Takagi, K. (1969b): Electron microscopical and biochemical studies of the elastogenesis in embryonic chick aorta. II. On elastins isolated from the subcellular fractions of embryonic chick aorta. *Kumamoto med. J.* **22**, 15.

Takagi, K., Kawase, O. (1967): An electron microscopic study of the elastogenesis in embryonic chick aorta. I. *J. Electron Microscopy* **16**, 330.

Takagi, K., Ogata, T., Kawase, O. (1967a): An electron microscopic study of the elastogenesis in embryonic chick aorta. II. *J. Electron Microscopy* **16**, 360.

Takagi, K., Ogata, T., Kawase, O. (1968): An electron microscopic study of the elastogenesis in embryonic chick aorta. *J. Electron Microscopy* **17**, 272.

Takagi, K., Ogata, T., Takagi, T., Kawase, O. (1967b): An electron microscopic study on the elastogenesis in embryonic chick aorta. III. *J. Electron Microscopy* **16**, 215.

Takatama, M. (1960): cit. Kosimahara. *Proc. Soc. Path. Jap.* **49**, 494.

Takebayashi, Sh. (1970): Ultrastructural studies on arteriolar lesions in experimenta-hypertension. *J. Electron Microscopy* **19**, 17.

Talbot, N. B., Sobel, E. H., McArthur, J., Crawford, J. D. (1960): *Functional Endocrinology from Birth through Adolescence.* Harvard Univ. Press, Cambridge, 1952, p. 271.

Tallgren, L. G., Knorring, J. (1969): Renal vascular involvement in a case of polymyalgia rheumatica with temporal arteritis. *Acta med. scand.* **185**, 421.

Taylor, C. D., Trueheart, R. E., Cox, G. E. (1963): Atherosclerosis in rhesus monkeys. III. The role of increased thickness of arterial walls in atherogenesis. *Arch. Path.* **76**, 14.

Taylor, H. E., Shepherd, W. E., Robertson, C. E. (1961): An immunohistochemical examination of granulation tissue with glomerular and long antiserums. *Amer. J. Path.* **38**, 39.

Terry, B. E., Jones, D. B., Mueller, C. B. (1970): Experimental ischemic renal arterial necrosis with resolution. *Amer. J. Path.* **58**, 69.

Tessenow, W. (1965): Intracellulare Lokalisation und sukzedaner Nachweis von unspezifischer Esterase und saurer Phosphatase in den proximalen Tubuli der Urniere von *Xenopus. Acta histochem. (Jena)* **20**, 234.

Texon, M. (1960): The haemodynamic concept of atherosclerosis. *Bull. N. Y. Acad. Med.* **36**, 263.

Texon, M. (1967): Mechanical factors involved in atherosclerosis. In, Breast, A. N., Moyer, J. H. (Eds): *Atherosclerotic Vascular Disease.* Butterworths, London, p. 23.

Texon, M., Imparato, A. M., Helpern, M. (1965): The role of vascular dynamics in the development of atherosclerosis. *J. Amer. med. Ass.* **194**, 1226.

Thoma, R. (1883): Über die Abhängigkeit der Bindegewebsneubildung in der Arterien-Intima von den mechanischen Bedingungen des Blutlaufes. *Virchows Arch. path. Anat.* **93**, 443.

Thomas, W. A., Florentin, R. A., Nam, S. Ch., Kim, D. N., Jones, R. M., Lee, K. T. (1968): Preproliferative phase of atherosclerosis in swine fed cholesterol. *Arch. Path.* **86**, 621.

Thomas, W. A., Jones, R., Scott, R. F., Morrison, E., Imai, H. (1963): Production of early atherosclerosis lesions in rats characterized by proliferation of modified smooth muscle cells. *Exp. molec. Path. Suppl.* **1**, 40.

Thomas, W. A., O'Neal, R. M. (1960): Electron microscopic studies on butter and corn oil in jejunal mucosa. *Arch. Path.* **69**, 121.

Thorban, W. (1961): Gefässveränderungen beim experimentellen Sudeck-Syndrom. *Metabolismus Parietis Vasorum* Praha, p. 579.

Tjawokin, W. W. (1969): Experimentelle Koronarsklerose durch Bewegungseinschränkung beim Kaninchen. Ein neues Modell der Arteriosklerose. *Virchows Arch. path. Anat.* **346**, 29.

Tobian, L., Janáček, J., Tomboulian, A., Tereire, D. (1961): Sodium and potassium in the walls of arteries in experimental renal hypertension. *J. clin. Invest.* **40**, 1922.

Tobian, L., Olson, R., Chesley, G. (1969): Water content of arteriolar wall in renovascular hypertension. *Amer. J. Physiol.* **216**, 22.

Tranzer, J. P. (1967): Filling gaps in the vascular endothelium with blood platelets. *Nature* **216**, 1126.

Tranzer, J. P., Thoenen, H. (1968): An electron microscopic study of selective acute degeneration of sympathetic nerve terminals after administration of 6-hydroxydopamine. *Experientia (Basel)* **24**, 155.

Trillo, A., Renaud, S., Haust, M. D. (1970): Ultrastructure of aortic lesions in normotensive hyperlipemic rats. *Fed. Proc.* **29**, 487 (Abstract).

Ts'ao, C. H. (1968): Myointimal cells as a possible source of replacement for endothelial cells in the rabbit. *Circulat. Res.* **23**, 671.

Tuttle, R. S. (1966): Age related changes in the sensitivity of rat aortic strips to norepinephrine and associated chemical and structural alterations. *J. Geront.* **21**, 510.

Uchida, E., Bohr, D. F. (1969): Myogenic tone in isolated perfused resistance vessels from rats. *Circulat. Res.* **25**, 549.

Vassalli, Pl., McCluskey, R. T. (1964): The pathogenetic role of the coagulation process in rabbit Masugi-nephritis. *Amer. J. Path.* **45**, 653.

Vassalli, Pl., Simon, G., Rouiller, Ch. (1963): Electron microscopic study of glomerular lesions resulting from intravascular fibrin formation. *Amer. J. Path.* **43,** 579.

Vazquez, J. J., Dixon, F. J. (1957): Immunohistochemical study of lesions in rheumatic fever, systemic lupus erythematodes and rheumatoid arthritis. *Lab. Invest.* **6,** 205.

Vazquez, J. J., Dixon, F. J. (1958): Immunohistochemical analysis of lesions associated with 'fibrinoid change'. *Arch. Path.* **66,** 504.

Vegge, T. (1969): Ultrastructure of the wall of human iris vessels. *Z. Zellforsch.* **94,** 19.

Velican, C. (1967): Topochemistry of acid carbohydrates in the human aortic and coronary intima. *J. Atheroscler. Res.* **7,** 517.

Velican, C. (1968): Histochemical analysis of the structural stability of biopolymers (preliminary data). *Acta histochem. (Jena)* **31,** 261.

Velican, C. (1969): Relationship between regional aortic susceptibility to atherosclerosis and macromolecular structural stability. *J. Atheroscler. Res.* **9,** 193.

Velican, C., Velican, D. (1970): *Organizarea macromoleculara a tesutului conjunctiv* (Macromolecular structure of connective tissue). Editura Academiei Republicii Socialiste România.

Velican, D., Velican, C. (1970): Structural heterogeneity of kidney basement membranes. *Nature* **226,** 1259.

Venable, J. H., Coggeshall, R. (1965): A simplified lead citrate stain for use in electron microscopy. *J. Cell. Biol.* **25,** 407.

Virágh, Sz. (1968): Sejtkapcsoló struktúrák funkcionális morphológiája (Functional morphology of cell linking structures). *MTA Biol. Oszt. Közl.* **11,** 327.

Virágh, Sz., Papp, M., Törő, I., Rusznyák, I. (1966): Cutaneous lymphatic capillaries in dextran induced oedema of the rat. An electron microscopic study. *Brit. J. exp. Path.* **47,** 563.

Virágh, Sz., Pozsonyi, T., Dine, R., Gerő, S. (1968): Uptake of ^{125}I labelled beta lipoprotein by the aortas of animals different to cholesterol induced atherosclerosis. *J. Atheroscler. Res.* **8,** 859.

Virchow, R. (1856): Phlogose und Thrombose im Gefäßsystem. In, *Gesammelte Abhandlungen zur wissenschaftlichen Medizin.* Meidinger Frankfurt am Main.

Voltera, M. (1925): Einige neue Befunde über die Struktur der Kapillaren und ihre Beziehungen zur sogenannten Kontraktilität derselben. *Zbl. inn. Med.* **46,** 876.

Voorhees, A. B. (1963): First decade of experience in the use of permeable arterial prostheses: from inception to practice. In, Wosolowski, S. A., Dennis, C. (Eds): *Fundamentals of Vascular Grafting.* McGraw-Hill, New York–London, Toronto, p. 157.

Voorhees, A. B., Jaretzki, A., Blakemore, A. H. (1952): Use of tubes constricted from vinyon "N" cloth in bridging arterial defects; preliminary report. *Ann. Surg.* **135,** 332.

Voorhees, A. B., Wosolowski, S. A. (1963): In, Wosolowski, S. A., Dennis, C. (Eds): *Fundamentals of Vascular Grafting.* McGraw-Hill, New York–London–Toronto, p. 174.

Wachstein, M., Meisel, E. (1960): Histochemistry of 'thiolacetic acid esterase' in relation to DeDuwe's lysosomes. *J. Histochem. Cytochem.* **8,** 317.

Waisman, J. (1968): The action of elastase on the fine structure of native vascular components. *Fed. Proc.* **27,** 475.

Wakerlin, G. E., Moss, W. G., Kiely, J. P. (1957): Effect of experimental renal hypertension on experimental thiouracil cholesterol atherosclerosis in dogs. *Circulat. Res.* **5,** 426.

Wallace, G., Campbell, M. D. (1968): Localization of adenosine 5'-triphosphatase in vascular and cellular synovium of rabbits. *Lab. Invest.* **18,** 304.

Walton, K. W., Williamson, V. (1968): Histological and immunofluorescent studies on the evolution of the human atheromatous plaque. *J. Atheroscler. Res.* **8,** 599.

Warren, R., McCombs, H. L. (1965): Morphologic studies on plastic arterial prostheses in humans. *Ann. Surg.* **161,** 73.

Watts, H. F. (1961): Pathogenesis of human coronary artery arteriosclerosis. Demonstration of serum lipoprotein in the lesions and of localized intimal enzyme defects by histochemistry. *Circulation* **24,** 1066.

Watts, H. F. (1963): The mechanism of arterial lipid accumulation in human coronary artery atherosclerosis. In, Likoff, W., Moyer, J. H. (Eds): *7th Hahnemann Symposium on Coronary Heart Disease.* Grune and Stratton, New York, p. 98.

Waugh, W. H. (1962): Adrenergic stimulation of depolarized arterial muscle. *Circulat. Res.* **11**, 264.

Weibel, E. R., Palade, G. E. (1964): New cytoplasmic components in arterial endothelia. *J. Cell. Biol.* **23**, 101.

Wegener, F. (1967): Die pneumogene allgemeine Granulomatose (P.G.) — sog. Wegenersche Granulomatose. In, Kaufmann, E., Staemmler, M. (Eds): *Lehrbuch der speziellen pathologischen Anatomie.* Walter der Gruyter, Berlin, p. 225.

Weiss, P. (1968): Submikroskopische Charakteristika und Reaktionsformen der glatten Muskelzelle unter besonderer Berücksichtigung der Gefässwandmuskelzelle. *Z. mikr. anat. Forsch.* **78**, 305.

Weller, R. I. (1966): The ultrastructure of intracellular lipid accumulations in atheroma. *J. Atheroscler. Res.* **6**, 184.

Weller, R. I., Clark, R. A., Oswald, W. B. (1968): Stages of the formation and metabolism of intracellular lipid droplets in atherosclerosis. An electron microscopic and histochemical study. *J. Atheroscler. Res.* **8**, 249.

Wernze, H., Flujy, J., Sembach, B. (1965): Der Lymphfluss im Ductus thoracicus unter Angiotensin und Noradrenalin. *Z. Ges. exp. Med.* **139**, 70.

Wertheimer, H. E., Ben-Tor, V. (1961): Physiologic and pathologic influences on the metabolism of rat aorta. *Circulat. Res.* **9**, 20.

Werthessen, N. T., Milch, L. J., Redmond, R. F., Smith, L. L., Smith, E. C. (1954): Biosynthesis and concentration of cholesterol by intact surviving bovine aorta *in vitro. Amer. J. Physiol.* **178**, 23.

Westlake, G., Grundy, S. M., O'Neal, R. M. (1963): The effect of atherogenic diet on pre-existing aortic intimal thickening in old dogs. *Exp. Molec. Path. Suppl.* **1**, 1.

Westman, I., Nylander, G. (1965): Electron microscopy of the human gastroepiploic artery. *Angiology* **16**, 292.

Wetzstein, R., Schwink, A., Stanka, P. (1963): Die periodisch strukturierten Körper in Subkommissuralorganen der Ratte. *Z. Zellforsch.* **61**, 493.

Wexler, B. C. (1968): Carotid artery occlusion in rats with and without arteriosclerosis. *Angiology* **19**, 554.

Whereat, A. F. (1961): Incorporation of acetate into fatty acid and cholesterol by normal and atherosclerotic intima (P). *Circulation* **24**, 1070.

Whereat, A. F (1966): Fatty acid synthesis in cell-free system from rabbit aorta. *J. Lipid Res.* **7**, 671.

Whereat, A. F. (1967): Atherosclerosis and metabolic disorder in the arterial wall. *Exp. molec. Path.* **7**, 233.

Whitaker, A. N., McKay, D. G., Csaudssy, I. (1969): Studies of catecholamine shock. Disseminated intravascular coagulation. *Amer. J. Path.* **56**, 153.

White, F. N., Grollman, A. (1964): Experimental periarteritis nodosa in the rat. *Arch. Path.* **78**, 31.

Wiener, J., Lattes, R. G., Meltzner, B. G., Spiro, D. (1968): Vascular permeability in experimental hypertension. *Amer. J. Path.* **52**, 52/a.

Wiener, J., Lattes, R. G., Meltzner, B. G., Spiro, D. (1969): The cellular pathology of experimental hypertension. IV. Evidence for increased vascuar permeability. *Amer. J. Path.* **54**, 187.

Wiener, J., Spiro, D., Lattes, R. G. (1965): The cellular pathology of experimental hypertension. II. Arteriolar hyalinosis and fibrinoid change. *Amer. J. Path.* **47**, 457.

Wilbrandt, R., Neuhaus, G., Sellin, D., Fritz, K. W. (1969): Zum Krankheitsbild der perakuten nekrotisierenden Angiitis. *Dtsch. med. Wschr.* **84**, 657.

Wilens, S. L. (1943): The effect of postural hypertension on the development of atheromatosis in rabbits fed cholesterol. *Amer. J. Path.* **19**, 293.

Wilens, S. L., Elster, S. K. (1950): The role of lipid deposition in renal arteriolar sclerosis. *Amer. J. med. Sci.* **219**, 183.

Wilens, S. L., McClurkey, R. T. (1954): The permeability of excised arteries and other tissue to serum lipid. *Circulat. Res.* **2**, 175.

Wilens, S., L., Sproul, E. E. (1938): Spontaneous cardiovascular disease in the rat. II. Lesions of the vascular system. *Amer. J. Path.* **14**, 201.

Williams, A. W. (1961): Relation of atheroma to local trauma. *J. Path. Bact.* **81**, 419.

Williams, G. (1956): Experimental studies in arterial ligation. *J. Path. Bact.* **72**, 569.

198

Williamson, J. R. (1964): Adipose tissue: morphological changes associated with lipid metabolisation. *J. Cell. Biol.* **20**, 57.

Wilson, C., Byrom, F. B. (1939): Renal changes in malignant hypertension; experimental evidence. *Lancet* i, 136.

Wilson, C., Byrom, F. B. (1941): The vicious circle in chronic Bright's disease. Experimental evidence from the hypertensive rat. *Quart. J. Med.* **10**, 65.

Winsor, T. (1958): *Peripheral Vascular Diseases, an Objective Approach.* Thomas, Springfield.

Winternitz, M. C. (1954): The blood supply of the wall. In, *Symposium on Atherosclerosis.* Nat. Acad. Sci., Washington, D. C., p 14.

Wissler, R. W. (1967): The arterial medial cell, smooth muscle or multifunctional mesenchyma. *Circulation* **36**, 1.

Wissler, R. W. (1968): The arterial medial cell, smooth muscle or multifunctional mesenchyma. *J. Atheroscler. Res.* **8**, 201.

Wissler, R. W., Eilert, M. L., Schroeder, M. A., Cohen, L. (1954): Production of lipomatous and atheromatous arterial lesions in the albino rat. *Arch. Path.* **57**, 333.

Wissler, R. W., Kao, V. (1962): Immunohistochemical studies of the human aorta. *Fed. Proc.* **21**, 95.

Woerner, C. A. (1959): Vasa vasorum of arteries, their demonstration and distribution. In, Lansing, A. (Ed.): *The Arterial Wall.* Williams and Wilkins, Baltimore, p. 1.

Wolf, R. L., Mendlowitz, M., Gitlow, S. E., Naftchi, N. (1962): The metabolism of angiotensin. *Circulat. Res.* **11**, 195.

Wolinsky, H. (1967): A lamellar unit of aortic medial structure and function in mammals. *Circulat. Res.* **20**, 99.

Wolinsky, H., Glagov, S. (1964): Structural basis for the static mechanical properties of the aortic media. *Circulat. Res.* **14**, 400.

Wolinsky, H., Glagov, S. (1967): Nature of species differences in the medial distribution of aortic vasa vasorum in mammals. *Circulat. Res.* **200**, 409.

Woolf, N., Crawford, T. (1960): Fatty streaks in the aortic intima studied by an immunohistochemical technique. *J. Path. Bact.* **80**, 405.

Woolf, N., Pilkington, T. R. E. (1965): The immunochemical demonstration of lipoproteins in vessel walls. *J. Path. Bact.* **90**, 459.

Wosolowski, S. A. (1962): *Evaluation of Tissue and Prosthetic Vascular Grafts.* Thomas, Springfield.

Wosolowski, S. A., Dennis, C. (1963): *Fundamentals of Vascular Grafting.* McGraw-Hill, New York–Toronto–London.

Wosolowski, S. A., Fries, C. C., Domingo, R. T., Liebig, W. J., Sawyer, P. N. (1963): The compound prosthetic vascular graft. A pathologic survey. *Surgery* **53**, 19.

Wosolowski, S. A., Fries, C. C., Karlson, K. E., DeBakey, M., Sawyer, P. N. (1961): Porosity: Primary determinant of ultimate fate of synthetic vascular grafts. *Surgery* **50**, 91.

Wosolowski, S. A., Fries, C. C., Sabini, A. M., Sawyer, P. N. (1965): The significance of turbulence in hemic system and in the distribution of the atheroslerotic lesion. *Surgery* **57**, 155.

Wurzel, M., Zweifach, B. W. (1966): Contracting principles of arterial smooth muscle in rabbit and dog plasma. *Arch. int. Pharmacodyn.* **162**, 1.

Wyllie, J. C., More, R. H., Haust, M. D. (1964): Demonstration of fibrin in yellow streaks by the fluorescent antibody technique. *J. Path. Bact.* **88**, 335.

Yarygin, N. E., Nikolaev, G. M. (1961): Pathomorphology of the vascular system in acute radiation sickness. *Arch. Patologii (Moscow)* **238**, 24.

Yasamura, A. (1967): Experimental studies on the role of a vascular permeability factor of kidney cortex. *Jap. Circulat. J. (Ni.)* **31**, 1457.

Yoffey, I. M., Coirtice, F. C. (1956): *Lymphatics, Lymph and Lymphoid Tissues.* Arnold, London.

Yokota, H. (1957): Histochemical and electron microscopic studies on elastic fibers. I. Electron microscopic observation of bovine ligamentum nuchae in ultrathin sections after elastase treatment. *Komamoto med. J.* **10**, 25.

Zahn, F. (1966): cit.: French, J. E.: Atherosclerosis in relation to the structure and function of the arterial intima with special reference to the endothelium. *Int. Rev.*

exp. Path. Richter G. W., Epstein, M. A (Eds): Academic Press, New York–London, p. 297.

Záhoř, Z., Vanecek, R., Czabanová, V., Müller, J., Komárková, A. (1967): The origin and development of the post-reproduction arteriopathy in female rats. *J. Atheroscler. Res.* **7**, 25.

Zeek, M. (1952): Periarteritis nodosa. A critical review. *Amer. J. clin. Path.* **22**, 777.

Zeek, M., Smith, C. C., Weeter, J. C. (1948): Studies on periarteritis nodosa. III. The differentiation between the vascular lesions of periarteritis nodosa and hypersensiti-vity. *Amer. J. Path.* **24**, 889.

Zelander, T., Ekholm, R., Edking, Y. (1962): The ultrastructural organization of the rat exocrine pancreas. III. Intralobular vessels and nerves. *J. Ultrastruct.* **7**, 84.

Zemplényi, T. (1962): Enzymes of the arterial wall. *J. Atheroscler. Res.* **2**, 2.

Zemplényi, T. (1968): *Enzyme Biochemistry of the Arterial Wall as Related to Atherosclerosis.* Lloyd-Luke, London.

Zilversmit, D. B., McCandless, E. L., Jordam, P. H., Henly, W. S. Ackerman, R. M. (1961): The synthesis of phospholipids in human atheromatous lesions. *Circulation* **23**, 370.

Zimmermann, B. G. (1962): Effect of acute sympathectomy on responses to angiotensin and norepinephrine. *Circulation* **11**, 780.

Zlateva, M. D. (1960): Changes in aorta in hypertensive disease. *Arkh. Pat.* **22**, 23.

Zollinger, H. U. (1959): Die hypertensive Arteriolopathie. *Schweiz. Z. allg. Path.* **22**, 262.

Zollinger, H. U. (1960): *Handbuch für allgemeine Pathologie.* Springer, Berlin–Göttingen–Heidelberg.

Zollinger, H. U. (1967): Adoptive Intima-Fibrose der Arterien. *Virchows Arch. path. Anat.* **342**, 154.

Zugibe, F. T. (1963): Mucopolysaccharides of the arterial wall. *J. Histochem. Cytochem.* **11**, 35.

PLATES

PLATE I

1. Electron micrograph of normal rat aorta. Arrow points to basement membrane-like granular-filamentous substance in the narrow subendothelial space below the endothelial cell row (E). The internal elastic lamina (IEL) is homogeneously electronlucent. The smooth muscle cells of the media (SC) have cytoplasmic processes and their cytoplasmic membrane carries many pinocytotic vesicles.

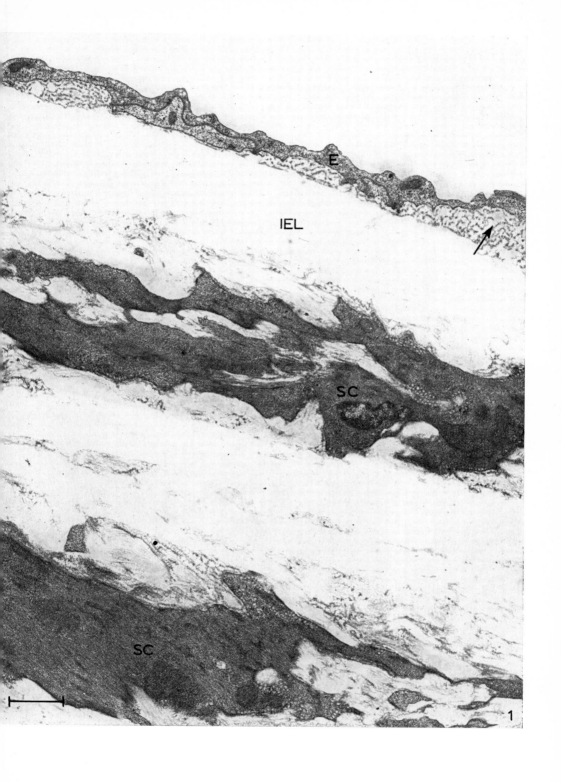

PLATE II

2. Electron micrograph of normal coronary artery of rat. Elastic fibres (EF) occur in islets below the endothelial cell row and the islets are connected by a basement membrane-like (BM) granular substance which is double-layered in places (arrow). Two smooth muscle cells (SC) lie under the BM. FC = fibrocyte; HMC = heart muscle fibre.

3. Section of normal rat aorta after fixation in ruthenium red. Note the distinctly positive reaction of the endothelial cell's (E) external coat; pinocytotic vesicles, intercellular junction and delicate granules in the narrow subendothelial space (arrow) also show the reaction. IEL = internal elastic lamina. Ruthenium red was applied after purification according to Brooks (1969); no counterstain was used.

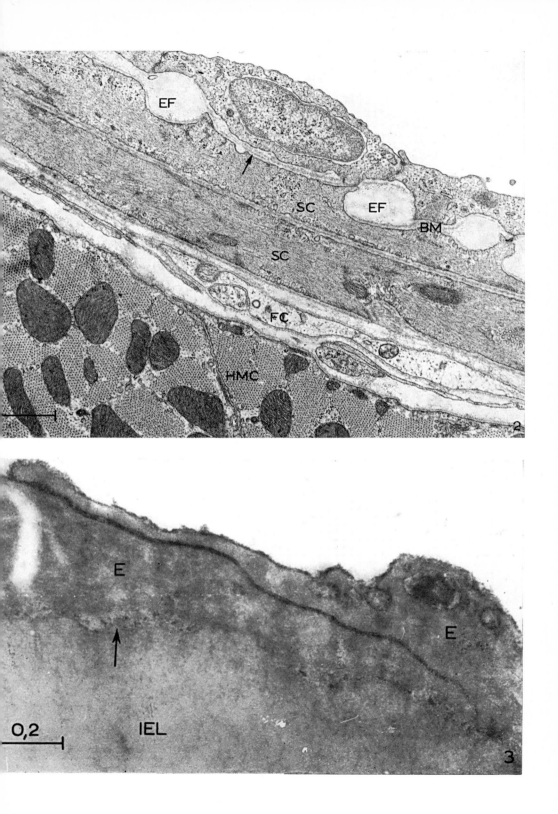

PLATE III

4. Section of aorta 3 months after painting with acid. The original media contains an elastic fibre (EF), the process of a fibrocyte (FB) and scross-sections of many collagenous fibres (C).

5. Aortic IP 3 months after painting with acid. Note lymph channel (LC) of varying cross-section between adventitial collagenous fibres (C).

6. Aortic wall 261 days after painting with acid. (*a*) Semi-thin section: the original media is thin and cicatrized and empty spaces (in part artefacts) in the IP represent chalk depositions. L = lumen; E = endothelium (toluidine blue stain). (*b*) Rounded smooth muscle cells (SC) with widened endoplasmic reticulum; (*c*) calcium apatite crystals at a higher magnification.

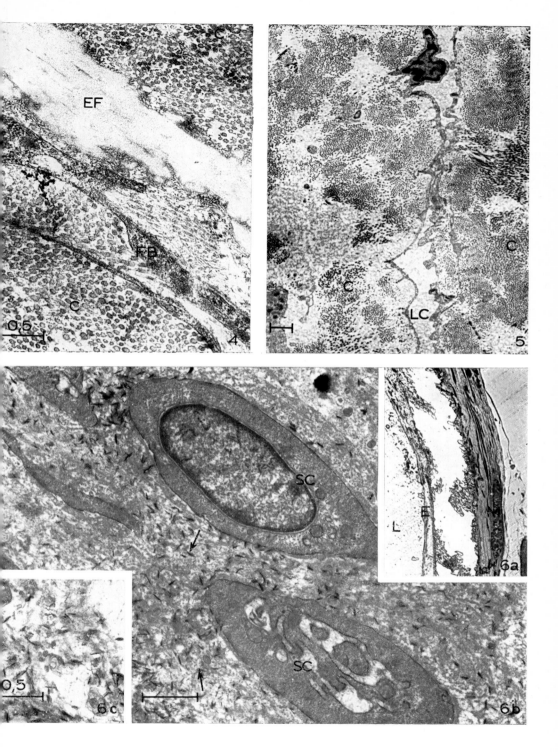

PLATE IV

7. Aortic wall 3 months after painting with acid. The nucleus (N) of the endothelial cell (E) is long, the chromatin aggregates along the nuclear membrane and the pinocytotic vesicles (arrow) contain a meshwork of a granular substance. L = lumen.

8. Aortic wall 3 months after painting with acid. The dark endothelial cell comprises a well-developed Golgi apparatus (G) and many pinocytotic vesicles, either closed or in various phases of opening.

9. Aortic wall one month after painting with acid. Abundant rough endoplasmic reticulum with widened ductules, free ribosomes and mitochondria with a dense matrix are present in the endothelial cell. Dense granules, 600–800 Å in diameter (arrow), lie along the luminal surface (L) of the cytoplasmic membrane.

10. Aortic wall 20 days after painting with acid. Dense granules, 400–600 Å in diameter (arrow), lie on surface of endothelial cell. Ribosomes and vesicles abound in the pale hyaloplasm. The nuclear membrane appears widened in places and the chromatin aggregates peripherally.

11. Aortic wall 3 months after painting with acid. Two adjacent endothelial cells connect with interdigitated processes. A loose, granular substance fills the 150–300 Å wide intercellular space.

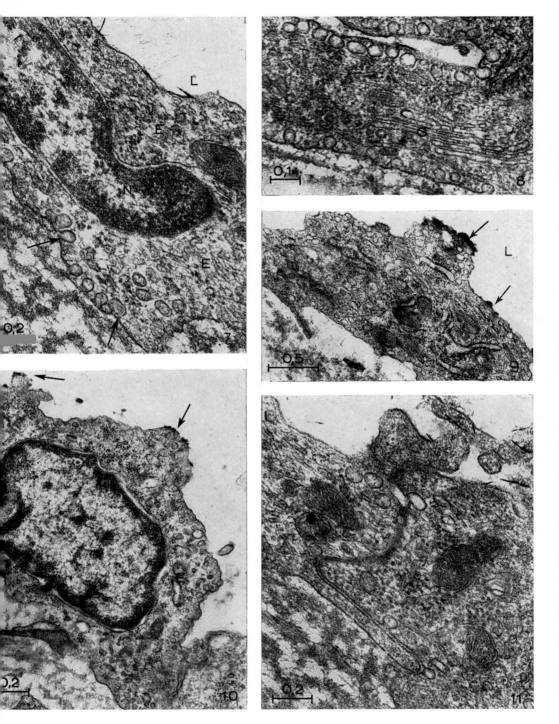

PLATE V

12. Aortic wall 12 days after painting with acid. Endothelial cells connected by interdigitated processes carry pinocytotic vesicles with granular contents on both surfaces. IEL = internal elastic lamina.

13. Aortic wall 12 days after painting with acid. Processes of dark and light endothelial cells. Pinocytotic vesicles aggregate in clusters (arrow) in places. IEL = internal elastic lamina.

14. Aortic wall 2.5 months after painting with acid. The endothelial cells contain lipid droplets (F) surrounded by a unit membrane. The mitochondrial matrix is electron dense and a few microfilaments (CF) and vesicles lie in the hyaloplasm.

15. Aortic wall 4 months after painting with acid. A granular 200–300 Å thick basement membrane (BM) of a low electron density is associated with the endothelial cells. Smooth muscle cell (SC) processes extend at bottom.

16. Aortic wall 1 month after painting with acid. A monocyte-like pale cell (MO) attaches to the endothelial cell row (E) above the damaged vessel wall portion.

17. Aortic wall 2 months after painting with acid. Dark and light endothelial cells. Dark cells comprise an abundant membrane system. Osmiophilic granules (arrow) lie at cell surfaces.

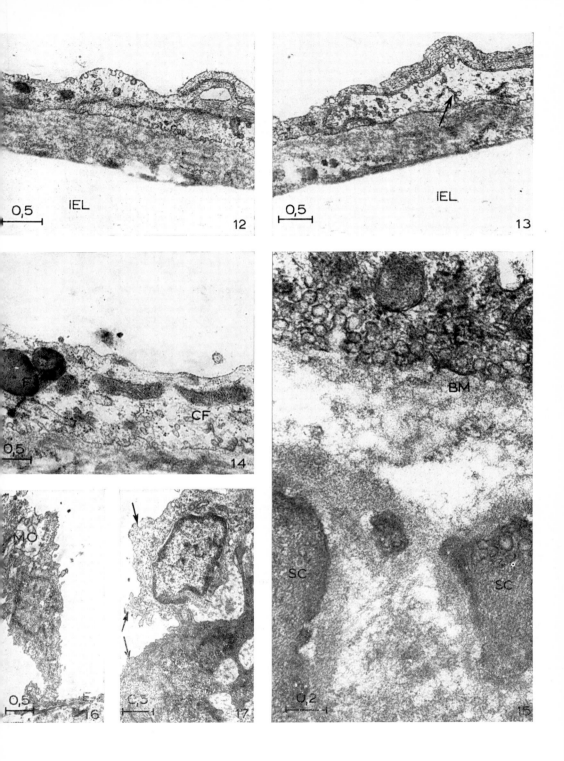

0,5   IEL   12

0,5   IEL   13

F
                        CF

0,5   14

BM

MO

SC   SC

0,5   16   0,3   17   0,2   15

PLATE VI

18. Aortic IP 3 months after painting with acid. Smooth muscle cells carrying processes are circularly oriented directly below the media and longitudinally oriented in a deeper location. The degenerated media is acellular and the elastic fibres are stretched (H. and E. stain).

19. Aortic IP 3 months after painting with acid. Note newly formed ground substance (GS), elastic units (EA) and smooth muscle cell processes (SC) associated with a multi-layered basement membrane below the endothelial cell (E).

20. Aortic IP 3 months after painting with acid. Part of an endothelial cell (E) with a well-developed Golgi apparatus is seen at top right. Cells composing the proliferation are associated with a 250–400 Å thick basement membrane (arrow), many pinocytotic vesicles lie inside the cells and the hyaloplasm of cell processes is filled by myofilaments (MF).

21. Aortic IP 2.5 months after painting with acid. The nuclei and organelles aggregate at the centre of smooth muscle cells. The Golgi apparatus (G) is well developed, the small mitochondria (arrow) lie in a dense matrix and there are abundant free RNA granules. Cross-sections of myofilaments are seen at the periphery. E = endothelium; IEL = damaged internal elastic lamina; N = nucleus.

22. Aortic IP 158 days after painting with acid. The basement membrane of smooth muscle cells (arrow) and the myofilamentous (MF) structure are clearly visible. E = endothelium.

23. Aortic IP 158 days after painting with acid. Note attachment bodies (AB) along the smooth muscle cell membrane and between the undulating myofilaments.

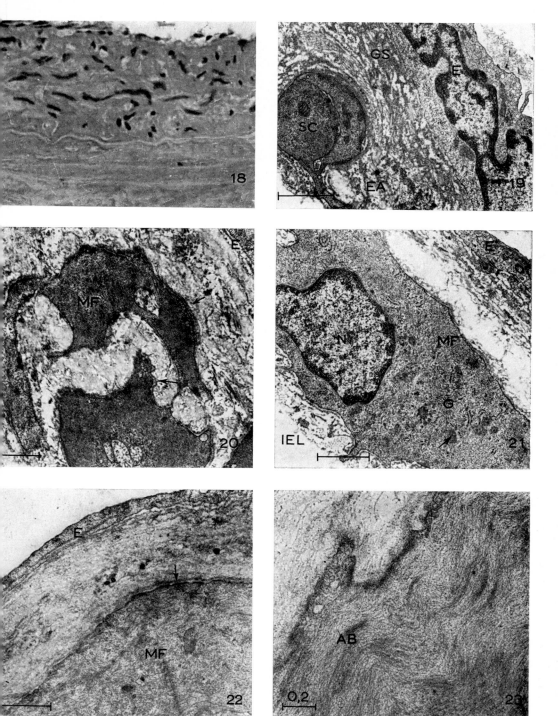

PLATE VII

24. Aortic IP 3 months after painting with acid. Golgi apparatus (G) and mitochondria have a perinuclear location, in the centre of the smooth muscle cell and widened cisternae of endoplasmic reticulum are seen in places. N = nucleus.

25. Aortic IP 3 months after painting with acid. The smooth muscle cells associate with a granular or filamentous, 350 Å thick, multilayered basement membrane (arrow), lifted above the cell membrane in places.

26. Aortic IP 5 months after painting with acid. Myelin figures (arrow) lie inside smooth muscle cells and in the extracellular space. E = endothelial cell.

27. Aortic IP 5 months after painting with acid. A neutral lipid droplet (F) is seen below the endothelial cell (E) in the extracellular space. SC = smooth muscle cell.

28. Aortic IP 18 days after painting with acid. Smooth muscle cell processes (SC) extend into widened stomas of the internal elastic lamina (IEL). Newly formed endothelial cells (E) cover the luminal surface.

29. Aortic IP 28 days after painting with acid. A smooth muscle cell process (SC) extends into a gap of the original internal elastic lamina (IEL). M = original media; P = proliferation.

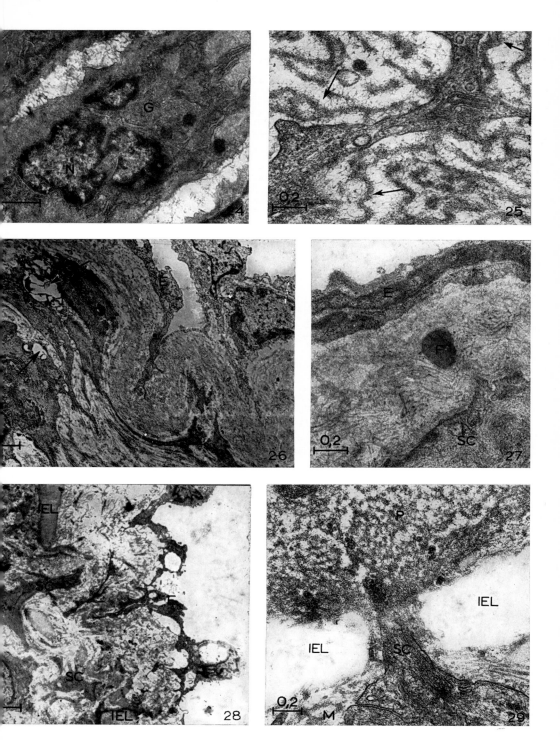

PLATE VIII

30. Aortic IP 56 days after painting with acid. Several layers of smooth muscle cells (SC) form a proliferation between endothelium (E) and original internal elastic lamina (IEL). Newly formed elastic elements (EA) lie in the intercellular space of the proliferation and many collagenous fibres (C) appear at the bottom. Cross-sections of elongated smooth muscle cells (SC) are seen immediately below the IEL of the damaged media (M) and multiplication of collagenous fibres and accumulation of degeneration products are apparent.

31. Aortic IP 96 days after painting with acid. An oedematous process (O) of a smooth muscle cell (SC) extends between the newly formed elastic fibres (EF) of the IP. E = endothelium; IEL = internal elastic lamina.

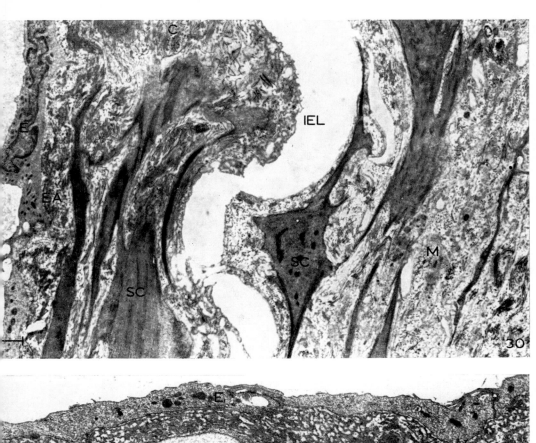

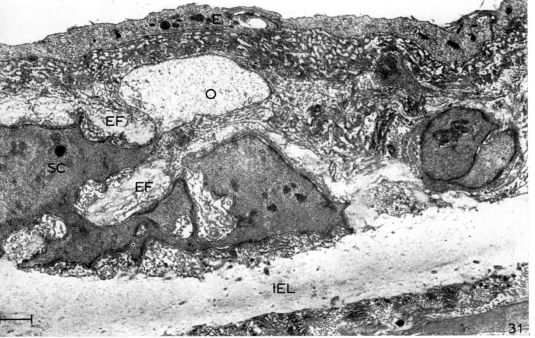

PLATE IX

32 and *33*. Aortic wall 3 months after painting with acid. Polarization micrograph of intimal proliferation (reverse compensation). Aniline reaction visualizes a delicate meshwork of elastic fibrils around the smooth muscle cell components of the proliferation.

34. Aortic IP one month after painting with acid. Small PTA-positive elastic aggregates (EA) lie in the extracellular space, and elastic granules, averaging 70 Å in diameter, appear at the marginal parts of the larger clumps.

35. Aortic IP 56 days after painting with acid. Large PTA-positive elastic clumps (EA) hold elastic granules at their periphery. Microfilaments (arrow) pass between, or into, the elastic granules. The basement membrane (BM) of the smooth muscle cell (SC) is bilayered.

36. Aortic IP 56 days after painting with acid. Note aggregation of PTA-positive elastic clumps (EA). SC = smooth muscle cell.

37. Aortic IP 56 days after painting with acid. Elastic clumps (EA) between smooth muscle cells are in the process of fusion to elastic fibres, and elastic granules and microfilaments are at their marginal parts (PTA stain).

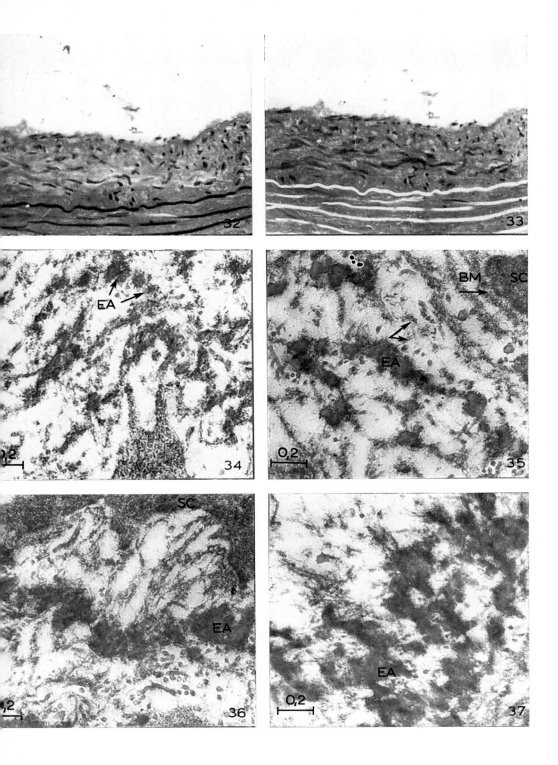

PLATE X

38–41. Elastic clumps and fibres in different stages of maturation. Immature clumps (EA) bind PTA firmly, while mature fibres (EF) do not bind it. SC = smooth muscle cell (*38* and *39* show a 56-day IP, *40–41* a 96-day IP, induced by painting with acid).

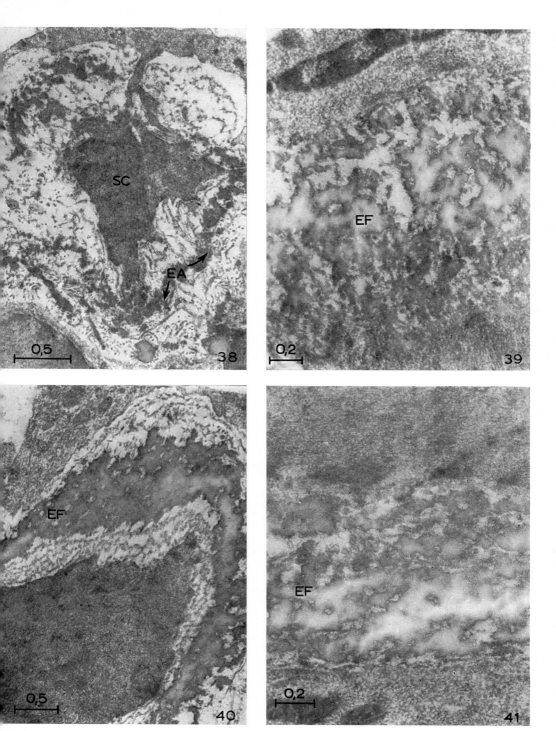

PLATE XI

42. Aortic IP one month after painting with acid. Counterstaining with uranyl acetate reveals the extracellular aggregation (arrow) of granules, on average 70 Å in diameter.

43. Aortic IP 56 days after painting with acid. Apart from electron-lucent aggregations of elastic granules, there are some larger elastic clumps (EA) showing only a marginal binding of uranyl acetate.

44. Aortic IP 56 days after painting with acid. Elastic clumps (EA) with elastic granules at their periphery; note microfilaments between the granules.

45. Aortic IP 3 months after painting with acid. The large elastic clump did not bind the counterstaining uranyl acetate.

46. Aortic IP 5 months after painting with acid. An almost mature internal elastic lamina (IEL) lies between newly formed endothelial cells (E) and smooth muscle cells (SC) of the proliferation.

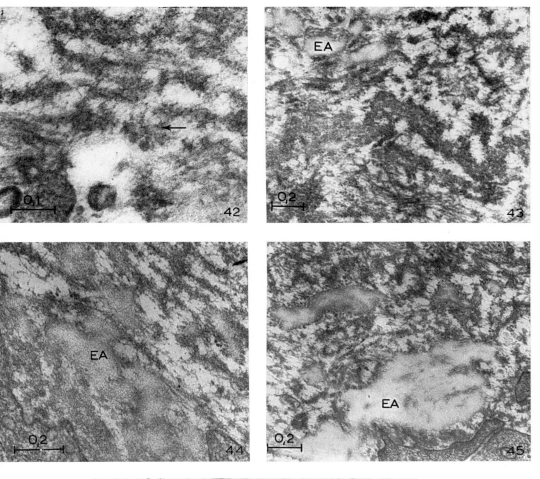

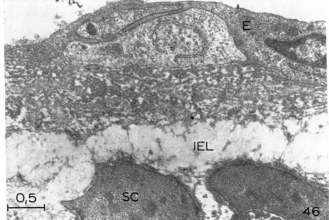

PLATE XII

47. Foetal aorta from 18-day embryo. PTA-positive elastic clumps (EA), lying near smooth muscle cells (SC) carry elastic granules and between them microfilaments (arrow) at their margins (PTA stain).

48–49. Foetal aorta from 18-day embryo. Islets of elastic clumps (EA) lie between smooth muscle cells (SC) (PTA stain).

50–51. Elastic fibres in various phases of development. The cores of the larger fibres (arrow) have already lost affinity to PTA. SC = smooth muscle cell; EA = elastic aggregations (clumps).

52. Almost mature internal elastic lamina (IEL) from 3-day-old newborn. Only the marginal zone of the fibre is electron-dense (PTA-positive).

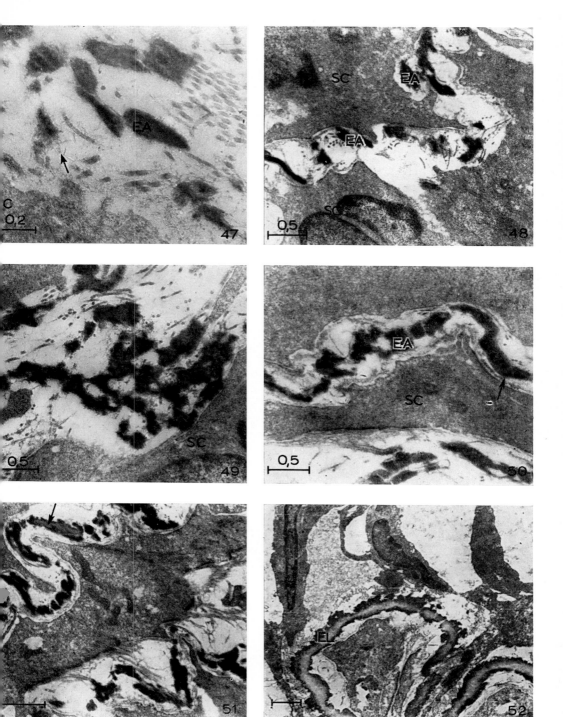

PLATE XIII

53–54. Immature elastic clumps (EA), counterstained with uranyl acetate, from aorta of 2-day-old embryo.

55. Elastic fibre (EF) surrounded by microfibrils from rat embryonic aorta, counterstained with uranyl acetate.

56. Part of evolved internal elastic lamina (IEL) from aorta of 5-day-old baby rat.

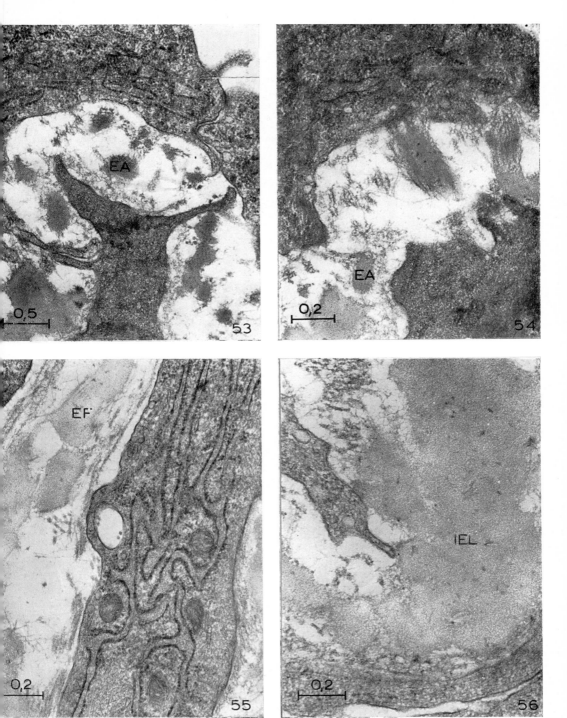

PLATE XIV

57. Semi-thin section of aorta from 8-day chick embryo. Subendothelially localizing cells are round or oval (M) and around them lies a sparse orcein-positive aggregation (EA). No elastic substance is present directly below the endothelium. Large orcein-positive elastic fibres (EF) lie at the outer part of the media, where also the appearance of the cells changes. SC = smooth muscle cell; E = endothelial cell.

58. Aorta from 10-day chick embryo. Elastic clumps (EA) have increased in the inner third of the intima, but they have not yet reached the subendothelial space. Cells also change appearance near the subendothelium (orcein stain, semi-thin section).

59. Aorta from 12-day-old chick embryo. Elongated smooth muscle cells (SC) form a coherent layer in the media. The oval nuclei comprise one or two nucleoli, and organelles are continuous with the nucleus. Elongated muscle cells are also seen immediately below the endothelium (semi-thin section, toluidine blue stain).

60. Aorta from 17-day-old chick embryo. Elastic clumps (EA) and fibres have multiplied considerably and occur up to the subendothelial extracellular space (semi-thin section, orcein stain).

61. Abdominal aorta of newly hatched chick. A fully developed meshwork of elastic lamellae is already present between the smooth muscle cell layers. An elastic lamella (IEL), interrupted by gaps (arrow) lies immediately below the endothelium (semi-thin section).

62. Durcupan-embedded semi-thin section of abdominal aorta from newly hatched chick, after digestion with elastase. The cellular structures are preserved, but the orcein-positive elastic fibres (DE) have completely disappeared from the spaces between medial smooth muscle cells (SC) (elastase digestion, orcein stain).

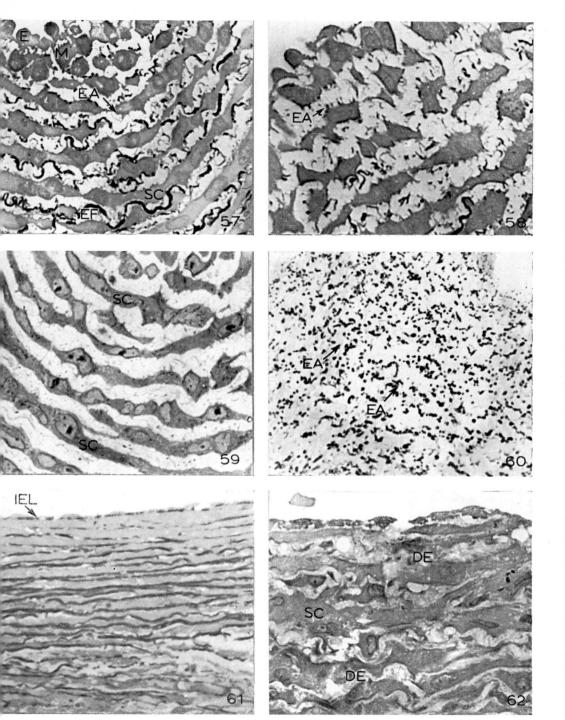

PLATE XV

63. Electron micrograph of thoracic aorta from 6-day-old chick embryo. Only a small amount of PTA-negative amorphous substance is present in the extracellular space. E = endothelial cell; M = mesenchymal cell (section counterstained with PTA).

64. Aorta from 8-day-old chick embryo. Small electron-dense aggregations lie below the endothelial cells and a similar structure is seen between two smooth muscle cells (SC). EA = elastic aggregations (section counterstained with PTA).

65. Aorta from 9-day-old chick embryo. At a high magnification, elastic granules (GR) and elastic microfibrils (MI) are seen in the extracellular space. The basement membrane (BM) of the smooth muscle cell shows a similar structure (section counterstained with PTA).

66. Aorta from 9-day-old chick embryo. PTA-positive elastic clumps (EA) are surrounded by elastic granules (GR) and elastic microfibrils (MI) pass into the clumps (section counterstained with PTA).

67. Elastic clumps in the process of fusion to fibres. Note system of irregularly ordered microfibrils (MI) in the extracellular space (section counterstained with PTA).

68. Aggregation of elastic elements in the process of fibre formation. Larger clumps gradually lose affinity to PTA. The large clump or fibre portion (EF) shown in the Figure binds PTA weakly at the core, but strongly at the marginal parts; accordingly, electron density is low at the centre, but still high at the margins. Note close association of collagenous fibres (C) with the elastic fibril.

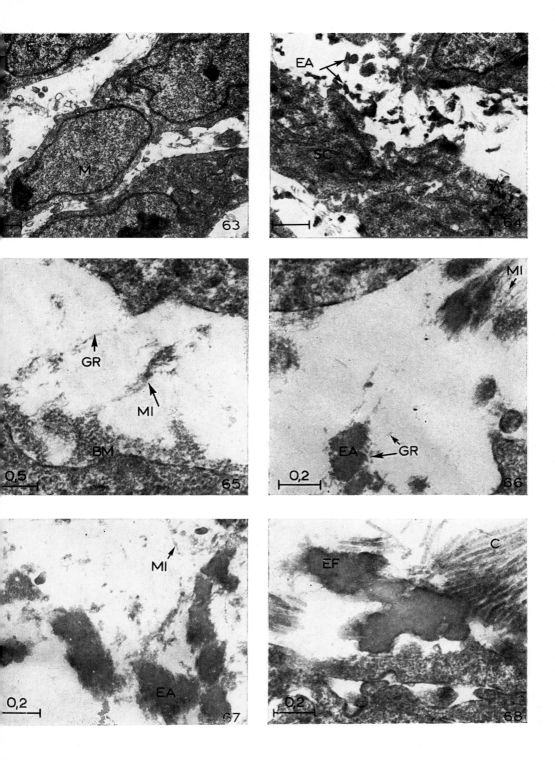

PLATE XVI

69. Aorta from 10-day-old embryo. An oval mesenchymal cell (M), equipped with processes, lies below the endothelial cell row (E); cells of the next row (SC) are longer and contain myofilaments, like smooth muscle cells.

70. Subendothelial mesenchymal cell (M) at a higher magnification. Cytoplasmic processes extend from the cell surface, the organelles are irregularly ordered and ergastoplasm and mitochondria are abundant.

71. Subendothelial mesenchymal cell. Apart from endoplasmic reticulum and mito-chondria, it contains many free ribosomes and vesicles of lipid density (LD).

72. Aorta from 12-day-old chick embryo. Below the endothelial cell row (E) linked by regular intercellular junctions lie elongated smooth muscle cells (SC), associated with a basement membrane (BM). Note myofilaments (MF) in the hyaloplasm and attachment bodies (AB) on cell surface. An elastic clump (EA) is present extra-cellularly.

73. Structure of smooth muscle cell (SC) at a higher magnification. A basement membrane (BM) surrounds the cell and the organelles are arranged perinuclearly; bundles of myofilaments (MF) lie parallel to the cell surface.

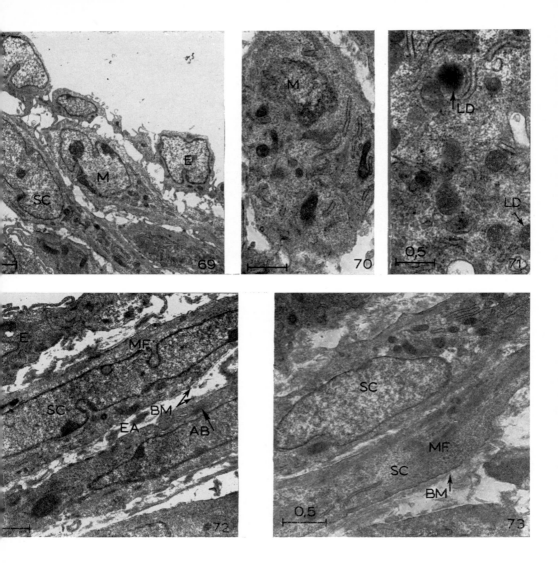

PLATE XVII

74. Electron micrograph of an elastic fibre (EF) with a low affinity to PTA. C = collagenous fibre.

75. Same after treatment of ultra-thin section with elastase. Marginal parts of fibre are preserved and bound PTA renders them electron dense; core rendered electron lucent by elastase action, but a continuous less mature portion of fibre resisted elastase. Microfibrillar structure (MI) at margin of fibre and surrounding small elastic clumps (EA) and granules (GR) are also preserved.

76. Ultra-thin section of aorta from 12-day-old chick embryo after direct exposure to elastase action. Elastic clumps seen in cross-section have electron-lucent cores owing to enzyme action, but elastic microfibrils (MI) at margins of clumps and in extracellular space are preserved, having resisted elastase. DE = digested elastic clump.

77. Intracellular membrane-coated vesicles (V) are similarly affected by elastase, as extracellular clumps (DE). MI = elastic microfibril.

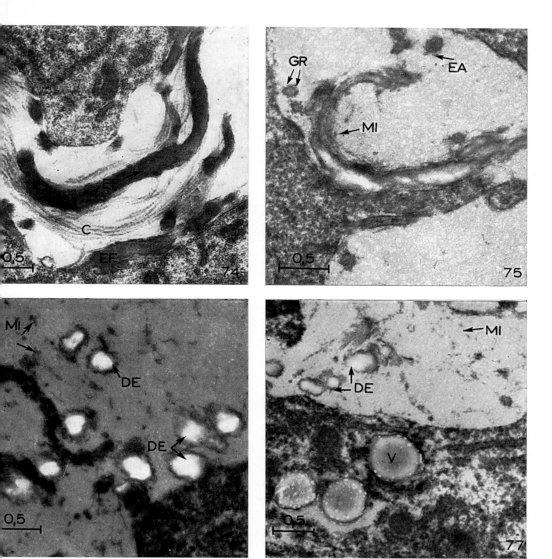

PLATE XVIII

78. Mature elastic fibres (EF) from aorta of 14-day chick embryo. PTA-negative cores are framed by narrow dark zones signifying a marginal PTA-positivity. Collagen fibres (C) and microfibrils (MI) lie in the extracellular space. EA = elastic clump; SC = smooth muscle; C = collagenous fibre.

79. Ultra-thin section after digestion with elastase. The elastic fibre (DE) between the smooth muscle cells (SC) became digested, thus appearing as an electron-lucent area, but marginal PTA-positivity is clearly visible. Other structures, such as collagenous fibres, microfibrils, cell components and immature PTA-positive elastic aggregations resisted the action of elastase.

80. Thoracic aorta of newly hatched chick. Mature undulating elastic lamella (EL) is PTA-negative, but the electron-dense, PTA-positive margins are clearly visible. SC = smooth muscle cell.

81. Ultra-thin section of aorta from newly hatched chick after digestion with elastase. The undulating elastic lamella became digested *in toto*, appearing as an electron-lucent area (DE), but all other extracellular structures, such as collagenous fibre (C), microfibrils and cell structures are preserved. SC = smooth muscle cell (section counterstained with PTA).

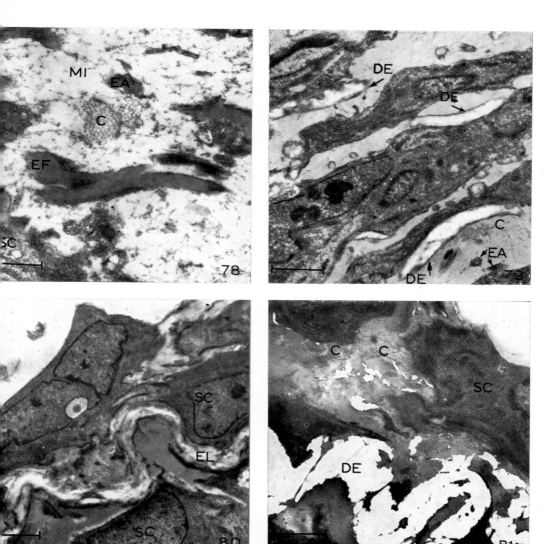

PLATE XIX

82. Aorta from 6-day chick embryo after fixation in ruthenium red-containing glutaraldehyde and osmium tetroxide. Only a small amount of ruthenium red-positive (RR)
substance is present extracellularly, in the third and fourth layers. E = endothelial
cell.

83. Extracellular space of aorta from 8-day-old chick embryo; it is filled by many
ruthenium red-positive granules or clumps. A dividing endothelial cell (E) at top is
coated by a ruthenium red-positive (RR) substance over the luminal surface.

84. Aorta from 12-day-old chick embryo after counterstaining with ruthenium red.
The endothelial cells are coated by a ruthenium red-positive substance. Fewer
ruthenium red-positive granules and clumps are seen in the extracellular space than
at 8 days: part of the extracellular space is filled by electron-lucent elastic clumps
(EA) and fibre (EF), with ruthenium red-positive bodies along their marginal parts.

85. Aorta from newly hatched chick. The extracellular space has diminished and
cells lie closer to one another than in early prenatal life. Almost the entire extracellular space is filled by an elastic fibre or lamella, with ruthenium red-positive
particles appearing inside and at the margins. EF = elastic fibre.

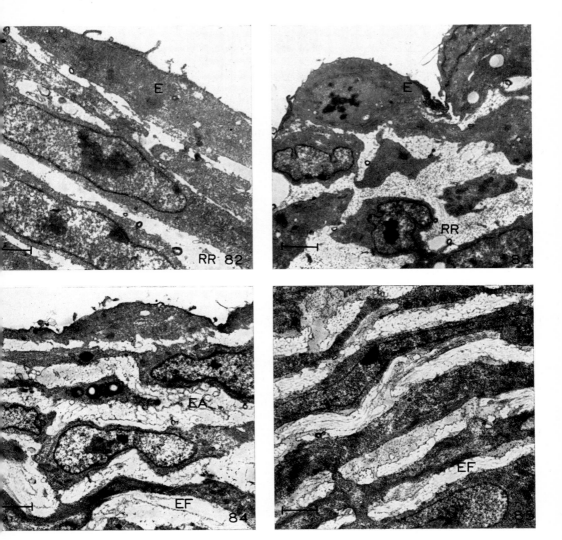

PLATE XX

86. Same at a higher magnification. Ruthenium red-positive spheres lie along the marginal parts of elastic clumps (EA); particles, fibrils (threads) and a meshwork of delicate filaments (EF) lie in the extracellular space.

87. Magnified portion of elastic fibre (EF); a ruthenium red-positive meshwork becomes visible inside the fibre after treatment with the stain. Ruthenium red-positive spheres (SP) and threads (TH) are seen at the surface of the fibre, forming a meshwork in the extracellular space.

88. Aorta of 14-day-old chick embryo after counterstaining with ruthenium red. Extracellular elastic aggregations (EA) enclose ruthenium red-positive mucopolysaccharide structures. TH = threads; SP = spheres.

89. Ultra-thin section from *88* after digestion with elastase. The enzyme has digested part of the elastic fibre, but it has not affected the internal ruthenium red-positive structures, nor the electron-dense marginal zone. The extracellular ruthenium red-positive structures and collagenous fibres (C) also appear to be intact.

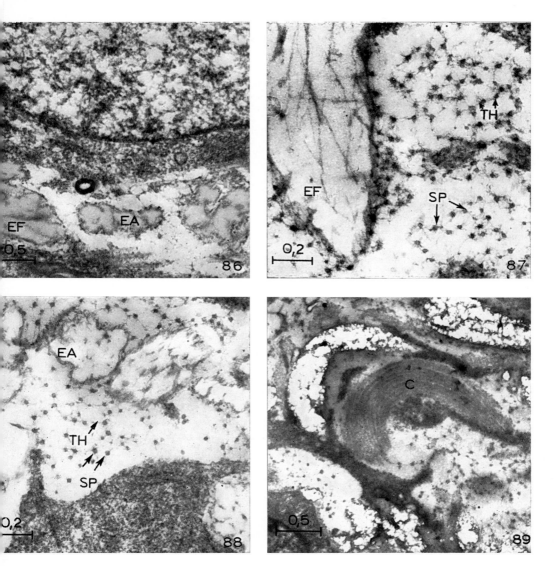

PLATE XXI

90. Smooth muscle cells of the proliferation have a well-developed Golgi apparatus (G).
91. Cisternae of the endoplasmic reticulum (ER) of muscle cells are widened and contain a granular substance of medium electron density. PTA stain.
92. The mitochondria (M) of smooth muscle cells have a dense matrix. The basement membrane is 300–400 Å wide (arrow).
93. The basement membrane of smooth muscle cells (SC) is composed of granules and filaments (arrow) averaging 80 Å in diameter. C = collagen.

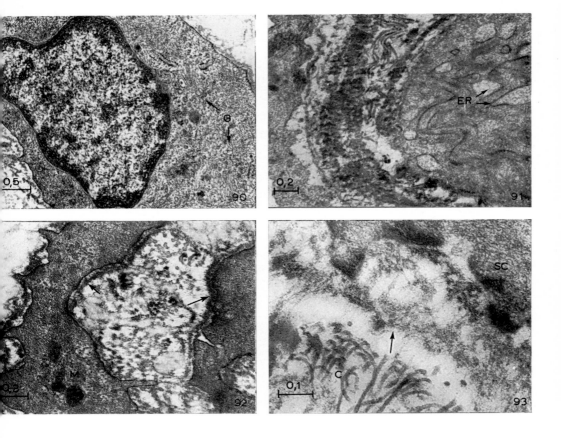

PLATE XXII

94. Tangential section of smooth muscle cell-associated basement membrane. The granular-filamentous structure of the basement membrane and its connection with the intercellular ground substance are clearly visible.

95–99. Smooth muscle cells (SC) of the proliferation associated with a multilayered, partly detached basement membrane; in places islet-like fragments of newly formed immature basement membrane accompany the cells (arrow).

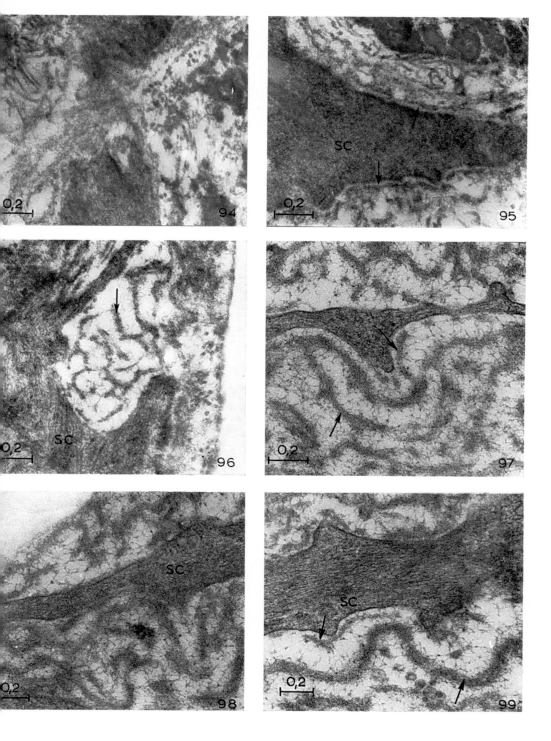

PLATE XXIII

100–102. 50-day IP. Newly formed elastic fibres (EF) and smooth muscle cells (SC) lie below the endothelial cell layer (E).

103. 50-day IP. The smooth muscle cells associate with a 300 Å thick basement membrane and many pinocytotic vesicles and attachment bodies (AB) lie along the cytoplasmic membranes.

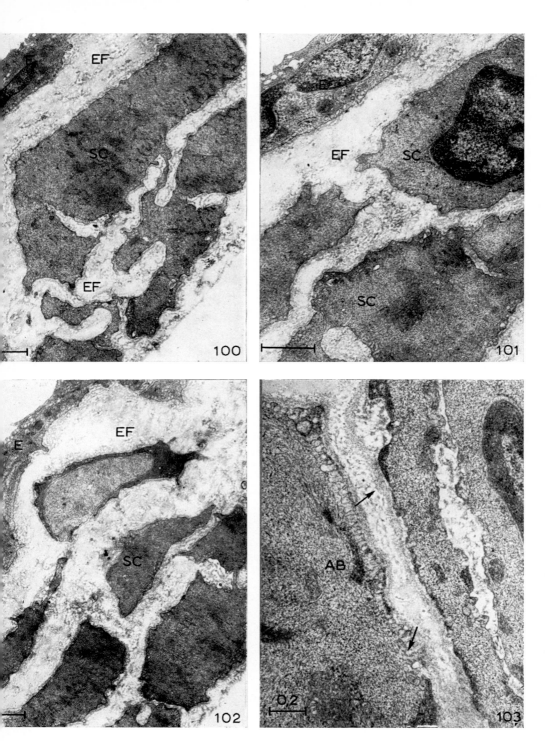

PLATE XXIV

104. 50-day IP. Newly formed elastic elements (EF) are seen extracellularly and the basement membrane shows a granular-filamentous structure. E = endothelium; SC = smooth muscle cell.

105. 95-day IP. Myelin figures and simple lipid membrane formations appear between the nearly mature elastic fibres (EF).

106. 95-day IP. Myelin figures (arrow) also appear in smooth muscle cells.

107. 95-day IP. Various circumscribed degenerative membrane formations and unsaturated lipid droplets lie in intercellular space. E = endothelium; SC = smooth muscle cell.

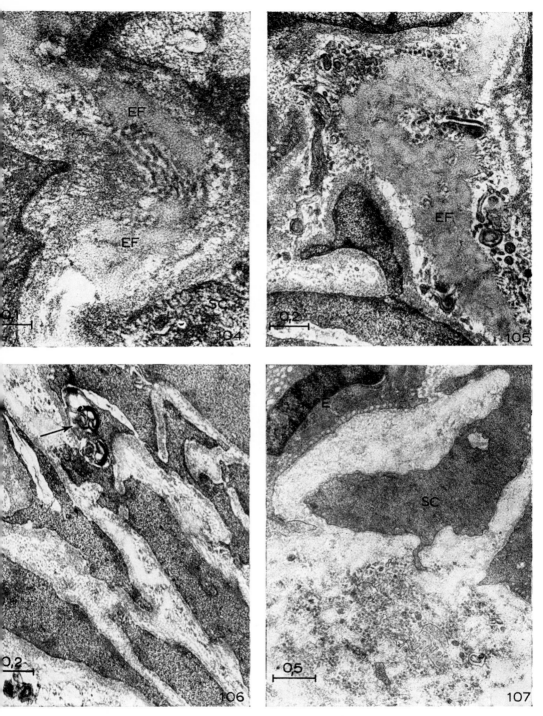

17

PLATE XXV

108–109. Porous vascular graft 4 years after implantation. Muscle cell components (SC) of the neo-intima associate with a 200 Å thick basement membrane (BM). The cells enclose many pinocytotic vesicles, myofilaments (MF) lie at the periphery of the hyaloplasm; the nucleus is centrally placed and organelles aggregate above it in a cap-like manner. N = nucleus.

110. Porous vascular graft 4 years after implantation. A well-developed Golgi apparatus, with a centrosome (arrow) and some widened cisternae of endoplasmic reticulum, lies centrally above the nucleus.

111. Less porous vascular graft 4 years after implantation. Fibroblast containing a widened rough endoplasmic reticulum (ER) filled by a granular substance.

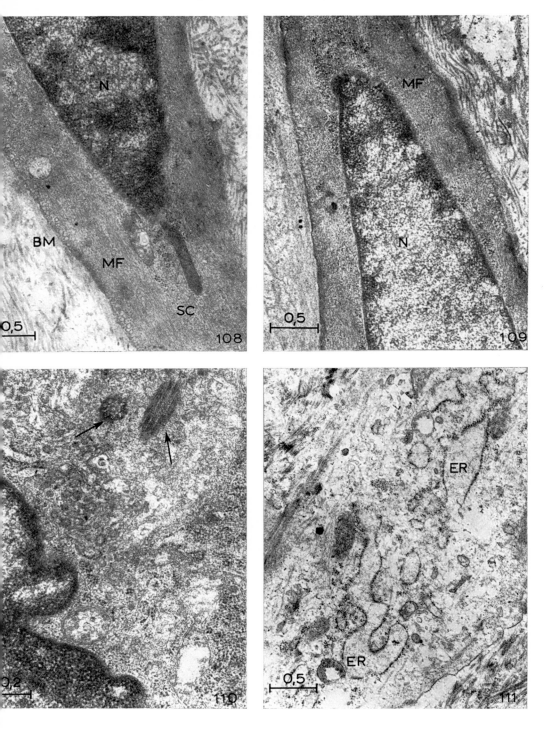

PLATE XXVI

112. Porous vascular graft 4 years after implantation. Smooth muscle cells (SC) equipped with cytoplasmic processes lie between many collagenous fibres (C). Myelin figures and degenerated membrane structures (arrow) lie at bottom left.

113. Less porous vascular graft 4 years after implantation. The thick collagenous tissue (C) lining the units of the prosthesis (PU) contains degenerated cell processes along with myelin figures and electron-dense particles (arrow).

114. Less porous vascular graft 4 years after implantation. The rounded chondrocyte carries small processes and contains lipofuscin pigment (LF), many glycogen granules (GL) and filamentary structures (CF). Apatite crystals (arrow) deposited on fibres lie in the lacunae between cell processes and intercellularly.

115. Less porous vascular graft 4 years after implantation. Part of an elastic fibre (EF), degenerated cell residues (arrow) and granular filamentary structures characteristic of the intercellular tissue of cartilage are seen in the Figure.

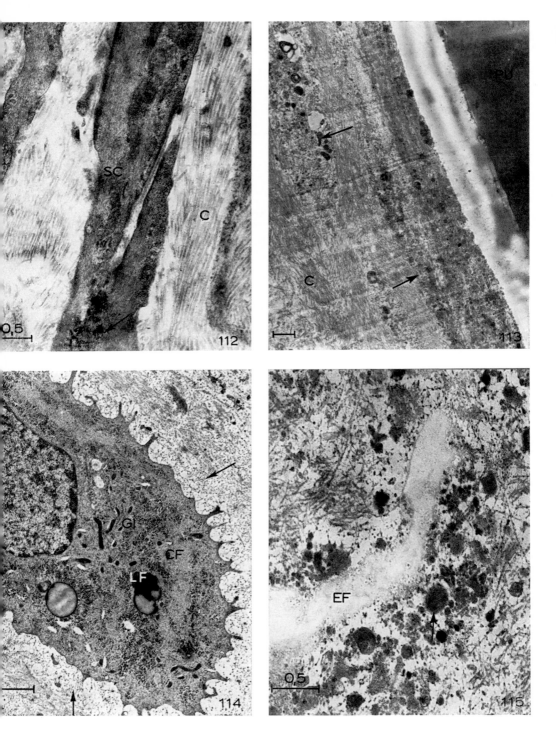

SC

C

0,5

112

PU

C

113

Gl

CF

LF

114

EF

0.5

115

PLATE XXVII

116. Aortic specimen from rat, kept hypertensive for 41 days. Cells with round nuclei (arrow) lie at the luminal side of the fibrinoid and the latter structure is no longer seen in the cell-populated area (Lőrincz–Gorácz's experimental hypertension model, M-stain).

117. Detail of aorta from rat kept hypertensive for 41 days. Note anisotropic clumps in the subendothelial fibrinoid (aniline reaction).

118. Rat aorta two days after induction of hypertension. A granular substance (GM) is accumulating in the widened subendothelial space. E = endothelial cell; IEL = internal elastic lamina; SC = smooth muscle cell.

119. 19-day hypertension. Fibrin (FI) bundles of a fibrillar structure and degenerative membrane formations (arrow) lie in the subendothelial space. E = endothelium; IEL = internal elastic lamina.

120. 2-day hypertension. A granular substance and polymerized fibrin (FI) lie in the subendothelial space. E = endothelial cell; IEL = internal elastic lamina.

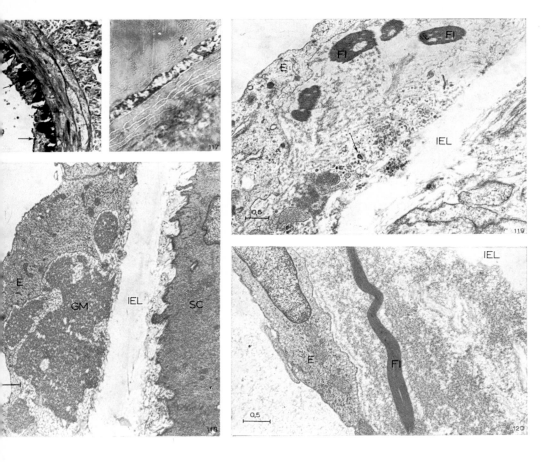

PLATE XXVIII

121. 41-day hypertension. Crystalline fibrin formations (CR) and a ground substance-like material (GM) have accumulated below the endothelium. E = endothelium; MP = macrophage.

122. 2-day hypertension. Processes of a lymphocyte (LY) and a macrophage (MP) are seen subendothelially (E = endothelium; IEL = internal elastic lamina.

123. 65-day hypertension. The multilayered IP is composed of smooth muscle cells (SC). In places the basement membrane appears stratified (arrow) and a ground substance-like granular material (GM) and newly formed elastic elements (EF) can be seen between the cells. E = endothelium; IEL = internal elastic lamina.

124. 65-day hypertension. Smooth muscle cell components (SC) of the IP have a bilayered or trilayered basement membrane (arrow). Elastic elements in different stages of maturation. (EF), a granular material (GM) and fibrin crystals (CR) lie in the subendothelial space. E = endothelium.

256

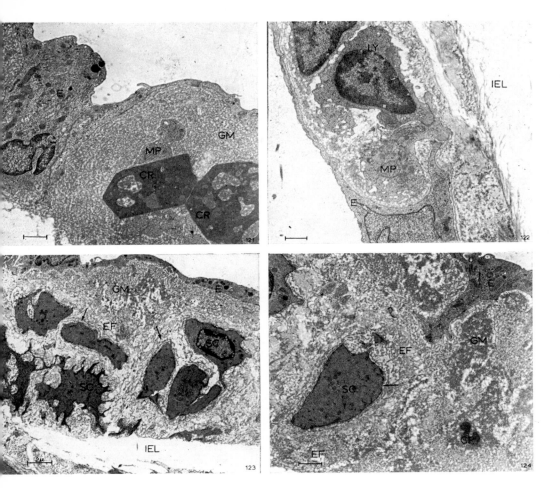

PLATE XXIX

125. Aorta after a 6-week atherogenic diet. A granular plasma material and chylo-micron droplets (arrow) lie in the aortic lumen (L). The endothelial cell (E) carries many pinocytotic vesicles on both surfaces and a ground substance-like material has accumulated below it EF = elastic fibre; N = nucleus.

126. Aorta after a 6-week atherogenic diet. Part of a macrophage (MP) is seen to attach to surface of endothelial cell (E). Double ring-like structures (arrow) lie below pinocytotic vesicles. The mitochondrial matrix (M) is dense and many RNA granules are scattered through the cytoplasm. L = lumen.

127. Aorta after a 6-week atherogenic diet. Endothelial cells (E) contain neutral lipid droplets (F). The widened subendothelial space is filled by a ground substance-like granular, filamentous material. L = lumen; IEL = internal elastic lamina.

128. Aorta after a 3-week atherogenic diet. Coalescent pinocytotic vesicles extend into depth of endothelial cell body. IEL = internal elastic lamina; L = lumen.

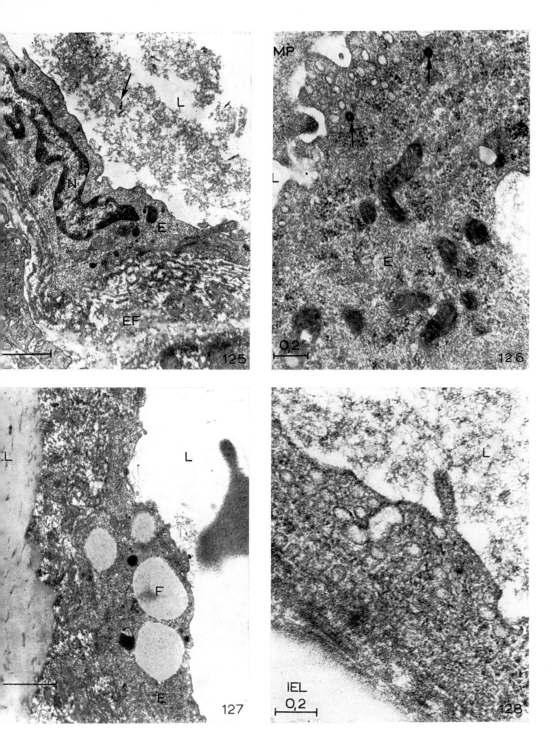

PLATE XXX

129. Aorta after a 3-week atherogenic diet. A lipid-laden macrophage (MP), processes of smooth muscle cells (SC) and a chylomicron droplet (arrow) can be seen in the widened space below the endothelium (E). IEL = internal elastic lamina.

130. Aorta after a 6-week atherogenic diet. The interendothelial junctions (double arrow) are patent and a chylomicron (simple arrow) lies subendothelially. The process of a smooth muscle cell (SC) extends into the stroma of the internal elastic lamina (IEL). E = endothelial cell.

131. Aorta after a 3-week atherogenic diet. The subendothelial space is widened only moderately and a few lipid membrane formations lie in it (arrow). L = lumen.

132. Aorta after a 9-week atherogenic diet. The wide subendothelial space is filled by lipid membranes between which lie released lipids and collagenous fibres. E = endothelium; IEL = internal elastic lamina.

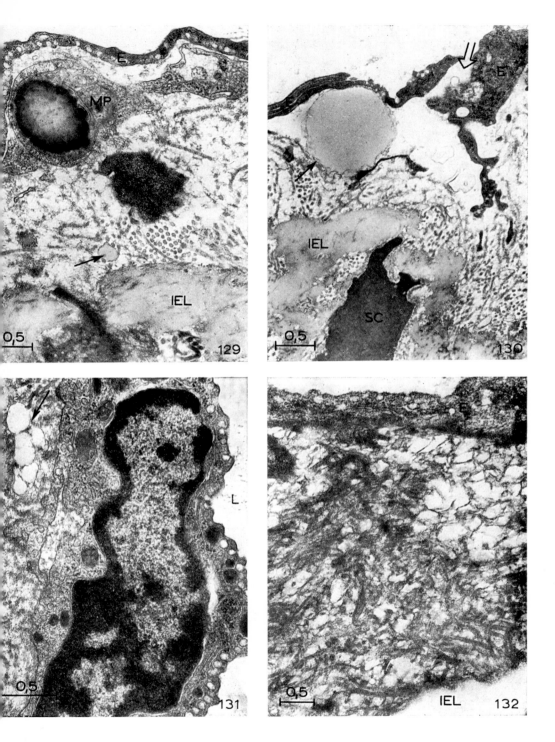

E

MP

IEL

0,5

129

E

IEL

SC

0,5

130

L

0,5

131

IEL

0,5

132

PLATE XXXI

133. Aorta after a 6-week atherogenic diet. The smooth muscle cells (SC) lie immediately below the internal elastic lamina (IEL). E = endothelium.

134. Aorta after a 6-week atherogenic diet. Processes of smooth muscle cells (SC) extend into the stomas of the internal elastic lamina (IEL). E = endothelium.

135. Aorta after a 9-week atherogenic diet. Newly formed elastic clumps (EF) lie below the endothelial cell (E).

136. Aorta after a 6-week atherogenic diet. Processes of smooth muscle cells (SC) extend into the widened subendothelial space. Electron-dense, ground substance-like elements in a fibrillar order, and a less dense granular substance fill the intercellular spaces. E = endothelial cell.

137. (*a*) Aorta after a 9-week atherogenic diet. IP composed of several rows of foam cells and smooth muscle cells. (*b*) Aorta after a 9-week atherogenic diet. The endothelial cell (E) contains many neutral lipid droplets and below it lie a lipophage (LI) and a smooth muscle cell process (SC), comprising two lipid droplets. Newly formed elastic elements are seen above the process. IEL = internal elastic lamina.

138. Aorta after a 9-week atherogenic diet. The endothelial cell contains lipid droplets and under it are seen a portion of a smooth muscle cell (SC) and elastic clumps (EF) in different stages of maturation, with a corresponding variation of electron density.

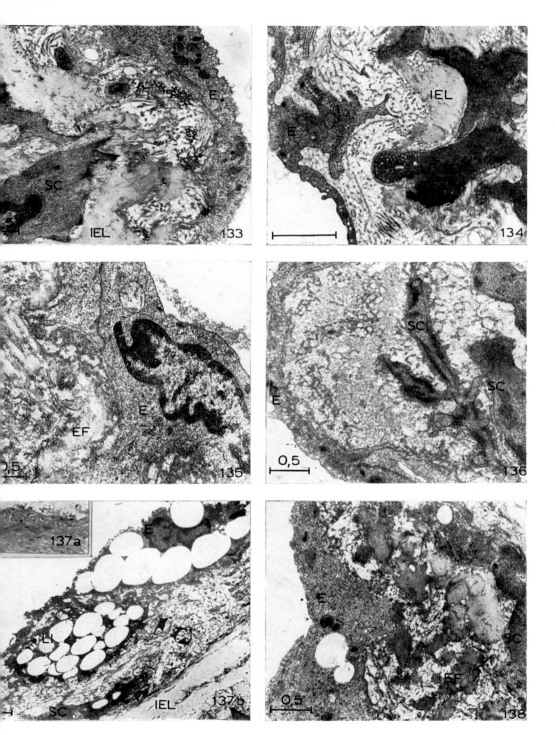

PLATE XXXII

139. Aorta after a 6-week atherogenic diet. A lipophage (LI) attaches to the surface of endothelial cells (E) and extends a process (arrow) between two cells. IEL = internal elastic lamina.

140. Aorta after a 6-week atherogenic diet. A lipophage (LI) lies in the subendothelial space. The process of a foam cell (arrow) extends into the patent intercellular junction. E = endothelial cell; IEL = internal elastic lamina.

141. Aorta after a 6-week atherogenic diet. A macrophage, equipped with processes (LI) contains lipid droplets of varying electron density; the interendothelial junctions (E) are preserved. IEL = internal elastic lamina.

142. Aorta after a 3-week atherogenic diet, from an animal treated with Ferrlecit 3 hours prior to termination. Iron particles, partly coated by membrane, lie within endothelial cell and lumen (L).

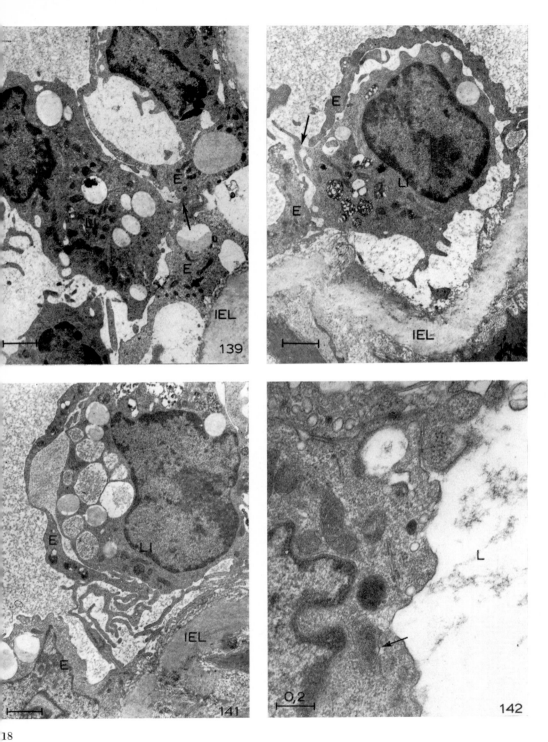

18

PLATE XXXIII

143. 9-week atherogenic diet. Lymph channels (arrow) have widened in the periarterial connective tissue of the abdominal aorta.

144. Abdominal aorta after a 9-week atherogenic diet. Cells of lymphatic vessel endothelium extend fixing processes (arrow) into adventitial interstitium and are connected by interdigitated processes. L = lumen; C = collagenous fibre.

145. Abdominal aorta after a 9-week atherogenic diet. The interendothelial junctions have opened (arrow). Collagenous fibres end directly at lymph endothelium. EF = elastic fibre; C = collagen; L = lumen.

146. Thoracic aorta after a 9-week atherogenic diet. The processes of endothelial cells overlap like a tiled roof and the collagenous fibres end at the basement membrane. L = lumen.

147. Abdominal aorta after a 9-week atherogenic diet. The lumen of the lymph channel passing between adventitial collagenous fibres appears collapsed at top, but widened at bottom. Many pinocytotic vesicles (arrow) are attached to both outer and inner surface of the cytoplasmic membrane. L = lumen.

148. Abdominal aorta after a 9-week atherogenic diet. A macrophage filled by neutral lipid droplets lies nearby the distended lymph channel. F = lipid droplet; N = nucleus.

149. Abdominal aorta after a 9-week atherogenic diet. Two gaps (arrow) are seen between processes of a lymph capillary endothelial cell. C = collagenous fibre; L = lumen; EF = elastic fibre.

150. Abdominal aorta after a 9-week atherogenic diet. The endothelial cell of the distended lymph capillary contains a neutral lipid droplet surrounded by a narrow cytoplasmic margin. The endothelial cells extend fixing processes (arrow) into the interstitium. F = lipid droplet.

151. Abdominal aorta after a 9-week atherogenic diet. The lymphatic endothelial cell encloses a lipid droplet, surrounded by a narrow cytoplasmic margin. The collagenous fibres attach to microfilaments associated with the endothelium. L = lumen.

152–153. Abdominal aorta after a 9-week atherogenic diet. A granular substance of medium electron density fills the lumina of the lymph channels. The endothelial cells contain neutral lipid droplets and the arrow points to a myelin figure. F = lipid droplet; L = lumen.

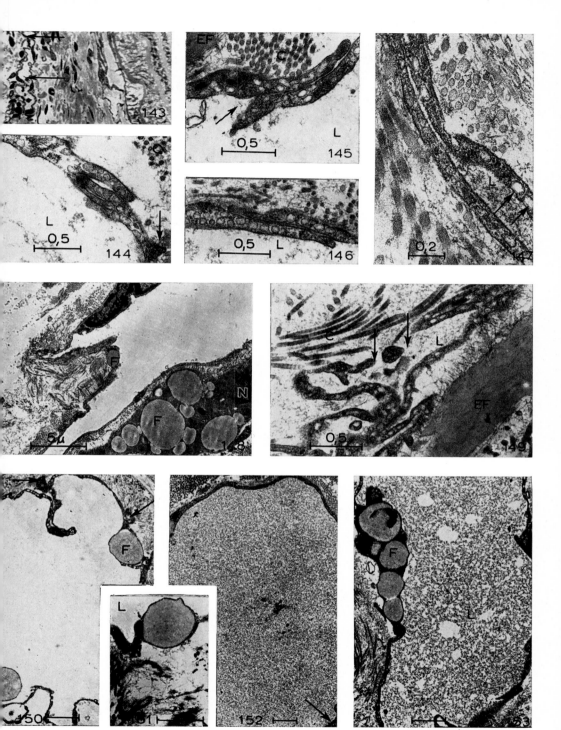

PLATE XXXIV

154–155. Comparison of coronary artery from a control rat (*154*) with that from a rat kept hypertensive for 3 days (*155*). Note hypertrophy of both endothelial (E) and smooth muscle cells (SC) and abundant organelles in *155*. Both preparations originate from the right ventricle. IEL = internal elastic lamina: L = lumen; HM = heart muscle; BE = basement membrane; FC = fibrocyte (Lőrincz–Gorácz experimental hypertension model).

156–157. Accumulation of a floccular substance of basement membrane density below endothelial junction (E) in mesenteric artery, after 40 days of hypertension (Lőrincz–Gorácz model). IEL = internal elastic lamina; BE = basement membrane; SC = smooth muscle; L = lumen.

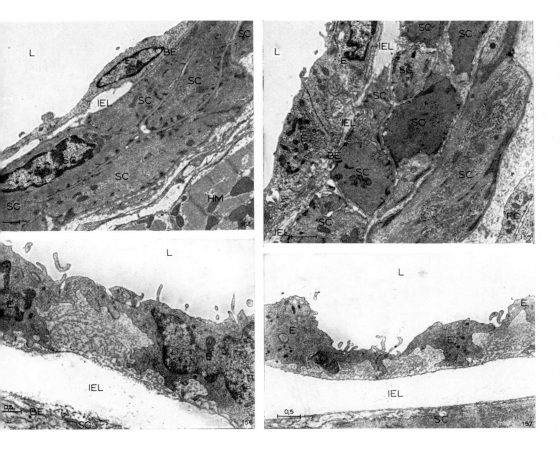

PLATE XXXV

158. Wall of small coronary artery after 7 days of hypertension. The widened subendo-thelial space between endothelium (E) and internal elastic lamina (IEL) contains loose bundles of fibrin (FI) (longitudinal and cross-sections), surrounded by a delicate granular, in places filamentous, substance (Lőrincz–Gorácz experimental hypertension model). L = lumen; SC = smooth muscle.

159. Another mural portion of small coronary from *158.* Fibrin bundles with defined contours lie in the subendothelial space in a granular substance of plasma density. The latter substance also surrounds degenerated medial smooth muscle cells (SC) below the internal elastic lamina (IEL), and forms a broad zone under the degenerated media. Loose fibrin bundles (FI) appear everywhere in the plasma-like material. *Inset*: magnified fibrin bundle from media. Note transverse striation of 165 Å periodi-city (Lőrincz–Gorácz model; 7-day hypertension). E = endothelial cell; L = lumen.

160. Mesenteric artery after 19 days of hypertension. Many crystalline fibrin (CR) bundles (FI) lie in the subendothelial space surrounded by a sparse material of plasma density (Rojo-Ortega–Gonest experimental hypertension model). L = lumen; E = endothelial layer; IEL = internal elastic lamina; SC = smooth muscle cell.

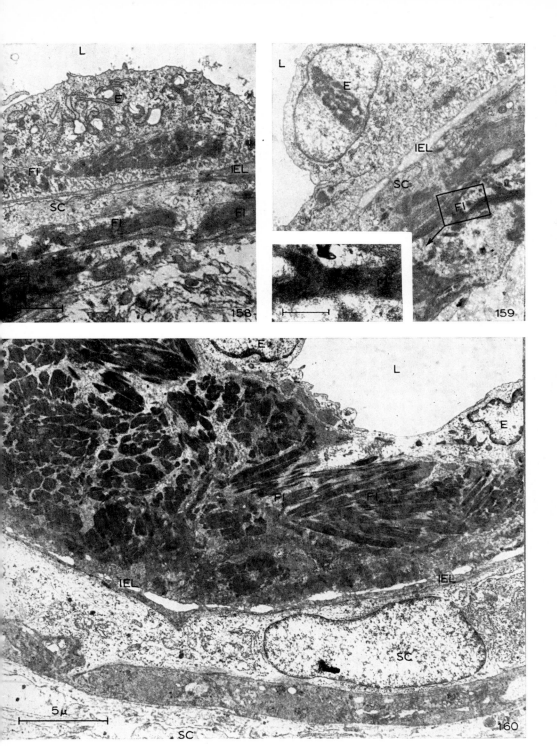

PLATE XXXVI

161. Arterial wall after 42 days of hypertension. Dense, sharply demarcated, fibrin bundles (FI) show a transverse striation of 207 Å periodicity, and a linear structure of 103 Å periodicity, enclosing a 60° angle with the former. The crystal-like hexagonal body with stripes of 103 Å periodicity (CR) presumably corresponds with the cross-section of a fibre (Lőrincz–Gorácz experimental hypertension model).

162. Arterial wall after 42 days of hypertension. Sharply demarcated fibrin bundles (FI) with a transverse striation of 218 Å periodicity. A crystalline (CR) fibrin formation (periodicity: 92 Å) lies adjacent (Lőrincz–Gorácz experimental hypertension model).

163. Arterial wall after 42 days of hypertension. Fibrin crystals (CR) with a broad periodicity and a clearly visible basal structure lie in a loose, granular, medium electron-dense substance in the subendothelial space. The hexagonal structure of the bundles is visible in places. *Inset*: part of a fibrin crystal showing a periodicity of 95 Å (Lőrincz–Gorácz experimental hypertension model). L = lumen; IEL = internal elastic lamina.

164. Wall of mesenteric artery after 42 days of hypertension. Exlusively crystal-like fibrin formations (CR) of a broad periodicity are seen in the subendothelial space in a granular material of plasma density. The cytoplasm of endothelial cells (E) shows varying degrees of electron density and a lymphocyte (LY) adheres to the luminal surface. Medial smooth muscle cells (SC) show degenerative changes (Lőrincz–Gorácz experimental hypertension model). IEL = internal elastic lamina; L = lumen.

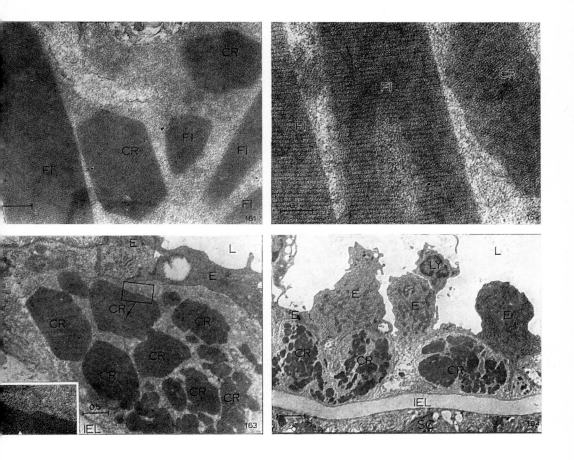

PLATE XXXVII

165. Coronary artery after 18 days of hypertension. Medial smooth muscle cells (SC) are surrounded by abundant ground substance, in the midst of which lie many bundles (FI) and crystalline formations (CR) of fibrin (Rojo-Ortega–Gonest experimental hypertension model). L = lumen; IEL = internal elastic lamina; (FC) oedematous muscle cell necrosis; E = endothelial cells.

166. Small pancreatic artery of rat kept hypertensive for 19 days. Oedematous necrobiosis (arrow). Cells are surrounded by an abundant plasma-like substance. Fibrocytes arrowfibroblasts (FB) and plasma cells (PL) surround the vessel wall (Rojo-Ortega–Gonest experimental hypertension model). IEL = internal elastic lamina; L = lumen; E = endothelial cell.

167. Necrobiotic muscle cells (SC) from mesenteric artery of rat kept hypertensive for 8 days. Cell at top contains osmiophilic granules, in places blackberry-like, originating from organelle degeneration; cell at bottom contains degenerated mitochondria and residual bodies more or less laden with lipids (to different degrees) (UL). Cells have lost basement membrane in whole or in part and a material of plasma density surrounds them (Lőrincz–Gorácz experimental hypertension model).

168. Smooth muscle cells (SC) from mesenteric artery of rat kept hypertensive for 8 days. The myofilaments are slightly aggregated, the mitochondria appear damaged. Muscle cell in centre shows state of oedematous necrobiosis: the smooth endoplasmic reticulum is increased, the myofilamentary structure has lost definition and the cytoplasmic process has lost its basement membrane. The interstitial space contains collagenous fibres (C) and small osmiophilic granules, presumably originating from muscle degeneration (Lőrincz–Gorácz experimental hypertension model).

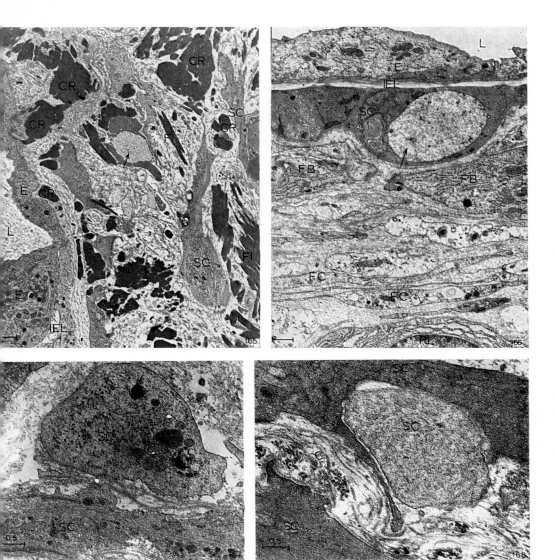

PLATE XXXVIII

169. Coronary artery from right ventricle of a rat kept hypertensive for 3 days. The adventitial fibroblasts (FB) are swollen and their rough endoplasmic reticulum system is hypertrophic. HM = heart muscle; C = collagen; SC = smooth muscle (Lőrincz–Gorácz experimental hypertension model).

170. Dense lead precipitate signifies alkaline phosphatase activity in pinocytotic vesicles (arrow) of adventitial fibroblast (FB) and peripheral medial muscle cells (SC). Control specimen (Majahara's alkaline phosphatase reaction, modified). C = collagen.

171. Birefringence of subendothelial fibrinoid persists after treatment with Canada balsam (*a*), phenol (*b*) and aniline (*c*), but it disappears after digestion (*d*) with 0.3% trypsin for 60 minutes (Carnoy's fixative). (*e*) Strong birefringence of subendothelial fibrinoid after treatment with noradrenalin (reverse compensation). (*f*) Necrotic smooth muscle cells of the media show an increased birefringence. (*g*) Vacuolized and necrotic smooth muscle cells can be visualized in the vessel wall by repeated treatment with Bupatol (M-stain).

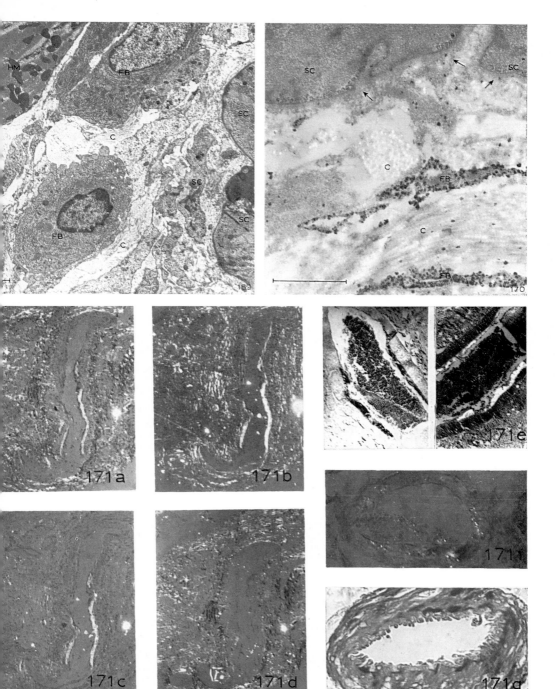

PLATE XXXIX

172. Endothelial cells (E) differ in density and a loose floccular substance lies below them in the subendothelial space. Dark endothelial cell shows a vigorous pinocytotic activity; interendothelial junctions are stretched (mesenteric small artery after 40-day hypertension; Lőrincz–Gorácz hypertension model). IEL = internal elastic lamina; L = lumen.

173. Mesenteric small artery after 40-day hypertension. Overlapping processes of endothelial cells (E) show different pinocytotic activity and density. A floccular material lies subendothelially (Lőrincz–Gorácz experimental hypertension model). L = lumen; IEL = internal elastic lamina.

174. Mesenteric small artery after 40-day hypertension. Part of an osmiophilic necrotic endothelial cell is seen between two endothelial cells (E) of normal density. Multiple layers of basement membrane (BM) lie between processes of medial smooth muscle cells (SC) below the internal elastic lamina (IEL); (Lőrincz–Gorácz experimental hypertension model). L = lumen.

175. Mesenteric small artery after 28-day hypertension. A leukocyte (LE) lies below the junction between hypertrophic endothelial cells (E) and a floccular material is seen above the internal elastic lamina (IEL). Endothelial cells enclose unsaturated lipid droplets (UL). Medial smooth muscle cells (SC) are herniated (arrow) (Lőrincz–Gorácz experimental hypertension model + long-term treatment with BTF). L = umen; BM = basement membrane.

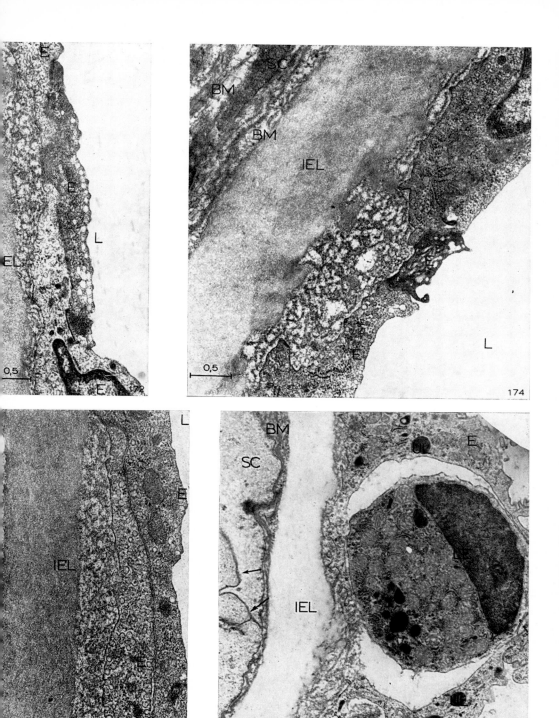

PLATE XL

176. Mesenteric small artery after 40-day hypertension. A floccular material of basement membrane-density has accumulated subendothelially, especially below the
junctions, above the non-uniform internal elastic lamina (IEL). Basement membrane
(BM) layers, comprising fragments of necrotic smooth muscle cells (SC) (arrow), lie
between IEL and media (Lőrincz–Gorácz experimental hypertension model). E =
endothelium; L = lumen.

177. Mesenteric small artery after 40-day hypertension. A floccular material, comprising cell debris, lies below the pale endothelial cell (E). Necrobiotic endothelial cell (E)
at top has a dark cytoplasm (Lőrincz–Gorácz experimental hypertension model).
IEL = internal elastic lamina; SC = smooth muscle cell; L = lumen.

178. Mesenteric small artery after 40-day hypertension and long-term BTF-treatment.
Hypertrophic endothelial cells enclose a multiplied endoplasmic reticulum, degenerated
mitochondria and occasional lipid droplets (UL). A floccular material arranged in
basement membrane-like rows lies in subendothelial space. Medial muscle cells (SC) are
herniated (arrow). (JEM 6C electron micrograph). L = lumen; IEL = internal elastic
lamina.

179. Mesenteric small artery after 40-day hypertension and long-term BTF-treatment.
Detail of hypertrophic endothelial cell. The rough endoplasmic reticulum (ER) has
increased around the nucleus and there are free ribosomes and lipid-laden residual
bodies (UL). A floccular material lies subendothelially (Lőrincz–Gorácz experimental
hypertension model). CC = centrosome.

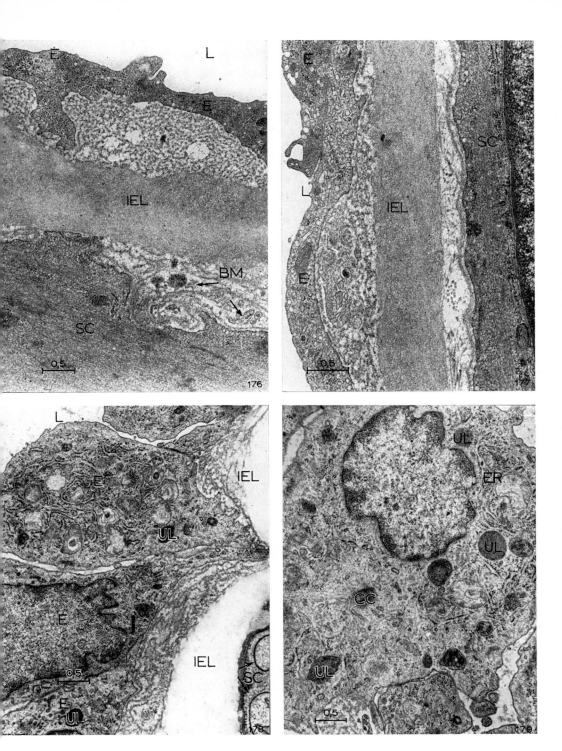

19

PLATE XLI

180. Subserosa artery after 9-day hypertension. A floccular material of plasma density surrounds two leukocytes (LE) in the subendothelial space; one leukocyte is in the process of phagocytizing fibrin (FI). *Inset*: Fibrin bundle from leukocyte, showing the characteristic axial periodicity of 190 Å (Lőrincz–Gorácz experimental hypertension model). E = endothelium; L = lumen.

181. Mesenteric small artery after 32-day hypertension. The widened subendothelial space below the hypertrophic endothelial cell layer (E) contains a partly differentiated smooth muscle cell (SC) and an undifferentiated pale cell. A floccular or in places homogeneous material of medium density lies between IEL and cellular elements and comprises in addition to osmiophilic clumps a few necrotic smooth muscle cell residues (arrow) (Lőrincz–Gorácz experimental hypertension model). BM = basement membrane-like substance. IEL = internal elastic lamina; L = lumen.

182. Mesenteric small artery after 32-day hypertension. Cytoplasmic organelles of endothelial cells aggregate along the luminal side. The differentiated smooth muscle cell (SC) lying below the endothelium (E) shows signs of hypertrophy. Cloudy floccular plasma lying at bottom of subendothelial space is seen to penetrate the media through the fenestrae of the internal elastic lamina (IEL). Osmiophilic clumps are seen in the plasma. L = lumen.

183. Circumscribed intimal thickening, consisting of mature smooth muscle cells (SC) with cytoplasmic processes and varying in electron density; abundant basement membrane (BM) surrounds the cells. (Mesenteric small artery after 42-day hypertension; Lőrincz–Gorácz model + chronic bleeding). E = endothelium; L = lumen.

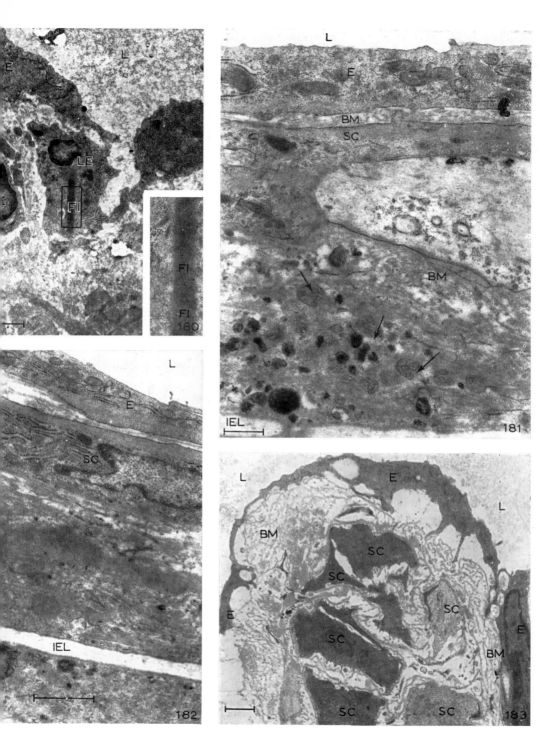

PLATE XLII

184. Mesenteric artery after 42-day hypertension. Part of a preserved smooth muscle cell (SC) is seen at bottom, showing a regular myofilamentous structure and a vigorous pinocytotic activity. At top right, part of an oedematous, necrotic smooth muscle cell (SC) is seen with a hypertrophic Golgi apparatus and smooth endoplasmic reticulum. The myofilaments have disintegrated into granules and the cell membrane shows no pinocytotic activity. A shrunken, osmiophilic muscle cell (SC) lies at bottom right (Lőrincz–Gorácz experimental hypertension model).

185. Mesenteric small artery after 42-day hypertension. Crystal-like masses of fibrin with a broad periodicity (CR) have aggregated in the subendothelial space. The hypertrophic endothelial cell (E) shows a vigorous pinocytotic activity; the contents of the pinocytotic vesicles are highly electron-dense (arrow) (Lőrincz–Gorácz experimental hypertension model). L = lumen; IEL = internal elastic lamina; SC = smooth muscle cell.

186. Mesenteric small artery after 42-day hypertension. The subendothelial fibrinoid is in the process of homogenization and the pale endothelial cells (E) above it contain bundles of cytofilaments (CF), most of which lie close to the cell bottom. The pinocytotic vesicles and the rough endoplasmic reticulum contain electron-dense material. A highly electron-dense, granular-filamentous material also lies between cells and fibrinoid (Lőrincz–Gorácz experimental hypertension model).

187. Mesenteric small artery after 42-day hypertension. Some endothelial cells (E) above the homogenizing fibrinoid are rich in ribosomes and organelles, and have a granular-filamentous (CF) cytoplasmic margin at bottom. The bottom surface of the cells shows a vigorous pinocytotic activity and the vesicles contain a dense material (arrow) (Lőrincz–Gorácz experimental hypertension model). L = lumen.

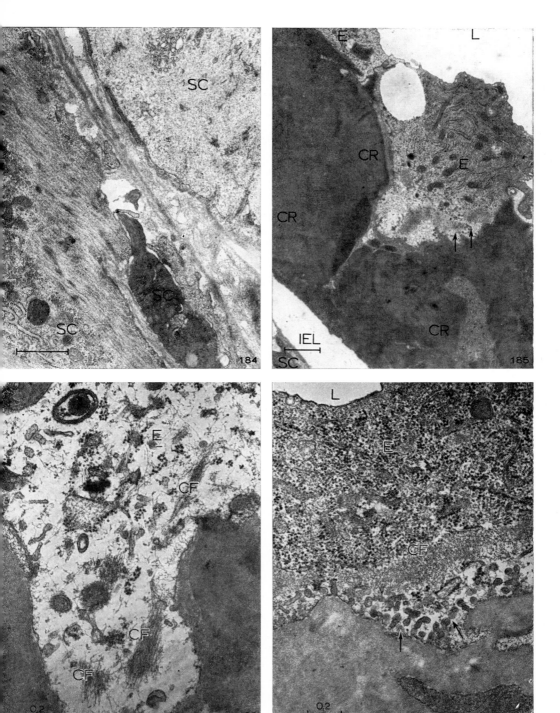

PLATE XLIII

188. Subserosa small artery after 42-day hypertension. A homogeneous, cloudy substance of medium electron density is seen below the thin endothelial cell layer (E), enclosing osmiophilic, in places lamellar, lipid inclusions. The substance has entered the media through the fenestrae of the IEL (Lőrincz–Gorácz experimental hypertension model). L = lumen.

189. Mesenteric small artery after 28-day hypertension and long-term BTF-treatment. Slightly hypertrophic smooth muscle cells (SC), showing herniation (arrow) are seen in the inner layer of the media (Lőrincz–Gorácz experimental hypertension model). IEL = internal elastic lamina.

190. Mesenteric small artery after 42-day hypertension. Distinctly hypertrophic smooth muscle cells (SC) are seen in the medial portion below the internal elastic lamina (IEL). Abundant basement membrane (BM) fills the intercellular space and a few myelin figures lie between the cells (Lőrincz–Gorácz experimental hypertension model). CR = crystalline fibrin.

191. Mesenteric small artery after 40-day hypertension. A necrotic cell, partly surrounded by basement membrane-like material (BM), lies between smooth muscle cells (SC) of the media. The cytoplasmic organelles and the myofilamentous structure of the necrotic cell are scarcely discernible and only fragments are left of its basement membrane (Lőrincz–Gorácz experimental hypertension model).

192. Hypertrophic smooth muscle cells (SC) with a widened ergastoplasm from media of mesenteric artery of rat kept hypertensive for 40 days (Lőrincz–Gorácz experimental hypertension model).

193. A hyaline-like material, containing lipid droplets and cell debris is seen in the subendothelial space and in the inner third of the media. The outer part of the media and the adventitia as well, are filled by a fibroblastic (FB) granulation tissue, also containing collagenous fibres (Lőrincz–Gorácz experimental hypertension model). IEL = internal elastic lamina; E = endothelium.

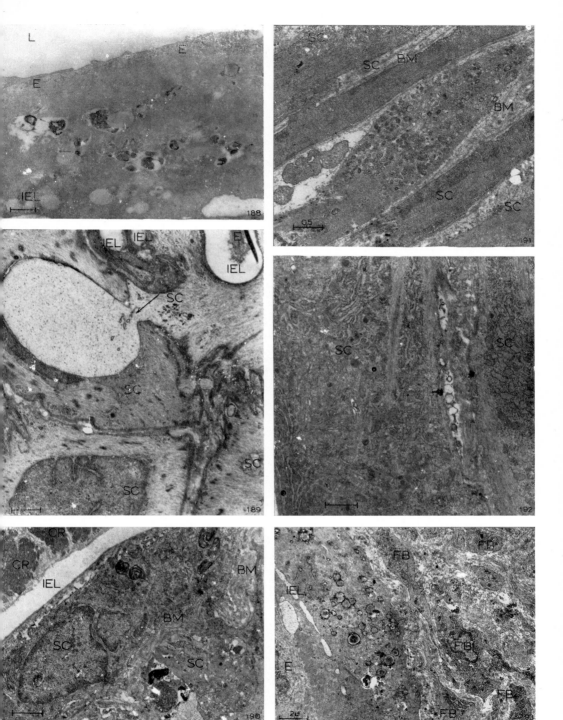

PLATE XLIV

194. Mesenteric artery after 40-day hypertension. Both endothelial (E) and smooth muscle cells (SC) contain lipofuscin-like (LF) osmiophilic residual bodies. The area below the endothelial junctions is filled by a floccular material of medium electron density, and an abundant basement membrane (BM) surrounds the smooth muscle cell, which shows signs of hypertrophy (Lőrincz–Gorácz experimental hypertension model). L = lumen; IEL = internal elastic lamina.

195. 7-day hypobaric hypoxia. The hypertrophic endothelial cell (E) compresses an unsaturated lipid droplet (UL) and shows a vigorous pinocytotic activity at the surface. A scarce substance of basement membrane density lies below the cell. The medial smooth muscle cell (SC) shows herniation (arrow). L = lumen; IEL = internal elastic lamina.

196. 50-day hypobaric hypoxia. Endothelial cells (E) extend processes from their surface and below the interendothelial junctions a substance of basement membrane density and occasionally stratified structure (BM) is seen. The process of an endothelial cell extends into the subendothelial space and an adjoining similar process, with pale cytoplasm, shows a vigorous pinocytotic activity. A floccular substance lies below these cells. Medial zones adjoining the internal elastic lamina (IEL) contain smooth muscle cell processes (SC) devoid of myofilamentous structure and basement membrane, and not showing a pinocytotic activity. Osmiophilic clumps originating from muscle degeneration are also present. L = lumen.

197. 7-day hypobaric hypoxia. A hypertrophic endothelial cell (E) encloses many osmiophilic, lipofuscin-like lipid inclusions (LF). Process formation and pinocytotic activity are seen at the surface. A slightly increased basement membrane lies below the cell. L = lumen; IEL = internal elastic lamina.

198. 50-day hypobaric hypoxia. Hypertrophic endothelial cell (E), carrying processes on the surface; Golgi apparatus and smooth endoplasmic reticulum inside the cell show a parallel lamellar structure. The basement membrane below the cell has slightly increased. The medial zone adjoining the internal elastic lamina (IEL) contains degenerated smooth muscle cell processes (SC), osmiophilic cell debris and many collagenous fibres (C). L = lumen.

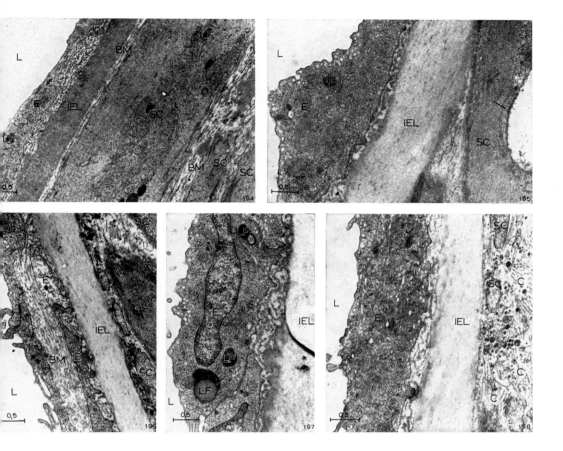

PLATE XLV

199. 7-day hypobaric hypoxia. Smooth muscle cell (SC) in media shows increased activity; Golgi apparatus and smooth endoplasmic reticulum have increased and the mitochondria appear slightly degenerated. A material of basement membrane density and collagenous fibres (C) surround the cell.

200. 50-day hypobaric hypoxia. Hypertrophic smooth muscle cell (SC) from border between media and adventitia. Details of smooth endoplasmic reticulum and free ribosomes are seen between many mitochondria. C = collagen.

201. Thread-like material in subendothelial fibrinoid, visualized by phase-contrast microscopy.

202. Dark colour differentiates necrotic smooth muscle cells from clumpy subendothelial substance under the phase contrast microscope.

203. Electrophoretogram of rat serum after intravenous administration of 1 ml per 100 g Ferrlecit. Iron-staining reaction is seen at sites corresponding to migrations of alpha$_1$-, alpha$_2$-globulin and prealbumin.

204. Immuno-electrophoretogram of rat serum after administration of colloidal iron. The latter does not show the Prussian-blue reaction, indicating that although the tracer moves along with the given plasma fractions, it does not bind to them.

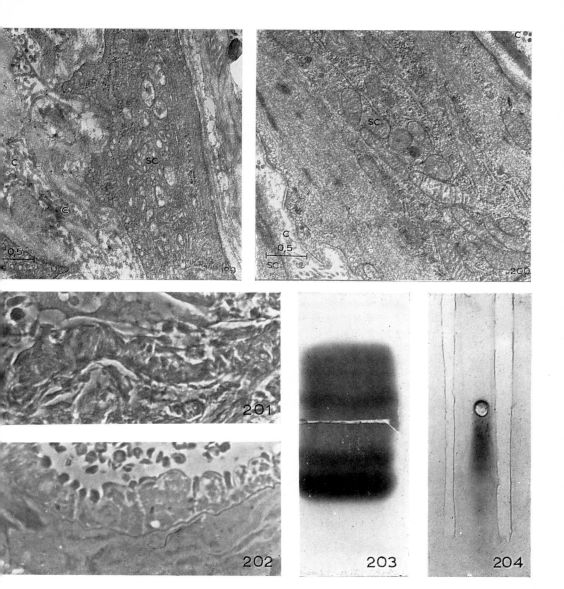

PLATE XLVI

205. Vascular changes associated with pancreatitis induced by injections of edible oil into pancreatic duct of pigeon. Ferrlecit was administered intravenously 2 hours before the birds were killed. Junctions widened to varying degrees (*a–f*) are seen in the inflamed area and the tracer has entered the junctions; pinocytotic vesicles (VE) surrounding the latter signify an increased transport activity (*c*). L = lumen; JU = junction; E = endothelial cell; N = nucleus; arrow = colloidal tracer substance.

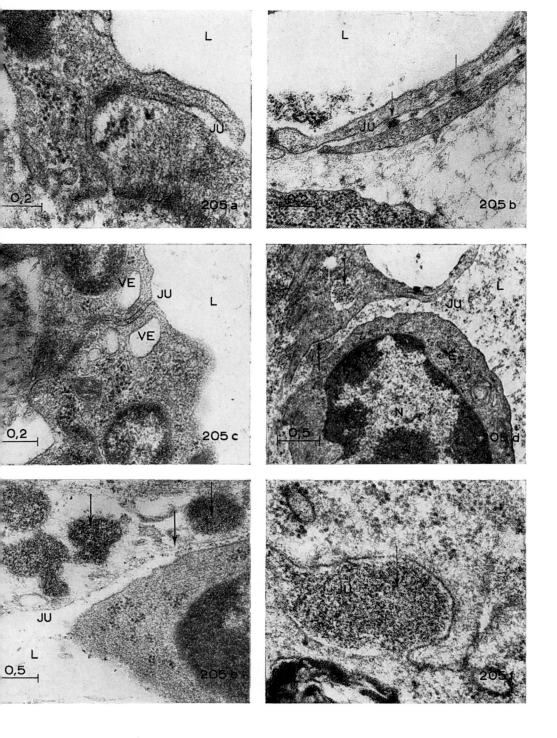

PLATE XLVII

206a, b. Injury of muscular-type arteriole in oil-induced pancreatitis of pigeon. Electron micrograph of areas showing a positive Prussian-blue reaction in semi-thin section. The endothelial cells are shrunken and patent gaps, filled by the colloidal tracer, are seen between them and also between smooth muscle cells. L = lumen; E = endothelial cell; IEL = internal elastic lamina; SC = smooth muscle cell; LD = oil droplet; arrow = colloidal tracer in gaps.

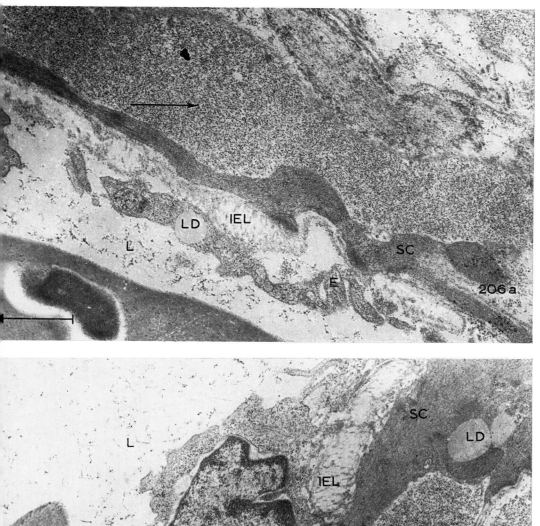

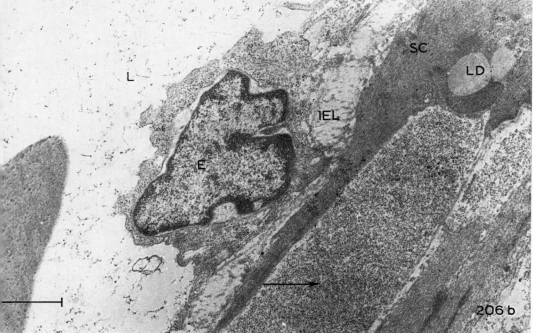

PLATE XLVIII

207. Cross-section of capillary from pancreas of pigeon with desoxycholate-induced pancreatitis. Colloidal iron tracer was administered intravenously 2 hours before the bird was killed. The tracer (*c*) is deposited on the luminal surface of the impaired endothelial cells. Note marked transcellular diffusion of tracer (*a, b*). SS = subendothelial space; FE = colloidal iron tracer; E = endothelial cell; N = nucleus; L = lumen; arrow = transport vesicles.

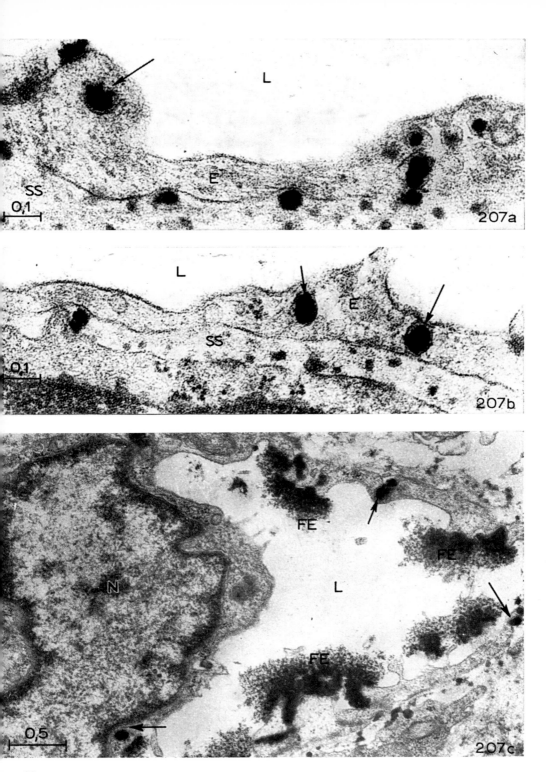

20

PLATE XLIX

208. Kupffer cells of rat given Ferrlecit intravenously after being kept hypertensive for 7 days (Lőrincz–Gorácz model). The colloidal tracer is easily identified by particle size within vesicles of Kupffer cells (*a*). Subserosa arteriole of the same rat. Colloidal tracer particles are seen in vesicles of endothelial cells and in the widened subendothelial space. The flap extending from endothelial surface into lumen signifies increased flow across the wall. Degenerated smooth muscle cells and fibrin crystals with a characteristic periodic structure lie below the internal elastic membrane (*b*). L = lumen; KC = Kupffer cell; V = vesicle; arrow = tracer substance; FL = cytoplasmic process; DB = dense body; E = endothelium; SC = smooth muscle cell; FI = fibrin crystal, IEL = internal elastic lamina.

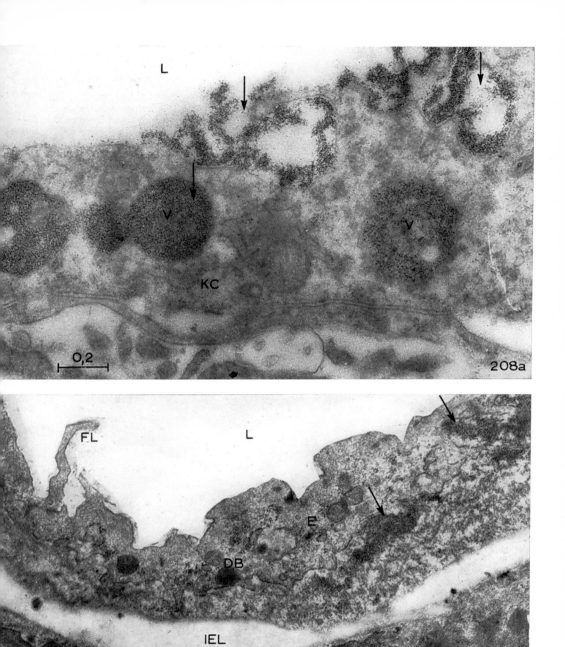

208a

208b

PLATE L

209. Wall of small artery of rat treated as in *208.* The subendothelial space is widened considerably below the junction and contains fibrin threads of a periodic structure, a loose floccular substance and tracer particles 50–70 Å in diameter. The two endothelial cells at the junction extend a cytoplasmic process toward the lumen (*a*). Same at a higher magnification. Fibrin crystals of different periodicity are seen at both sides of the internal elastic membrane, surrounded by tracer substance (*b*). L = lumen; FL = cytoplasmic process; E = endothelium; FI = fibrin; IEL = internal elastic lamina; arrow = tracer substance; CF = fibrin crystal.

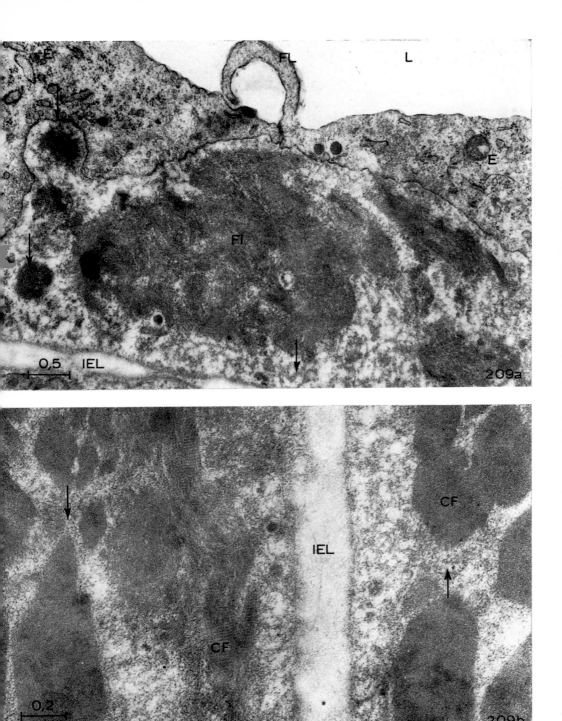

E

FL

L

FI

E

0,5   IEL

209a

CF

IEL

CF

0,2

209b

PLATE LI

210. Electron micrograph of aortic intima from a control rat. Only a thin layer of acellular connective tissue separates endothelial cells (E) and internal elastic lamina (IEL). Endothelial cell junction (JU) and plasmalemmal vesicles are indicated by arrows.

211 and *212*. Electron micrograph of aortic intima from rat kept hypertensive for two days. The widened subendothelial space between endothelial cells (E) and internal elastic lamina (IEL) contains a granular material (GM) corresponding with non-polymeric plasma proteins. Endothelial cells show a striking hyperplasia of the Golgi complex (G) and contain many ribosomes and dense bodies. The arrows point to endothelial junctions (JU) and plasmalemmal vesicles.

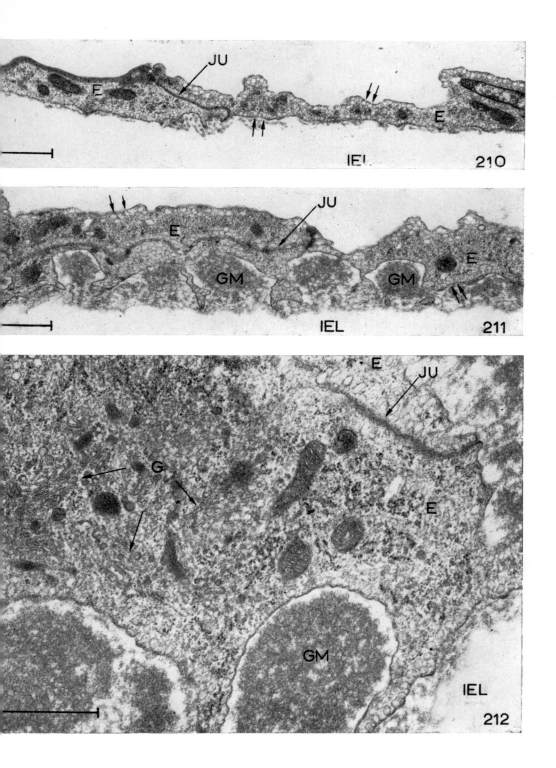

PLATE LII

213 and *214*. Details of aortic intima of rat kept hypertensive for two days. Apart from an accumulated granular material (GM), the subendothelial space contains a lymphocyte (LY; *213*) and polymerized fibrin (FI; *214*). Fibrin fibres show a characteristic axial periodicity of 200 Å. Electron micrograph of aortic endothelial cell (E) from control rat. Endothelial cell is flat, nuclear chromatin is concentrated close to nuclear membrane. L = aortic lumen.

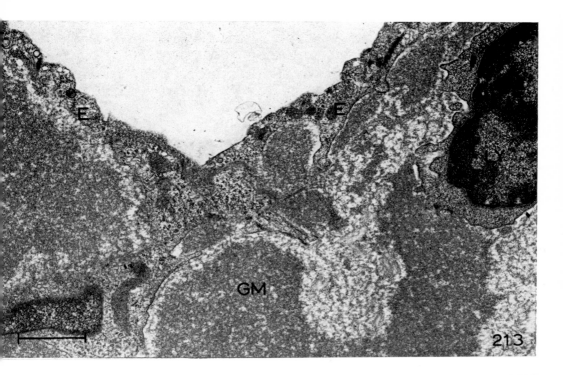

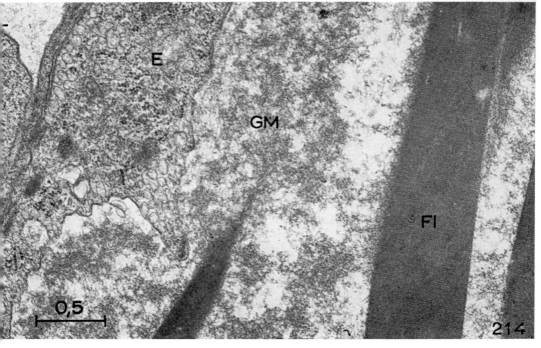

PLATE LIII

215. Electron micrograph of aortic endothelial cell from a control rat. The cell is flat, the nuclear chromatin is concentrated close to the nuclear membrane. L = lumen; IEL = internal elastic lamina.

216 and *217.* Electron micrographs of aortic endothelial cells from rat kept hypertensive for two days. Cytoplasm and nucleus appear enlarged. Nucleus is crenated, chromatin is uniformly dispersed and nucleolus (NO) is prominent. The cytoplasm contains much rough endoplasmic reticulum (RER) and many free ribosomes. Note granular material (GM) under endothelial cell, and within invaginations of subendothelial space in *216.* IEL = internal elastic lamina.

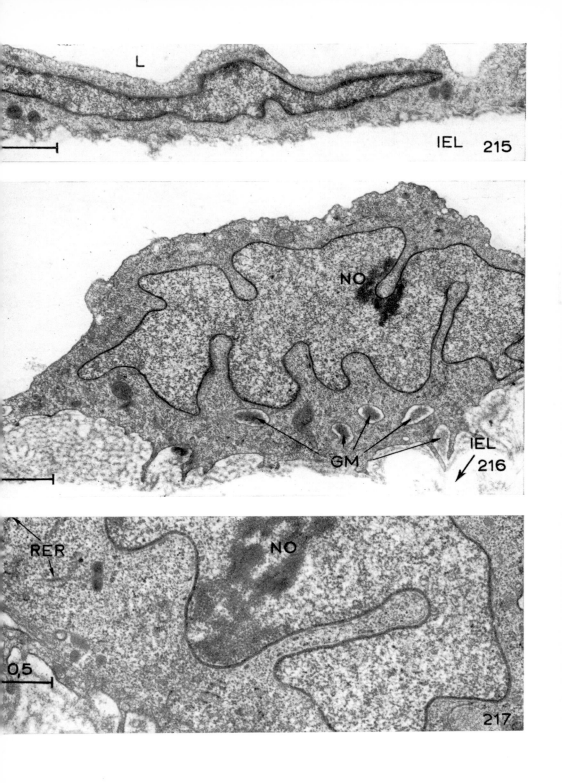

PLATE LIV

218. Detail of endothelial cell from rat kept hypertensive for two days. Large dense bodies (DB) are seen in the cytoplasm. GM = granular material in the subendothelial space. IEL = internal elastic lamina; LY = lymphocyte.

219. Electron micrograph of aortic intima from rat kept hypertensive for two days. Note lymphocyte (LY) passing through the cytoplasm of an endothelial cell (E). JU = interendothelial junction; IEL = internal elastic lamina.

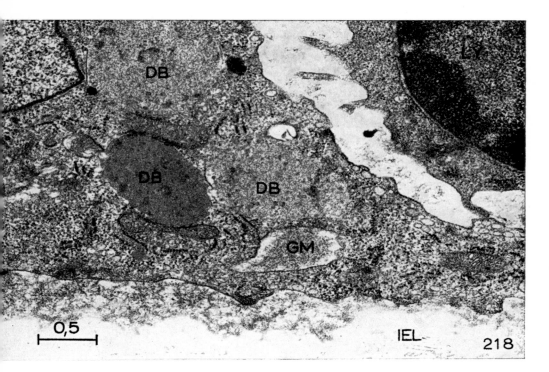

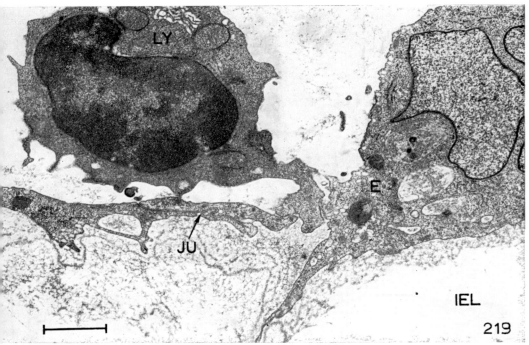

PLATE LV

220. Electron micrograph of smooth muscle cell in aortic media of control rat.

221. Electron micrograph of smooth muscle cell from aortic media of a rat kept hypertensive for two days. The nucleus (NO) is prominent and the nuclear chromatin is uniformly dispersed. Rough endoplasmic reticulum (RER) and Golgi complex (G) are strikingly increased in the cytoplasm compared to muscle cells from controls. Many dense granules (arrows) are apparent in the Golgi regions (G).

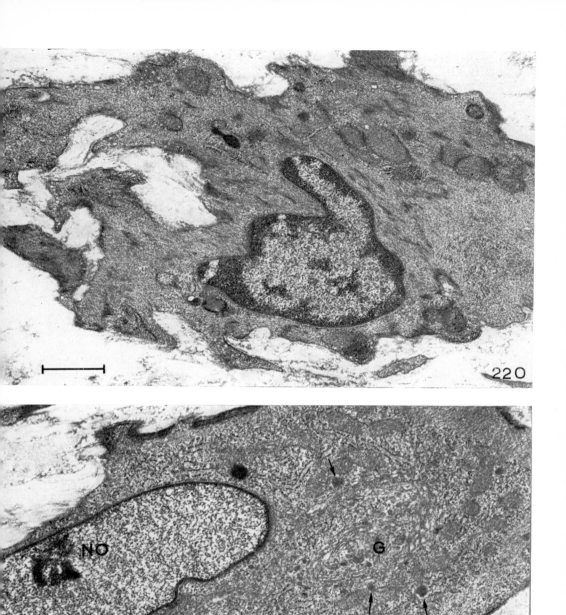

PLATE LVI

222. Electron micrograph of aortic intima of a control rat, 1.5 minutes after administration of horseradish peroxidase. The peroxidase reaction product appears on surface of endothelial cells, in interendothelial junctions (JU) and within some plasmalemmal vesicles near intercellular junctions (arrows). Low-density reaction product is seen in the subendothelial space (SS). No reaction product is seen in the aortic lumen, owing to fixation by perfusion. E = endothelial cell; IEL = internal elastic lamina. Unstained section.

223 and *224.* Electron micrograph of aortic intima from rat kept hypertensive for two days and killed 1.5 minutes after administration of horseradish peroxidase. As in controls, the peroxidase reaction product is deposited on surfaces of endothelial cell, in interendothelial junctions (JU) and within some plasmalemmal vesicles, especially in those communicating with the subendothelial surface of the cells (arrows). The widened subendothelial space (SS) and the medial side of the internal elastic lamina (IEL) also show an intensive peroxidase reaction. SC = smooth muscle cell.

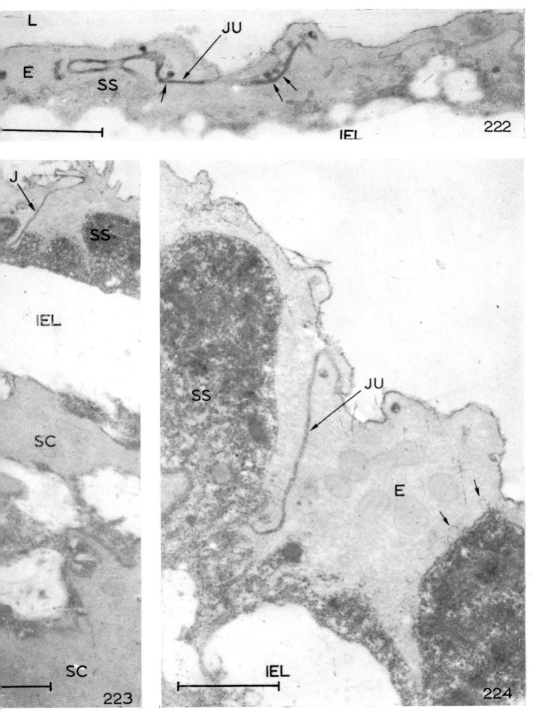

PLATE LVII

225. Electron micrograph of aortic intima from control rat 6 minutes after ferritin injection. A few ferritin molecules (F) are seen within plasmalemmal vesicles and in the subendothelial space (SS) between endothelial cells (E) and internal elastic lamina (IEL). No ferritin is present in the aortic lumen (L), however, owing to fixation by perfusion. Unstained section.

226. Detail of aortic intima from rat kept hypertensive for 2 days and killed 6 minutes after ferritin injection. A strikingly increased amount of ferritin (F) is seen in the widened subendothelial space (SS), as compared to controls, and many ferritin molecules lie within plasmalemmal vesicles of endothelial cell (E). N = nucleus of endothelial cell. Unstained section.

227. Other detail of aortic intima from *226*. Ferritin (F) accumulates in the subendothelial space (SS) around fibrin (FI) bodies and still more ferritin molecules than in *226* lie within plasmalemmal vesicles of endothelial cells (E). In the encircled areas each plasmalemmal vesicle contains 4 to 5 ferritin molecules. Unstained section.

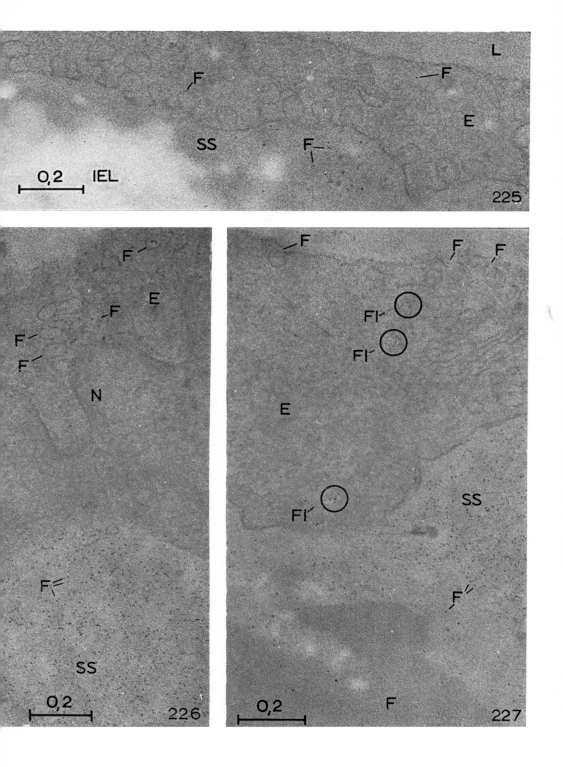

PLATE LVIII

228. Detail of aortic intima from rat kept hypertensive for 2 days. Multivesicular bodies (MV) in endothelial cells contain many ferritin molecules. SS = subendothelial space. Section slightly stained with ethanolic uranyl acetate.

229. Detail of aortic intima from rat kept hypertensive for two days. Ferritin molecules are concentrated within dense bodies (DB) of endothelial cells. SS = subendothelial space; IEL = internal elastic lamina. Section slightly stained with ethanolic uranyl acetate.

230. Junction (JU) between two endothelial cells of rat kept hypertensive for two days. No ferritin (F) molecules are seen within the junction. SS = subendothelial space. Section slightly stained with ethanolic uranyl acetate.

231. Detail of endothelial cell from rat kept hypertensive for 2 days. Almost every plasmalemmal vesicle contains one to several ferritin molecules. L = lumen. Section slightly stained with ethanolic uranyl acetate.

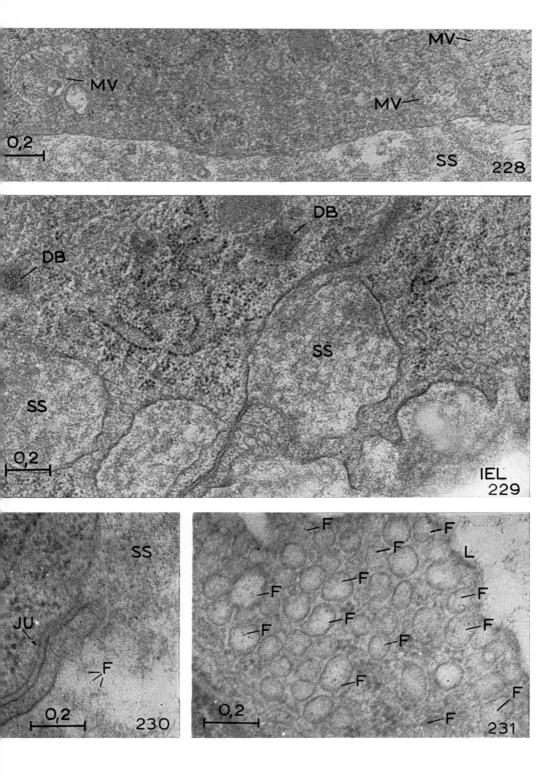

PLATE LIX

232. Single muscle cell necrosis in artery from a case of allergic granulomatosis (M-stain).

233. Single muscle cell necrosis from lupus erythematosus (M-stain).

234. Single muscle cell necrosis from periarteritis nodosa (M-stain).

235. Segmental muscle cell necrosis from human hypertension (azan stain).

236. Human periarteritis nodosa lesion surrounded by fibrin deposition and inflammatory reaction (azan stain).

237. Characteristic fibrinoid necrosis from Wegener's allergic granulomatosis (azan stain).

238. Small artery from hypertensive biopsy material. Note muscle necrosis and fibrin deposition inside and around the vessel wall (M-stain).

239. Muscle cell necrosis and perivascular fibrin deposition in periarteritis nodosa (M-stain).

240. Periarteritis nodosa lesion of large artery: subendothelial fibrinoid above the internal elastic membrane (M-stain).

241. Distinct IP of large artery in basilar meningitis (H. and E. stain).

242. Arterial lesion in Takayashu's disease: giant cell granulation tissue destroys medial elastic fibres (resorcin-fuchsin–van Gieson's stain)

243. Newly formed elastic fibre system in IP developing from inflammtory changes in Takayashu's disease (resorcin-fuchsin stain).

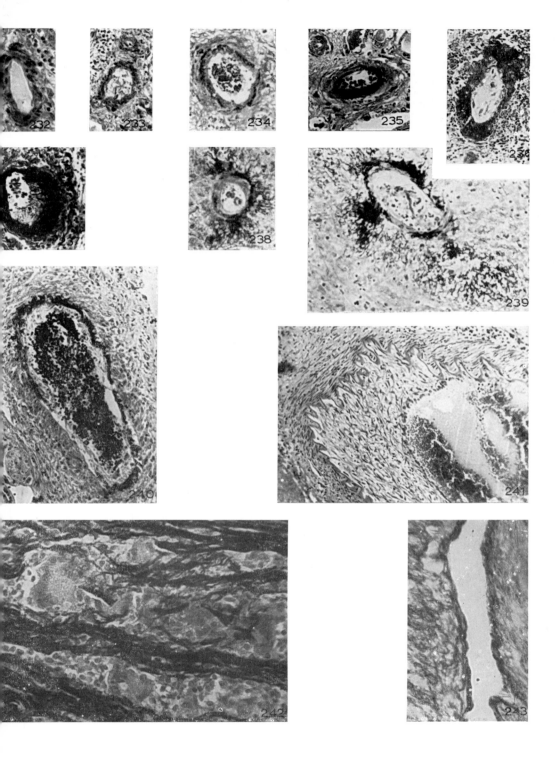

PLATE LX

244. Lőrincz–Gorácz operation for producing experimental renal hypertension: the opening of the rubber capsule is stretched and the casing is so placed on the kidney that its opening should lie is the area of the renal hilus.

245. Lőrincz–Gorácz operation for producing experimental renal hypertension: the two ends of the rubber capsule are bound together so as to keep it slightly taut and the kidney is then replaced back into the abdominal cavity.

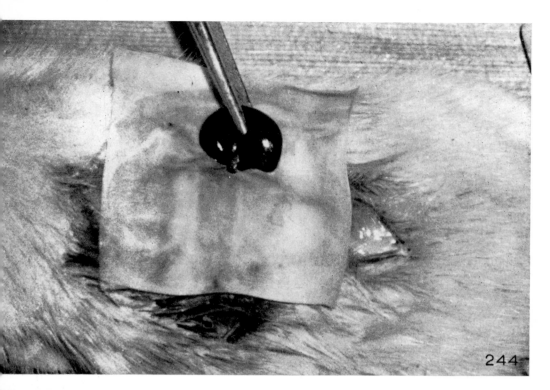

244

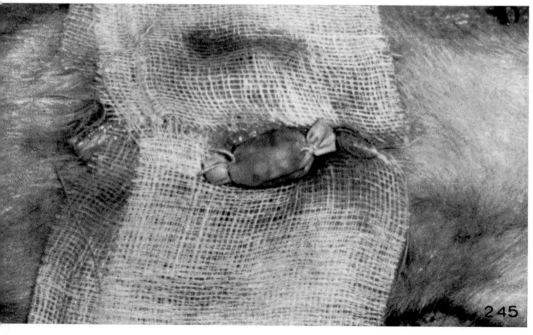

245

PLATE LXI (see p. 332)

1. Rat aorta 1 hour after painting with acid. The damaged mural portion becomes thinner, elastic fibres become stretched, and the nuclear staining reaction is seen (M-stain).

2. Non-specific esterase reaction 1 day after painting with acid. The necrotic mural segment shows no enzyme reaction at all, but adventitial cells at the border zone are strongly positive.

3. Alkaline phosphatase reaction one day after painting with acid. The meshwork-like alkaline phosphatase activity of the injured segment (see above) is no longer apparent.

4. Rat aorta 5 days after painting with acid. Part of the damaged IEL is covered by a single endothelial cell layer, in other parts only isolated mononuclear cells lie above it (arrow) (H. and E. stain).

5. Non-specific esterase reaction 5 days after painting with acid. Newly formed intimal cells show a much stronger reaction than the original ones. Marginal muscle cells of the media also show an increased activity.

6. Three months after painting with acid the cell components of the IP stain positively with M-stain, like normal smooth muscle cells.

7. Rat aorta 3 months after painting with acid. The cell components of the IP stain red (azan stain).

8. Non-specific esterase reaction 90 days after painting with acid. Cell components of the multilayered IP show a strongly positive reaction.

9. Dog aorta 60 days after painting with acid. Much AMP is present in the intercellular substance of the IP (PAS–alcian blue reaction).

10. Rat aorta 45 days after painting with acid. There is a newly formed IEL and below it delicate elastic elements are seen in the IP. The elastic fibres of the original media are stretched (resorcin-fuchsin stain).

11. Rat aorta from *10* at a higher magnification. Newly formed elastic fibres are easily visible between cells (resorcin-fuchsin stain).

12. Alkaline phosphatase reaction 90 days after painting with acid. A new rudimentary alkaline phosphatase-positive network is seen in the adventitial coat.

13. Regenerated aortic segment 45 days after painting with acid, from an animal fed cholesterol for 8 days. The lipid-like substance is clearly visible within newly formed endothelial cells (Sudan III stain).

14. Aortic wall 45 days after painting with acid, from an animal maintained on a high cholesterol diet for 6 weeks. Fat deposition is clearly visible in the broad aortic IP (Sudan black stain).

15. Aorta 45 days after painting with acid, from an animal fed lime + cholesterol for 10 weeks. Positive Kossa reaction signifies chalk deposition in IP.

16. IP in rat aorta, 360 days after painting with acid. Newly formed IEL is visualized by resorcin-fuchsin stain. Small resorcin-fuchsin-positive fibrils lie in extracellular space of IP between the original stretched elastic lamellae and the newly formed IEL (semi-thin section embedded in water-soluble Durcupan).

17. Section shown in *16* after digestion with elastase. The enzyme has digested the elastic fibres of the original media and the newly formed IEL as well, but the less mature fibrils located between the two structures have resisted the action of elastase.

18 and *19.* Rat aorta 50 days after constriction by double ligature. A multilayered IP, containing newly formed elastic elements (double arrow) is seen above the IEL (arrow) (toluidine blue stain, semi-thin section).

20. Vascular graft in abdominal aorta of dog 2 months after implantation. The neo-intima, composed chiefly of red-staining smooth muscle cells and a few connective tissue elements, and the neo-media, composed for the most part of connective tissue cells and fibres, are both clearly visible between the units of the prosthesis (azan stain).

21. Aortic graft 2 months after implantation. Elastic fibres lie intercellularly in the neo-intima (resorcin-fuchsin stain).

22. Large muscular artery after 28-day hypertension. Damaged smooth muscle cells of the media show an increased staining affinity (M-stain).

322

PLATE LXII (see p. 333)

23. Large muscular artery after 30-day hypertension. A brownish-black fibrinoid is seen between the stretched IEL and the lifted endothelial cell row. Damaged medial smooth muscle cells have disintegrated into clumps in places. Note perivascular cell infiltration (M-stain).

24. IP after 38-day hypertension. Some cell components and also damaged medial smooth muscle cells (M) as well show sudanophilia (Sudan IV stain).

25. IP after 44-day hypertension. In the broad IP, remnants of the fibrinoid are seen only above the IEL (arrow) (M-stain).

26. Aortic wall after 40-day hypertension. Pale plasma deposition (arrow) has lifted some endothelial cells from the IEL. Several smooth muscle cells of the media (M) show a vacuolar degeneration (H. and E. stain).

27. Aortic wall after 40-day hypertension. Single and confluent (arrow) smooth muscle cell necroses in the media show an increased staining affinity (M-stain).

28 and *29.* 44-day hypertension. The subendothelially deposited plasma materials give in their process of condensation the same colour reaction as the fibrinoid: M = media; FI = fibrinoid (M-stain and azan stain).

30. 40-day hypertension. The large muscular artery has become distended, and red-staining remnants of IP and fibrinoid are seen at the bottom of the subendothelial space. A blue-staining hyaline zone extends over this area. L = lumen; M = media (azan stain).

31. 44-day hypertension. An IP has already replaced part of the subendothelial fibrinoid in the large muscular artery (MA), while in the aorta (A) a narrow zone of subendothelial fibrinoid (arrow) has just appeared. The damaged wall of the small artery (SA) has already become transformed to scar tissue (M-stain).

32. Infiltration of endothelial cells by delicate lipid droplets after 3 weeks of an atherogenic diet (Sudan IV stain).

33. Same case as in *32.* Treatment with iron tracer after a 3-week atherogenic diet. Colloidal iron particles have entered aortic endothelial cells and subendothelial space of abdominal aorta, as signified by a positive Prussian-blue reaction.

34. Immediate vascular response to painting with acid. Smooth muscle cells have become swollen, endothelial cells have become hyperchromatic and detached from the internal elastic lamina and some leukocytes have appeared in the adventitia a few minutes after painting with acid (H. and E. stain).

35. Vascular response 20 minutes after painting with acid. Single muscle cell necroses, easily visualized by M-stain, have appeared below the undulating internal elastic lamina.

36. Cross-section of rabbit femoral artery 1 day after painting with acid. The wall has become very thin and stains homogeneously, because its cellular components have lost stain-binding capacity (H. and E. stain).

37. Vascular change on painting with acid. Injured and preserved mural segments are clearly distinguishable on treatment with elastic stain. The damaged portion of the wall has become reduced to one-fourth of its original width and the internal elastic lamina has become stretched.

38. Vascular change on painting with acid. Necrobiotic and regenerative muscle cells at the border between injured and preserved segments have a stronger affinity to azan than normal muscle cells. The injured area shows exclusively the blue colour of collagen.

39. An IP consisting of a few rows of cells also has appeared near the acid-painted area (H. and E. stain).

40. Same as in *39.* The internal elastic membrane has become fibrous and delicate elastic fibres have arisen in the proliferative zone of the IP (resorcin-fuchsin stain).

41. Phase of regeneration 10–15 days after painting with acid. An IP consisting of several rows of cells has developed on the surface of the injured segment, slightly overlapping the adjacent preserved areas. The cell components of the IP stain red with azan, like smooth muscle cells, and blue-staining collagen is apparent between them (azan stain).

Plate LXII continued

42. Regeneration after painting with acid. Newly formed elastic membranes, membrane systems and even an internal elastic membrane-like formation are seen in the injured area. Fragments of elastic fibres are also present (resorcin-fuchsin stain).
43. Coronary artery of rat kept hypertensive for 2 weeks. Medial muscle cells are slightly swollen (M-stain).
44. Same as in *43*; autoradiograph. Incorporation of $^{35}SO_4$ by medial smooth muscle cells is clearly visible (Kodak G5 emulsion; 3-week exposure time).

PLATE LXIII (see p. 334)

45. Necrotic smooth muscle cells are clearly visible in a semi-thin section (toluidine blue stain).
46. Mesenteric arteriole after a 3-day hypertension. Early coalescent muscle cell necroses are seen with the nuclear substance preserved (Feulgen reaction).
47. Segmental muscle cell necroses are seen over the entire width of the media after 5 days of hypertension (M-stain).
48. Mesenteric small artery after 3-day hypertension; both single and coalescent segmental muscle cell necroses are apparent (azan stain).
49. Detail of artery from *48* (M-stain).
50. Mesenteric small artery from hypertensive animal. Muscle cell necroses coalesce over entire circumference of the vessel and intermingle with intramurally diffused plasma (azan stain).
51. Intramural plasma deposition in the process of transformation to a circumferential media fibrinoid in mesenteric small artery of hypertensive animal (PAS–gallocyanin stain).
52. Small subserosa intestinal artery after 9-day hypertension. Necrotic smooth muscle cells and subendothelial fibrinoid are clearly visible (M-stain).
53. Circular media fibrinoid in mesenteric small artery, and perivascular granulation (PAS–gallocyanin stain).
54. Circular subendothelial and media fibrinoid in hypertensive vessel, and perivascular granulation tissue (resorcin-fuchsin–van Gieson stain).
55. Same vessel as in *54*. The subendothelial fibrinoid assumes a black colour on treatment with M-stain.
56. Subserosa intestinal artery after a 21-day hypertension. The subendothelial fibrinoid nearly obliterates the lumen (resorcin-fuchsin stain).
57. Mesenteric artery with a resistant internal elastic lamina (IEL) after a 21-day hypertension. The IEL is stretched and the circular subendothelial fibrinoid above it radiates through the pores of the IEL into media and adventitia (Endes' trichrome stain).
58. Coronary branch from heart wall 48 hours after the administration of noradrenalin. Necrotic muscle cells and fibres of both vessel wall and myocardium stain a vivid greenish-yellow with the modified Heutinger stain.
59. Alkaline phosphatase-active network at border between media and adventitia in abdominal aorta of non-hypertensive animal (alpha-naphthylphosphate–diasol blue B).
60. Extensive alkaline phosphatase-active network in abdominal aorta of animal kept hypertensive for 5 days (Lőrincz–Gorácz experimental hypertension model; alpha-naphthylphosphate–diasol blue B).
61. Low-intensity phosphatase activity at border between media and adventitia in intramural coronary branch of non-hypertensive animal (alpha-naphthylphosphate–diasol blue B).
62. Increased alkaline phosphatase activity in coronary branch of animal kept hypertensive for 5 days (Lőrincz–Gorácz experimental hypertension model; alpha-naphthylphosphate–diasol blue B).

Plate LXIII continued

63. Partially necrotized mesenteric artery from rat kept hypertensive for 5 days. The activity of the alkaline phosphatase meshwork has diminished, or ceased entirely in the damaged sectors (Lőrincz–Gorácz experimental hypertenison model; alpha-naphthylphosphate–diasol blue B).

64. Fibrinoid necrosis of mesenteric arteriole from rat kept hypertensive for 7 days. The ring-like subendothelial fibrinoid has reduced the lumen considerably and the alkaline phosphatase activity has vanished almost entirely above it (Lőrincz–Gorácz experimental hypertension model; alpha-naphthylphosphate–diasol blue B).

65. Broad arteritic perivascular granulation and fibrinoid necrosis in mesenteric small artery of rat kept hypertensive for 12 days. The reticular alkaline phosphatase-positive meshwork is no longer seen, but occasional alkaline phosphatase-positive cells occur in the granulation tissue (Lőrincz–Gorácz experimental hypertension model; alpha-naphthylphosphate–diasol blue B).

66. Rat aorta constricted by infrarenal ligature for 6 days. Alkaline phosphatase meshwork has disappeared from the border between media and adventitia in the segment distal from the ligature, but a distincly positive reaction is seen around a small collateral artery (alpha-naphthylphosphate–diasol blue B).

67. Mesenteric arteriole of rat kept hypertensive for 2 days. Some muscle cells already show a diffuse cytoplasmic non-specific esterase reaction, while unimpaired cells do not show it (Lőrincz–Gorácz experimental hypertension model; non-specific esterase reaction; naphthol AS acetate–fast blue, RR, pH 6.5).

PLATE LXIV (see p. 335)

68. Subserosa intestinal arteriole of rat kept hypertensive for 3 days. Non-specific esterase reaction is highly positive over the entire circumference of the vessel, showing in places a granular distribution (Lőrincz–Gorácz experimental hypertension model; non-specific esterase reaction; naphthol AS acetate–fast blue, RR, pH 6.5).

69. Mesenteric arteriole of rat kept hypertensive for 7 days. Deteriorating medial muscle cells show a highly positive, in places granular, non-specific esterase reaction; the subendothelial fibrinoid of the broadened vessel wall shows no reaction (Lőrincz–Gorácz experimental hypertension model; non-specific esterase reaction; naphthol AS acetate–fast blue, RR, pH 6.5).

70. Mesenteric arteriole of rat kept hypertensive for 12 days. The fibrinoid necrotic area of the vessel wall shows no reaction, only cells of the endothelium and perivascular granulation show a non-specific esterase activity (Lőrincz–Gorácz experimental hypertension model; non-specific esterase reaction; naphthol AS acetate–fast blue RR, pH 6.5).

71. Mesenteric artery of rat kept hypertensive for 2 weeks. The PAS-positive subendothelial fibrinoid is seen along the entire circumference of the vessel and AMPs have increased in media and adventitia (PAS–alcian blue stain).

72. Autoradiograph of artery from *71.* Incorporation of $^{35}SO_4$ into media and adventitia is clearly apparent, the fibrinoid itself is negative and detail of a vein near the artery shows a low intensity of activity (Kodak G5 emulsion; exposure: 3 weeks).

73. Mesenteric artery from rat with hypertension. The subendothelial fibrinoid does not bind Sudan black, but necrotic smooth muscle cells and periadventitial granulation have assumed a black colour from the lipid stain.

74 and *75.* Miliary-type muscle fibre necroses in myocardium after administration of noradrenalin (azan stain; PAS reaction).

76 and *77.* Small cardiac intramural artery 48 hours after noradrenalin infusion. Some muscle cells appear normal, others have pycnotic nuclei and swollen cytoplasm, indicating the prenecrotic phase (H. and E. stain).

78. Single and segmental coalescent muscle cell necroses in outer layer of media 48 hours after noradrenalin infusion (azan stain).

Plate LXIV continued

79. Single muscle cell necroses in outer zone of media 48 hours after noradrenalin infusion (PAS reaction).

80. Small intramural coronary branch 48 hours after noradrenalin infusion. Extensive plasma insudation develops to a media fibrinoid along the vessel's circumference (azan stain).

81. The media fibrinoid of artery from *80* appears homogeneous on staining with azan, but single necrotic muscle cells can still be visualized in it by M-stain.

82. Segmental coalescence of muscle cell necroses in outer zone of media 48 hours after noradrenalin administration (PAS reaction).

83. Muscle cell necroses and early intramural plasma diffusion 48 hours after noradrenalin administration (PAS reaction).

84. Group of necrotic smooth muscle cells in arterial wall 48 hours after noradrenalin administration. Positive reaction shows plasma insudation around preserved smooth muscle cells.

85. PAS-positive subendothelial fibrinoid, penetrating in places also between muscle cells, 48 hours after noradrenalin administration.

86. Medial muscle cell necrosis 1 day after painting with acid: necrotic cells show the red colour of the positive PAS reaction.

87. Single medial muscle cell necroses later coalesce and stain homogeneously black with M-stain.

88. Segmental muscle cell necroses intermingle with plasma insudation to form a segmental vascular wall necrosis 3–4 days after painting with acid (azan stain).

89. Small vessel-wall stains homogeneously red with azan within 2–5 days after painting with acid; this staining reaction is characteristic of the fibrinoid change.

90. Same vessel as in *89*; single necrotic muscle cells can still be visualized with M-stain.

91. Cellular elements are scarcely discernible in the vessel wall 5–6 days after painting with acid; the wall appears homogeneous and infiltrating cells are seen in the adventitia (H. and E. stain).

92. Subendothelial plasma deposition 1 week after painting with acid. Insudation has already reached the adventitia in which M-stain reveals the presence of fibrin.

93. Adventitial fibrin deposition, clearly distinguishable from necrotic smooth muscle cells, is seen in the fluorescence micrograph.

94. The media fibrinoid developing in response to painting with acid is still demonstrable by M-stain while the perivascular granulation develops.

95. Same vessel as in *94*. Staining with azan reveals a perivascular fibrinoid change which is associated with a granulation process and together they form a lesion in every respect similar to periarteritis nodosa.

96. Characteristic fibrinoid change of vessel wall after painting with acid: the entire wall stains homogeneously red with azan. Bottom right: cross-section of artery (detail); middle: longitudinal section of artery (detail).

97. Same as in *96*, on staining with M-stain. The two components of the lesion, the subendothelial and media fibrinoid are clearly visible on either side of the internal elastic lamina in both longitudinal and cross-section.

98. Coronary artery of rabbit sensitized with horse serum. A homogeneously eosinophilic plasma deposition is seen subintimally, below swollen endothelial cells. Some medial muscle cells show nuclear vacuolization (H. and E. stain).

PLATE LXV (see p. 336)

99. Coronary artery of rabbit sensitized with horse serum. The endothelial cells are swollen, medial muscle cells show a nuclear vacuolization. Note segmental homogenization of the media (H. and E. stain).

100. Coronary artery of rabbit treated with horse serum. Necrotic muscle cells of the media show a homogeneously red PAS-reaction.

Plate LXV continued

101. Coronary artery of rabbit treated with horse serum. M-stain permits the distinction of some single necrotic muscle cells within the media fibrinoid.
102. Coronary artery of rabbit treated with horse serum. Fibrinoid necrosis arising by coalescence of single medial muscle cell necrosis (azan stain).
103. Coronary artery of rabbit treated with horse serum. Periarteritis nodosa-like lesion. Endothelial cells are swollen, part of the media appears homogeneously eosinophilic, with a few infiltrating granulocytes. Note distinct periarterial inflammatory cell reaction (H. and E. stain).
104. Periarteritis nodosa-like lesion in intrahepatic small branch of hepatic artery of horse serum-treated rabbit. There is an IP, and an inflammatory cell reaction involves the intima, media and adventitia. The fibrinoid has developed subendothelially, because the vessel possesses a strong internal elastic lamina.
105. Same vessel as in *104*, after staining with M-stain. The subendothelial fibrinoid above the internal elastic lamina does not bind PTA; the periarterial fibrin deposition stains black and granulation tissue surrounds it.
106 and *107.* Mesenteric artery of rat kept hypertensive for 42 days. A broad, cell-rich IP is seen above the subendothelial fibrinoid. The area above the internal elastic lamina still stains like a fibrinoid. The greater part of the media has undergone a fibrous transformation (Lőrincz–Gorácz experimental hypertension model; azan, resorcin-fuchsin and van Gieson stains).
108. Mesenteric artery of rat kept hypertensive for 40 days. A semilunar, cell-rich IP has reduced the lumen. Detail of fibrinoid is seen above the internal elastic lamina. Medial muscle cells are pycnotic and vacuolized (Lőrincz–Gorácz experimental hypertension model; H. and E. stain).
109. Uneven, cushion-like IP in mesenteric artery of rat kept hypertensive for 40 days. Occasional necrotic smooth muscle cells are seen in the outer part of the media, and scar tissue has developed around the vessel (Lőrincz–Gorácz experimental hypertension model; Holt's formaline–glutaraldehyde–osmium fixation, Araldite embedding, semi-thin section, toluidine blue stain).
110. Segmental IP protruding into lumen of subserosa artery from rat kept hypertensive for 40 days. Fibroblast and muscle cell-like components of the proliferation and immigrating leukocytes are clearly distinguishable from one another in light micrograph. Note disseminated muscle cell necrosis in the media and perivascular scar tissue formation (Lőrincz–Gorácz experimental hypertension model; Holt's formaline–glutaraldehyde–osmium fixation; Araldite embedding; semi-thin section; toluidine blue stain).
111. Mesenteric arteriole of rat kept hypertensive for 40 days. Subendothelial fibrinoid, staining red with azan, is seen at top. The media has changed into scar tissue, consisting of connective tissue fibres and hyaline-like areas staining blue with azan (Lőrincz–Gorácz experimental hypertension model; azan stain).
112. Mesenteric artery of rat kept hypertensive for 40 days. A circular IP, rich in cells and fibres, has reduced the lumen. Concentrically arranged, fibrous connective tissue has replaced the deteriorated media (Lőrincz–Gorácz experimental hypertension model; azan stain).
113. Hyaline transformation of circular subendothelial fibrinoid in subserosa artery of rat kept hypertensive for 40 days. Endothelial cells are clearly visible on the surface of the hyaline tissue and occasional nuclear staining reactions are seen inside it. The media has become replaced by scar tissue (Lőrincz–Gorácz experimental hypertension model; PAS–gallocyanin stain).
114. Circular IP in mesenteric artery of rat kept hypertensive for 40 days. The upper layers of the IP contain many elastic fibres, but the less mature deeper layers contain none. The internal elastic lamina is stretched (resorcin-fuchsin stain).
115. Multilayered IP and perivascular cell infiltration developing after painting of the vessel wall with acid (H. and E. stain).
116. Hyaline connective tissue replaces the vascular muscle layer after painting with acid (azan stain).
117. Multilayered IP reduces the lumen after painting with acid. Note pycnotic muscle cells (H. and E. stain).

Plate LXV continued

118. Newly formed elastic fibres and yellow-staining muscle-like cells in semicircular IP after painting with acid (resorcin-fuchsin–van Gieson's stain).

119. Meshwork of newly formed elastic fibres between cells during regeneration after painting with acid (resorcin-fuchsin stain).

120. Mass of elasto-hyaline tissue in uterine artery 60 days after painting with acid (PAS reaction).

121. Recurrent fibrinoid in cicatrizing vessel wall damaged by painting with acid (azan stain).

122. Vessel wall one month after noradrenalin treatment. The homogeneous vessel-wall has become hyalinized, an IP reduces the lumen and perivascular scar tissue, still containing inflammatory elements, is seen (H. and E. stain).

PLATE LXVI (see p. 337)

123. Chronic change after noradrenalin treatment: an IP has evolved around the entire circumference of the severely damaged vessel wall (H. and E. stain).

124. Hyaline transformation and cicatrization of vessel wall in chronic stage of the change induced by treatment with horse serum (M-stain).

125. Mesenteric artery of medium calibre from rat kept hypertensive for 1 week and given subcutaneously 15 mg/kg Sanegyt daily. Note deposition of a small amount of fibrin in parts of the intima. The media has slightly broadened, muscle cells are moderately swollen, but there is no necrosis (M-stain).

126. Mesenteric artery of small calibre from rat kept hypertensive for 2 weeks and treated daily with 7.5 mg BTF through a gastric tube. The endothelial cell layer is preserved; enlargement and multiplication of muscle cells widen the media and also dividing cell forms are seen. Occasional lymphocytes, histiocytes and fibroblasts locate in the slightly widened adventitia (H. and E. stain).

127. Coronary artery of rat kept hypertensive for 3 weeks and treated with 15 mg/kg Sanotensin (guanethidine sulphate) daily. Note smooth muscle cell hypertrophy and hyperplasia in the widened media (M-stain).

128. Small-calibre mesenteric artery from rat kept hypertensive for 3 weeks, but not treated with drug (control). A subintimal fibrinoid lies at one side of the stretched internal elastic lamina and an IP lies on its other side. Clumps of fibrinoid are seen in the deep zone of the intima. Hypertrophic muscle cells and an inflammatory cellular reaction are seen in the media. An enormous perivascular granulation is associated with the adventitia (M-stain).

129. Small-calibre mesenteric artery from rat kept hypertensive for 2 weeks and treated with 20 mg/kg Vincamin daily. There is an IP and both media and adventitia show a distinct fibrosis. A marked reduction of the lumen has taken place (M-stain).

130. Vascular response 1–2 days after painting with acid. Van Gieson's stain reveals no aortic change, only the cellular elements of a collateral small arterial branch have lost staining affinity.

131. Same as in *130*, after treatment with M-stain. Necrotic muscle cells in detail of aorta and collateral small artery appear in black colour.

132. Same as in *130* after treatment with PAS. Detail of muscular artery shows homogenization and a fibrinoid mural change, while no plasma insudation is seen in the aorta.

133. Barrier role of the internal elastic lamina can be seen from this micrograph. The undulating black line (arrow) represents a row of muscle cells that became necrotic 1 day after painting with acid, but plasma insudation has been retarded by the IEL, thus no fibrinoid lesion is present.

134. Pancreatic small artery of pigeon with oil-induced pancreatitis. Colloidal tracer administered *in vivo* is visualized by Prussian-blue reaction of the semi-thin section. Blue areas represent mural depositions of either plasma or tracer, thus facilitating the orientation of ultra-thin sections.

Plate LXVI continued

135. Heart muscle of dog after 3 days of a mechanically induced lymph stasis. Blue areas signify the positive Prussian-blue reaction of colloidal iron particles in mural plasma depositions of the widened lymph capillaries.

136. Change of a small coronary vessel under the influence of mechanical lymph stasis. The intimal endothelial cells are vacuolized and plasma has become deposited in the subendothelial space (azan stain).

137. Effect of mechanical lymph stasis on small coronary branch of dog. Continuous plasma depositions, staining red with azan, lie subendothelially and the vessel wall is oedematous.

138. Same vessel as in *137*. Plasma depositions below the intima and in the media stain violet-black with M-stain.

139. Effect of regional mechanical lymph stasis on coronary artery of dog. Confluent areas below the intima and in the media uniformly show the characteristic staining properties of fibrin (azan stain) and vacuolized and PAS-positive areas are seen below the intima (PAS stain).

140. Coronary branch injured by regional mechanical lymph stasis. Endothelial cells and cushion are oedematous and vacuolized and PAS-positive areas are seen below the intima (PAS stain).

141. Lymph stasis-induced change of small coronary artery from Ferrlecit-treated animal. Deposition of the tracer in oedematous endothelial cells and cushion is signified by a discrete positive Prussian-blue reaction.

142. Effect of mechanical lymph stasis. Extensive subintimal plasma insudation also penetrates the media in places (PAS stain).

143. Same vessel, as in *142*. The location of Prussian blue-positive areas suggests that permeability increase and consequent plasma insudation took place after the intramural passage of colloidal iron.

144. Small muscular vessel from the area of a lymphoedema induced in hindleg of dog by ligation of regional lymph circulation. Colloidal particles of the iron tracer, administered prior to termination, have become deposited in the vessel wall (Prussian-blue reaction).

145. Dog coronary artery after perfusion with No-Spa and noradrenalin. The endothelial cells are vacuolized and plasma depositions are seen below the intima (PAS–alcian blue stain).

PLATE LXVII (see p. 338)

146. Subintimal plasma deposition reduces the lumen of a small coronary artery after perfusion with noradrenalin and No-Spa (H. and E. stain).

147. Same vessel as in *146*, after PAS reaction. The intimal cushion is PAS-positive, but muscle cells are preserved (non-staining).

148. Same vessel as in *146*, after treatment with M-stain. The subintimal plasma deposition stains black.

149. Small coronary artery of an animal killed 42 days after infusion of noradrenalin and No-Spa. The mural structure is loose at the site of the original oedema and scar tissue has formed in places (M-stain).

150 and *151*. Mesenteric small artery of rat rendered hypertensive by the method of Lőrincz and Gorácz and killed after 7 days. M-stain has revealed the presence of a subintimal fibrinoid above the stretched internal elastic lamina. The latter shows a single discontinuity: the colloidal tracer administered prior to termination entered the media through this fenestra (Prussian-blue reaction).

152. Subserosa small artery of control rat after treatment with elastic stain.

153. Section of small arteriole from control rat after digestion with elastase for 30 minutes. The internal elastic lamina has widened and transversal fragments are becoming detached from it (elastic stain).

Plate LXVII continued

154. Subserosa small artery of rat kept hypertensive for 7 days. A subintimal fibrinoid deposition lies above the stretched internal elastic lamina (Lőrincz–Gorácz experimental hypertension model; M-stain).
155. Same section as in *154*, after digestion with elastese for 30 minutes. The stretched internal elastic lamina resisted elastase action and stains as before; the ribbon-like widening is no longer seen.
156. Subserosa small artery of albino rat rendered hypertensive by the Lőrincz–Gorácz method and given India ink tracer before termination. The colloidal carbon particles are deposited chiefly below the intima, but in places have also entered the media, appearing as circumscribed areas in the ring-like fibrinoid (azan stain).
157. Deposition of colloidal iron tracer in fibrinoid change of subserosa small artery. A blue reaction indicates the presence of the tracer over the entire width of the fibrinoid, signifying a marked increase of vascular permeability.
158. Mesenteric artery of a rat kept hypertensive for 7 days. There is a subintimal fibrinoid, staining characteristically red with azan, and a perivascular granulation is present (Lőrincz–Gorácz experimental hypertension model).
159. Vessel of rat from *158* after treatment with M-stain.
160. Vessel of rat kept hypertensive for 7 days and given iron tracer prior to termination. The positive Prussian-blue reaction signifies the presence of tracer particles subintimally and in some areas of the media; entrance of tracer into greater part of media is inhibited by the stretched, but structurally still preserved, internal elastic lamina.
161. Subserosa small artery of rat kept hypertensive for 8 days. Severe fibrinoid necrosis has already involved part of the media (Lőrincz–Gorácz experimental hypertension model; azan stain).
162. Same vessel as in *161*, after Prussian-blue reaction. The colloidal tracer has gained access into the fibrinoid, signifying a severe permeability disturbance of the vessel wall.

PLATE LXVIII (see p. 339)

163. Arterial lesion in Wegener's granulomatosis. Single and sectorial muscle cell necroses are clearly visible after staining with azan.
164. Same artery as in *163*, after treatment with M-stain. Muscle cell necroses are easily recognized by their black colour.
165. Single and coalescent vascular muscle cell necroses in basilar meningitis (azan stain).
166. Uterine artery in the process of post-partum involution. Note homogeneous fibrinoid change of the vessel wall (azan stain).
167. Same uterine artery as in *166*, after treatment with M-stain; this enables the differentiation of the necrotic muscle cells from the plasma deposition.
168. Splenic arteries showing a homogeneous fibrinoid change of the wall; in one artery, only necrotic smooth muscle cells are present (azan stain).
169. Splenic artery from *168*, after treatment with M-stain: this visualizes the single muscle cell necroses not differentiated by azan.
170. Homogeneous fibrinoid necrosis of vessel-wall and perivascular cell infiltration in Wegener's granulomatosis (azan stain).
171. Black spots in the inflamed perivascular area signify extramural depositions of fibrin (M-stain).
172. Distinct subendothelial fibrinoid of large artery from a case of basilar meningitis (azan stain).
173. Muscle cell necrosis and subendothelial fibrinoid formation in arterial wall from Wegener's granulomatosis (PAS reaction).
174. Intimal proliferation in large artery from basilar meningitis (gallocyanin–PAS stain).

Plate LXVIII continued

175. Proliferative phenomena in small renal artery, observed in addition to acute hypertensive vascular lesions (azan stain).

176. Lumen-reducing IP reminiscent of Buerger disease lesion in periarteritis nodosa (azan stain).

177. Cell components of IP in Takayashu's disease assume a red colour on treatment with the azan staining technique, as modified by Krutsay. The aged proliferation nearby the media is rich in collagen and contains only a few cells.

178. Repeated elastic fibre synthesis is seen in IP from a hypertensive artery (resorcin-fuchsin stain).

179. Multiple elastic fibre synthesis in arterial IP from a pyelonephritis case (resorcin-fuchsin–van Gieson stain).

180. Artery from preserved portion of kidney in pyelonephritis shows no change on staining with resorcin-fuchsin and van Gieson stains.

181. Segment of artery shown in *180*, from inflamed area of the kidney: multiple elastic fibre formation is clearly seen (resorcin-fuchsin stain).

182. Mural hyalinization and lumen reduction of uterine artery (azan stain).

183. Two neighbouring arteries from a pyelonephritis case; the wall of one vessel has become transformed to hyaline and scar tissue, the other shows a fresh fibrinoid change, with an IP on the luminal side (azan stain).

184. Mesenteric artery from experimental hypertension. Several layers of fibrin overlap and organization phenomena are seen, as in Buerger disease lesions.

185–188. Vascular changes in SLE. *185*: Acute (azan–M-stain) and chronic periarteritis-nodosa-like changes (H. and E. stain) are simultaneously present in small arteries. *186*: Artery nearly obliterated by chronic proliferation simultaneously shows fresh fibrinoid changes (azan stain). *187*: Recurrent chronic lesions in large artery: tissue layers in varioust stages of proliferation overlap and collagenous fibres are abundant in the earliest ones. Periadventitial scar tissue represents the final stage of an earlier granulation process (azan stain). *188*: Aortic subendothelial fibrinoid and overlaying IP (M-stain).

PLATE LXI

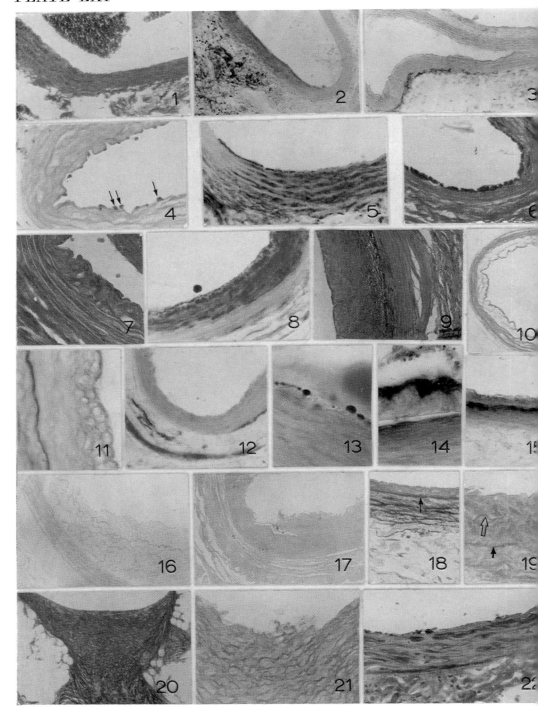

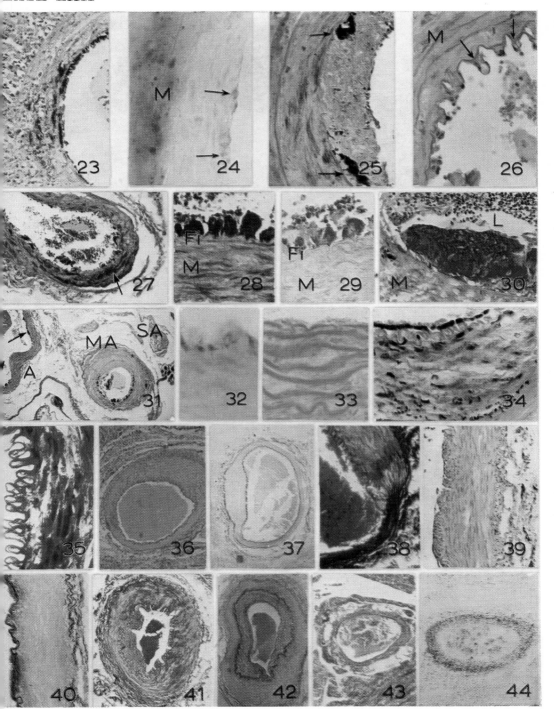

PLATE LXIII

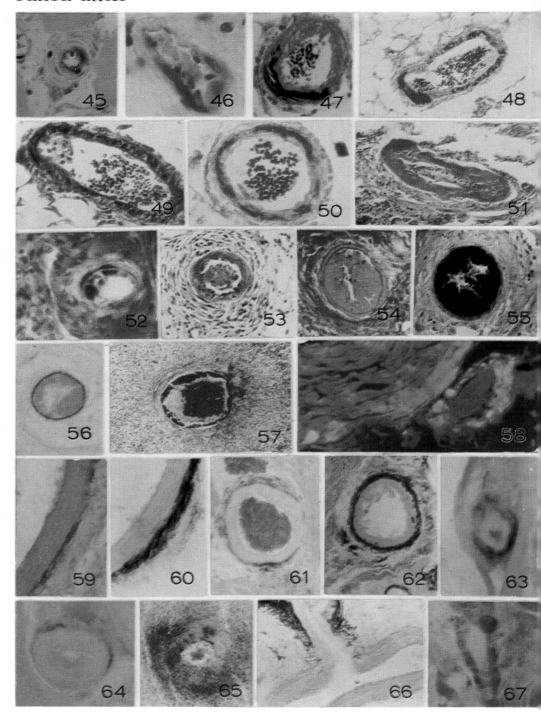

PLATE LXIV

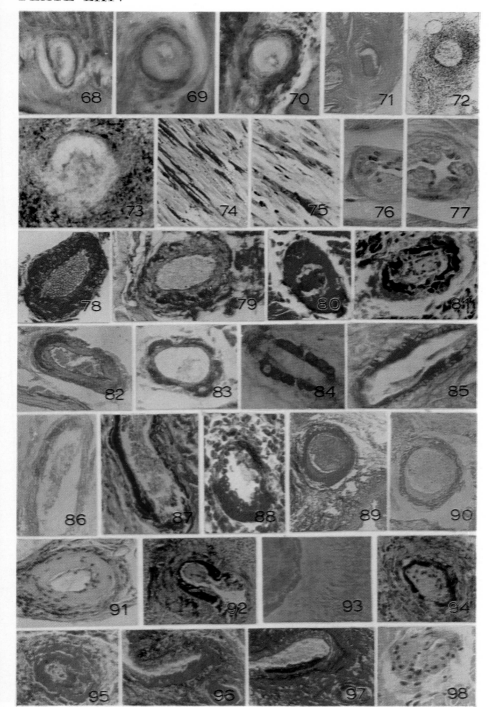

PLATE LXV

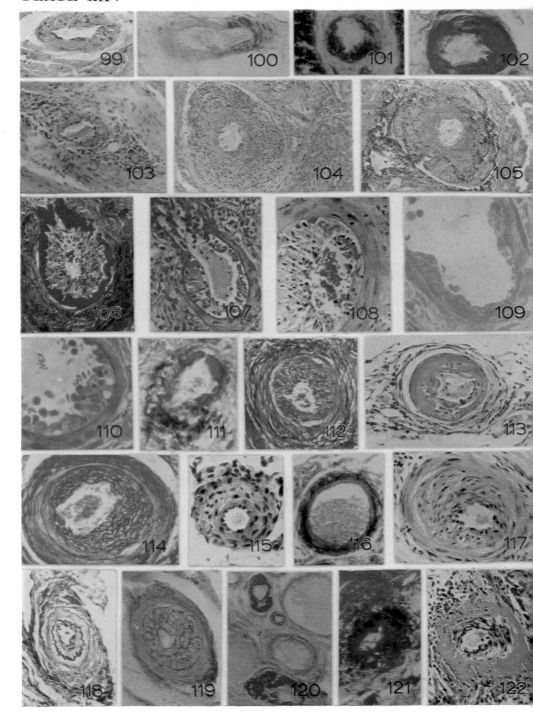

PLATE LXVI

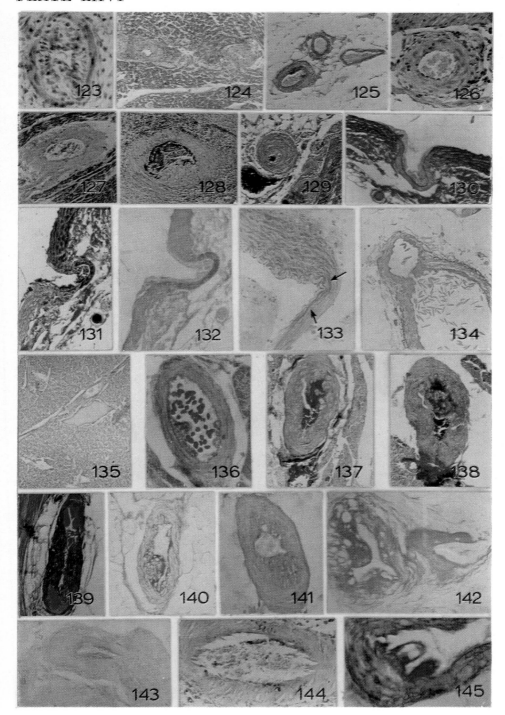

PLATE LXVII

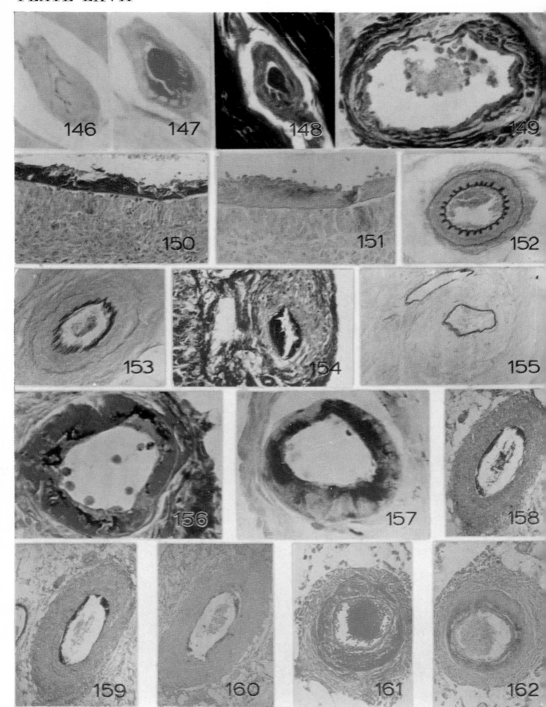

PLATE LXVIII

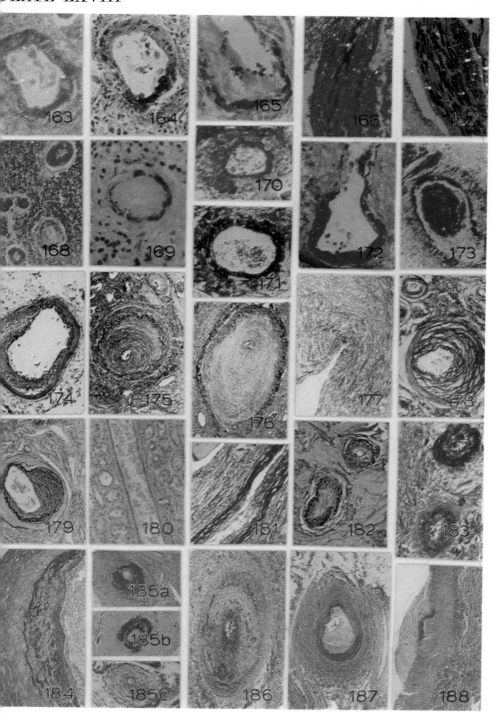